MRI and Ultrasound in Diagnosis and Management of Rheumatological Diseases

ANNALS OF THE NEW YORK ACADEMY OF SCIENCES
Volume 1154

MRI and Ultrasound in Diagnosis and Management of Rheumatological Diseases

Edited by
JAMES D. KATZ AND KATHLEEN BRINDLE

The George Washington University School of Medicine, Washington, DC

Published by Blackwell Publishing on behalf of the New York Academy of Sciences
Boston, Massachusetts
2009

The *Annals of the New York Academy of Sciences* (ISSN: 0077-8923 [print]; ISSN: 1749-6632 [online]) is published 32 times a year on behalf of the New York Academy of Sciences by Wiley Subscription Services, Inc., a Wiley Company, 111 River Street, Hoboken, NJ 07030-5774.

MAILING: The *Annals* is mailed standard rate. POSTMASTER: Send all address changes to *ANNALS OF THE NEW YORK ACADEMY OF SCIENCES*, Journal Customer Services, John Wiley & Sons Inc., 350 Main Street, Malden, MA 02148-5020.

Journal Customer Services: For ordering information, claims, and any inquiry concerning your subscription, please go to interscience.wiley.com/support or contact your nearest office:

Americas: Email: cs-journals@wiley.com; Tel: +1 781 388 8598 or 1 800 835 6770 (Toll free in the USA & Canada).
Europe, Middle East and Asia: Email: cs-journals@wiley.com; Tel: +44 (0) 1865 778315
Asia Pacific: Email: cs-journals@wiley.com; Tel: +65 6511 8000
Information for Subscribers: The *Annals* is published in 32 issues per year. Subscription prices for 2008 are:
Print & Online: US$4862 (US), US$5296 (Rest of World), €3432 (Europe), £2702 (UK). Prices are exclusive of tax. Australian GST, Canadian GST and European VAT will be applied at the appropriate rates. For more information on current tax rates, please go to www3.interscience.wiley.com/aboutus/journal_ordering_and_payment.html#Tax. The price includes online access to the current and all online back files to January 1, 1997, where available. For other pricing options, including access information and terms and conditions, please visit www.interscience.wiley.com/journal-info.

Delivery Terms and Legal Title: Prices include delivery of print publications to the recipient's address. Delivery terms are Delivered Duty Unpaid (DDU); the recipient is responsible for paying any import duty or taxes. Legal title passes to the customer on despatch by our distributors.

Membership information: Members may order copies of *Annals* volumes directly from the Academy by visiting www.nyas.org/annals, emailing membership@nyas.org, faxing +1 212 298 3650, or calling 1 800 843 6927 (toll free in the USA), or +1 212 298 8640. For more information on becoming a member of the New York Academy of Sciences, please visit www.nyas.org/membership. Claims and inquiries on member orders should be directed to the Academy at email: membership@nyas.org or Tel: 1 800 843 6927 (toll free in the USA) or +1 212 298 8640.

Printed in the USA.

The *Annals* is available to subscribers online at Wiley InterScience and the New York Academy of Sciences' Web site. Visit www.interscience.wiley.com to search the articles and register for table of contents e-mail alerts.

ISSN: 0077-8923 (print); 1749-6632 (online)
ISBN-10: 1-57331-736-5; ISBN-13: 978-1-57331-736-8

A catalogue record for this title is available from the British Library.

ANNALS OF THE NEW YORK ACADEMY OF SCIENCES

Volume 1154

MRI and Ultrasound in Diagnosis and Management of Rheumatological Diseases

Editors
JAMES D. KATZ AND KATHLEEN BRINDLE

CONTENTS

Section IV. Research Aspects

Preface

Inflammatory arthritis encompasses a rapidly destructive disorder of joints with associated systemic manifestations. A worrisome feature of this class of disorders is the fact that subclinical inflammation may persist even when there is an assessment of clinical remission. The advent of disease-modifying therapeutics that promise to halt rheumatoid arthritis (RA) disease progression has escalated the clinical importance of early diagnosis and subsequent assessment of remission. Magnetic resonance imaging (MRI) is an advanced imaging technique capable of identifying RA lesions before such changes become manifest on conventional radiographs. Where MRI excels is at soft tissue imaging. It enables detection of changes that are not seen on plain radiographs or even CT scanning procedures. For example, MRI may better define problems unique to RA such as tendon rupture. In this manner, it may refine the clinician's ability to not only diagnose RA but also to monitor the disease over time and consequently more deftly adjust the therapy.

Histochemical studies are beginning to shed light on the changes detected by MRI. Its bone edema pattern, for example, appears to reflect subchondral lymphocytic infiltration, a not-too-surprising finding in light of our current knowledge of the periarticular cytokine milieu of RA. The challenge to radiologists now is to correlate findings such as synovial thickening, glycosaminoglycan content, and the overall volume of erosive change with clinical prognosis.

The development of low- and medium-field-strength scanners has driven the recent phenomenon of office-based MRI. These easily installed, lower-cost machines are useful for imaging musculoskeletal conditions of the extremities. Moreover, office-based MRI is increasingly used as a data source justifying a clinical change in management. Therefore MRI in patients with inflammatory arthritis is a topic of interest not just to academics but also to clinicians in private practice.

Another rapidly growing area of musculoskeletal medicine entails imaging with ultrasonography. The obvious appeal of such a technique is the absence of ionizing radiation and the ease of "bedside" use. Studies already suggest that ultrasound (US) assessment rivals MRI for small-joint evaluation of inflammatory and destructive changes. Most promising is its ability to directly visualize the synovium and, possibly, synovial blood flow. The weaknesses of US in RA, however, center on the difficulty of imaging complex joints and the inability to detect bone changes such as bone marrow infiltration with immune cells.

A book on the subject of MRI and US for the imaging of patients with rheumatological disorders should be of interest to radiologists, rheumatologists, orthopedic surgeons, and neurologists, as well as academic institutions charged with training new doctors. We hope that the reference we have created will be of special use in geographical regions where musculoskeletal radiologists and rheumatologists are not adequately represented. Toward this goal, the reader will find within the pages of this book enough information to appreciate the basic physics behind advanced imaging techniques as well as the

MRI and Ultrasound in Diagnosis and Management: Ann. N.Y. Acad. Sci. 1154: vii–viii (2009).
doi: 10.1111/j.1749-6632.2009.04379.x © 2009 New York Academy of Sciences.

various "trade-offs" imposed by the balancing act necessitated by the tension between, for example, "signal" and "noise." We expect that the reader will also learn the clinical nuances of musculoskeletal imaging as well as derive an understanding of the research methodology surrounding issues such as the grading of lesions. Finally, the reader should gain insight into the future directions of MRI and US.

JAMES D. KATZ AND KATHLEEN BRINDLE
The George Washington University
Washington, DC

Section I. Magnetic Resonance Imaging and Ultrasound

Introduction: Arthritis and Myositis

James D. Katz and Geeta Nayyar

Rheumatology Division, The George Washington University, Washington, DC, USA

In this chapter background medical information pertinent to the use of MRI and/or ultrasound in various musculoskeletal conditions is presented. Appreciation of the genetic, biochemical, histological, and immunological features of rheumatic diseases will be of benefit to the technician responsible for performing and interpreting these types of interrogations. For example, recognizing that cartilage disorder predates bone findings in osteoarthritis will help identify early versus late degenerative findings. Similarly, understanding the fibrovascular nature of rheumatoid pannus will help guide the use of more sophisticated ultrasound techniques such as power Doppler.

Key words: arthritis; myositis; rheumatology

Degenerative Musculoskeletal Conditions

During development embryonic mesenchymal stem cells differentiate into muscle, adipose tissue, bone, and cartilage. Cartilage is a tissue with limited regenerative or repair capabilities and chondrocytes synthesize and maintain its extracellular matrix (ECM). Growth factors including TGF-beta, bone morphogenetic proteins, insulin-like growth factor, and basic fibroblast growth factor can improve chondrocyte proliferation as well as synthesis of the ECM.[1] An early event in osteoarthritis (OA) is a loss from the ECM of aggrecan,[2] which is a proteoglycan and is broken down by aggrecanases and other endoproteinases. Matrix metalloproteinases, which also play a role in proteoglycan breakdown, are collagenolytic as well. Collagenolysis takes place later in OA than aggrecanolysis. Other later events in the progression of OA include fibrillations, fissures, and ulcerations of the articular cartilage surface.

The frequency of OA increases with age, affecting more than 25% of individuals over the age of 60. OA is characterized by alterations in proteoglycan and collagen. Cartilage changes are characterized by an accumulation of advanced glycation end products, the result of nonenzymatic glycation of proteins, which happens with age. Proinflammatory cytokines and prostaglandins play roles in mediating OA.

The subchondral sclerosis commonly seen in OA reflects an abnormality in osteoblasts and is thought to be a "reaction" to the primary cartilage abnormalities. Symptomatic hand OA affects more than 13% of people over the age of 70 and is more common in women. OA of the 1st CMC (carpal metacarpal) is associated with reduced handgrip strength.[11] Prominent squaring of the base of the thumb has been termed the shelf sign. Thumb pain is reported when ringing a washcloth if 1st CMC OA is present. Subchondral sclerosis, independent of other radiological findings, may be a predictor for thumb pain. Other functional challenges may include opening jar tops or bottles. An MRI of hand OA will reveal cartilage loss, bone edema, synovial enhancement, osteophytes, and erosions. Age, gender, and genetics are risk factors for OA of the hand. In situations of both overuse and obesity, there is conflicting evidence regarding support of their potential respective roles in disease pathogenesis. Hypermobility may be protective for IP (interphalangeal), PIP (proximal interphalangeal),

Address for correspondence: Dr. Geeta Nayyar, 1111 Army Navy Drive, Apt 1106, Arlington, VA, USA 22202. geeta.nayyar@gmail.com

MRI and Ultrasound in Diagnosis and Management: Ann. N.Y. Acad. Sci. 1154: 3–9 (2009).
doi: 10.1111/j.1749-6632.2009.04380.x © 2009 New York Academy of Sciences.

and MCP (metacarpal phalangeal) joints, while it may be positively associated with OA of the CMC joints. Plain radiological hints that sometimes help distinguish erosive OA from psoriatic arthritis (PsA) include the fact that in PsA there is no significant osteophyte formation and PsA erosions tend to be marginal.

DISH (diffuse idiopathic skeletal hyperostosis) is ligamentous anteriolateral ossification that coexists with OA. In this syndrome, ligaments and entheses calcify with a predilection for the right side of the spine.[4] Nonspinal entheses such as the peripatellar ligaments and the Achilles tendon may be involved. The diagnosis is radiographic and defined as four or more contiguous ankylosed vertebrae in the absence of sacroiliitis and is often associated with preserved disc space height and with a complaint of stiffness. DISH is distinct from spondyloarthropathies (ossification of the outer layer of the annulus fibrosus), ossification of the posterior longitudinal ligament (OPLL), or ossification of the ligamentum flavum (OLF). The disease, which is more common and more severe in men, is associated with hyperinsulinemia, obesity, coronary artery disease, and isoretinol use.

The rotator cuff, which comprises the tendons of the supraspinatus, infraspinatus, teres minor, and subscapularis muscles, aids in shoulder rotation. The tendons attach at the humeral tuberosities and secure the humeral head against the tug of the deltoid. In essence they exert a downward-acting force. The rotator cuff separates the glenohumeral joint space from the subacromial bursa. Rotator cuff tendonitis, which is a common cause of pain, may or may not be associated with calcific deposits. In severe cases pain begins with the initiation of abduction. Clinical presentations often include complaints of difficulty in dressing and night pain. Pain may be increased with active abduction against resistance. A positive drop-arm sign may be seen with a large tear in the rotator cuff. Tears may go unrecognized and may be seen secondary to trauma, fracture, dislocation, and rheumatoid arthritis. The impingement theory

of rotator cuff disorders involves compressive injury to the tendons between the humeral head and the coracoacromial arch, which could result in either ischemia or increased intramuscular pressure and subsequently accelerate degeneration. MRI observed changes of degeneration correlate with histological changes.[5] Tendinopathy appears to precede rotator cuff tears. There is an exposure–response relationship between lifetime work with the upper arm elevated and supraspinatus tendinopathy.

Inflammatory Musculoskeletal Conditions

Rheumatoid arthritis (RA) is a systemic inflammatory condition of unknown etiology, which is characterized by a propensity to damage joints in the setting of persistent synovitis. Although all ages can be affected, the peak incidence occurs in the middle adult years. Patients with RA commonly complain of morning stiffness. Clinical signs of RA include warmth and swelling of joints. Cartilage loss and periarticular erosion, together, are responsible for structural changes such as ulnar deviation, swan neck deformity, or boutonniere deformity. Tenosynovitis of the transverse ligament of C1 may result in atlantoaxial instability. The extra-articular manifestations of RA include rheumatoid nodules, keratoconjunctivitis sicca, interstitial lung disease, pleurisy, anemia, and vasculitis.

A genetic influence is evidenced by virtue of both gender and HLA-DR haplotype. Within the HLA-DR4 haplotype is the HLA-DRB1 region, which helps determine RA disease severity. HLA-DRB1 alleles encode for the shared epitope, which is a common amino acid sequence. Specifically, HLA-DRB1 alleles encode for sequences found in the third hypervariable region of the DRB1 molecule, and the strongest allele associated with RA is HLA-DRB1*0401. In particular, these alleles are associated with a higher level of joint destruction, bone erosions, and rheumatoid vasculitis. Other predictors for poor prognosis include the presence of rheumatoid nodules and the rheumatoid factor. Nonspecific laboratory correlates of disease and disease activity may include the rheumatoid factor (RF), acute phase reactants (including the erythrocyte sedimentation rate and C-reactive protein tests), and the finding of anemia of chronic disease. The RF may be seen in as many as 85% of afflicted individuals but can also be a feature associated with other chronic inflammatory conditions. The RF encompasses a polyclonal group of autoantibodies directed against diverse epitopes of the Fc portion of IgG. RF production is under T-cell control.

Antibodies to citrullinated proteins (anti-CCP) include antiperinuclear factor, antikeratin antibodies, and antifilaggrin antibodies. These antibodies all target epitopes in which arginine residues have been converted to citrulline by posttranslational activity of deiminase enzymes. In humans, there is local production of antibodies to citrullinated proteins within the inflamed joint. These antibodies, which may be seen even before clinical symptoms develop, are associated with more severe joint destruction and greater disease activity. It has further been shown that smoking predisposes to CCP-positive RA only in the presence of shared epitope alleles; tobacco exposure increases the risk for such antibodies particularly in the presence of HLA-DRB1*01 and HLA-DRB1*10 shared epitope alleles.[10] In general, HLA-DRB1*0401 confers the highest risk for production of anti-CCP antibodies. Complicating the scientific interpretation of this phenomenon is the presence of citrullinated proteins in other inflammatory conditions. Hence, it has been suggested that protein deimination occurs as an associated phenomenon of nonspecific inflammation, so citrullination per se is probably not sufficient to trigger RA.

RA synovium becomes hypertrophic and edematous with villous fronds that expand into the joint cavity. Synovitis is characterized by the accumulation of many cell populations, including T cells, plasma cells, B cells, macrophages, neutrophils, mast cells, natural killer (NK) cells, and dendritic cells in the sublining layer. The dominant cellular components of the lining layer are fibroblast-like synoviocytes (FLS) and macrophages. The latter may also be seen in the sublining layer. T cells and plasma cells are prominent in the synovial sublining layer. Lymphocyte aggregates are observed in 50–60% of patients with RA and can be surrounded by plasma cells. In addition, macrophages and lymphocytes infiltrate the areas between the lymphocyte aggregates. Large numbers of T cells are also present in the synovial sublining. The majority of these cells reflect an oligoclonal expansion of CD4 cells, and CD4 T cells interact with macrophages within the rheumatoid synovium.

The histopathological manifestation of RA is a fibrovascular proliferation of synovium known as pannus, which may be characterized by multilayer synovial hypertrophy. This granulation tissue is associated with destruction of periarticular bone and cartilage. It often invades where the synovium reflects off of bone, resulting in the characteristic marginal erosions seen radiographically. The inflammation of RA is driven in large part by cytokines. Some examples of the mechanisms of cytokine-driven processes thought to be important in the joint damage wrought by RA include production of osteoclast-differentiation factor, IL-1, TNF-alpha, and matrix metalloproteinases. Various effector cells, including T cells, synovial fibroblasts, synovial macrophages, and chondrocytes, produce these chemical mediators. In turn, such cytokines lead to osteoclast differentiation/activation, decreased proteoglycan production, and the degradation of collagen, proteoglycans, lamin, fibronectin, and elastin. IL-6, a 184 amino acid glycoprotein, is another effector cytokine in RA. Macrophages, B cells, T cells, fibroblasts, and endothelial cells (among others) can produce IL-6, which regulates the hepatic acute phase response and stimulates the production of C-reactive protein while suppressing serum albumin production. IL-6 is elevated in the serum and synovial fluid of RA patients and plays a role in osteoclastogenesis, autoantibody production, and immune cell activation (e.g., it leads to T-cell differentiation). Anti-IL-6 receptor antibody may be a therapeutic intervention for RA.

Chemokines (chemotactic cytokines), small heparin-binding proteins that direct the movement of mononuclear cells to sites of inflammation, are also elevated in the joints of patients with RA. They activate surface receptors, which, in turn, initiate signaling cascades that culminate in cell shape change and cell movement. It is thought that they aid in the recruitment of monocytes and T cells into synovial tissues. Chemokine receptor 1 (CCR1) can be found on T cells, monocytes, eosinophils, and basophils and may play a role in RA.[7,8] Another type of chemokine, termed lymphotactin (XCL1), is found on T cells and NK cells and may also play a role in RA.

The main goal of therapy is to stop the destructive intra-articular process that leads to disability and death. Along with physical and occupational therapy, drug therapy includes nonsteroidal anti-inflammatory agents, corticosteroids (both local and systemic), disease modifying agents, and biological modifiers.[3] Combination therapy may be required in some cases. Methotrexate (MTX), which slows the progression of radiographic erosions, is the most commonly employed disease-modifying drug. Even though it has potential liver, marrow, and pulmonary toxicity, it is less toxic than corticosteroids. TNF-alpha antagonists are powerful but expensive interventions for both early and established RA. TNF inhibition improves ACR 20 (disease activity) scores in subjects compared to others receiving MTX alone. Use of TNF-alpha antagonists is contraindicated in patients with multiple sclerosis, congestive heart failure, or tuberculosis. TNF-alpha antagonist-associated TB cases are notable for a higher than usual incidence of extrapulmonary and disseminated disease.[6,9] In the United States, incidence rates for TB in RA patients treated with infliximab is estimated to be nearly 4 times that of baseline. Most cases

of TB occur within a few months of initiating treatment and hence are thought to represent reactivation TB. Successfully fending off TB requires macrophages, T cells, and cytokines, whereas TNF-alpha is required for proper formation of granulomas.

Juvenile rheumatoid arthritis (JRA, also called juvenile chronic arthritis or juvenile idiopathic arthritis) is a diagnosis of exclusion and involves various subtypes. Systemic-onset JRA is characterized by fevers, rash, lymphadenopathy, and hepatosplenomegaly. Polyarticular-onset JRA is characterized by five or more involved joints and may be either rheumatoid factor positive or negative. Pauci-articular JRA, which affects four or fewer joints, can be subdivided into two groups: early and late onset, depending upon the age at presentation. Early-onset JRA typically affects young girls who often are ANA-positive. Anterior uveitis is a special concern in this population. As many as 60% of youths who have a pauciarticular-onset JRA will go on to a polyarticular course. The therapy for children is similar to that for adult RA.

Ankylosing spondylitis (AS) is an ossifying inflammatory disease with a predilection for the spine.[14] The first radiographic areas of involvement are the sacroiliac (SI) joints. Erosions are first seen on the iliac side. Both the synovial and ligamentous aspects of the joint may ossify. In the spine, reactive sclerosis in response to erosion at the corner of the vertebral body gives rise to the "ivory" corner sign. Later this becomes a squared vertebral body. Ossification begins in the outer portion of the annulus fibrosus (Sharpley's fibers). This ossification may extend into the deep layers of the longitudinal ligaments. Syndesmophytes typically ascend the lumbar spine. The disc spaces may be preserved. A pseudoarthrosis within a bamboo spine is seen when there is an area of skipped ossification or a fracture. After the axial spine, the most commonly involved joint is the hip, followed by the shoulder. The knee is affected in 30% of cases. The symphysis pubis is affected in 23% of cases.

Psoriatic arthritis is another disease in the spondyloarthropathy category and occurs in up to 30% of individuals with psoriasis, a condition that affects an estimated 2% of the general population. PsA is characterized by activated T cells in synovial fluid and the synovium.[12] The combination of oligoarthritis, dactylitis, and heel pain is strongly suggestive of PsA. Dactylitis is seen in 16–24% of cases of PsA, and is associated with a poor prognosis for the affected digit in terms of erosive propensity. Although tenosynovitis and synovitis are the major underlying pathologies of dactylitis in PsA, other findings by MRI include circumferential soft tissue edema and bone edema. Flexor tenosynovitis appears to be more common than extensor tenosynovitis.[13] Even when the dactylitis is chronic and nontender, it may demonstrate such widespread abnormalities.

Miscellaneous Rheumatological Conditions

Calcium crystal arthritis is a process of matrix calcification. Calcification has been recorded in a variety of extra-articular tissues including the eye. Intercritical pseudogout (pyrophosphate arthropathy) joint fluid may demonstrate intracellular crystals just as has been recorded for intercritical gout patients. Calcium crystal arthritis is associated with changes in the concentrations of pyrophosphate and phosphate. There is also an alteration in the morphology of chondrocytes near CPPD (calcium pyrophosphate deposition disease) deposits, and they may become unusually large (chondrocyte hypertrophy). In some cases, crystal deposits may be seen by ultrasound. Arthroscopy is not reliable as it only detects surface deposits. MRI is similarly poor at distinguishing CPPD deposits, as they appear as signal voids.[15]

Pigmented villonodular synovitis (PVNS), a rare inflammatory synovitis of unknown etiology that has a predilection for the knee and hip,[16] is most commonly seen as a monoar-

ticular process. Histological features include hemosiderin deposits with villous transformation of the synovial lining. Plain radiography may reveal dense soft tissue masses and, later, bone changes. In general, however, plain radiography is normal in 32% of cases (54% of cases involving the knee). Plain X-rays may be difficult to distinguish from tuberculous and rheumatoid arthritides. Hemosiderin has ferromagnetic properties that support the superiority of MRI in depicting PVNS. Bone erosion, when seen, is due to pressure atrophy, invasion of bone, or a combination of both. The gradient-recalled echo sequence (GRE) is best for depicting hemosiderin deposits. Increased signal intensity obscures the hemosiderin on short inversion time inversion recovery sequence (fat suppression). It should be remembered that hemosiderin deposits in the soft tissue can be seen in hematomas, giant cell tumors, and pseudoaneurysms. Contrast enhancement does not appear to add to the diagnostic capability of MRI in this disorder.

The idiopathic inflammatory myopathies (IIM) are diverse diseases of the skeletal muscles in which striated muscle cells or connective tissue elements may be affected.

Myopathies can result from abnormalities of skeletal muscle proteins (Duchenne's muscular dystrophy), alterations of the sarcolemmal channels (hyperkalemic periodic paralysis), endocrine abnormalities (e.g., hypothyroidism, glucocorticoid excess states, adrenal insufficiency), mitochondrial alterations (mitochondrial myopathies), cell/humoral mediated autoimmune mechanisms (polymyositis, dermatomyositis), infections (pyomyositis, HIV-related polymyositis), or different toxins (e.g., colchicine, alcohol, statins, cocaine, D-penicillamine), just to name the most important categories.

Dermatomyositis, polymyositis, and inclusion body myositis are the three major categories of idiopathic inflammatory myopathy. These inflammatory myopathies are clinically, histologically, and pathogenically distinct. They may occur in isolation or accompanying other connective tissue diseases (e.g., overlap syndromes, mixed connective tissue disease). The incidence of idiopathic inflammatory muscle disease in general is approximately 1:100,000. These myopathies affect the upper and lower girdle muscles in a rather symmetric fashion. Sometimes, pharyngeal muscles and the myocardium are affected. Patients suffer from subacute (weeks to months), progressive and symmetric proximal muscle weakness of the upper and lower extremities. Patients characteristically have problems arising from a sitting position, shampooing their hair, or walking up or down stairs. Inclusion body myositis characteristically involves distal muscles, such as foot extensors and finger flexors. Weakness and atrophy can be asymmetric or may selectively involve the quadriceps in this latter syndrome.

In addition to the above clinical features, the diagnosis of inflammatory myopathies is supported by muscle enzymes, electromyography testing, and muscle biopsy, and MRI has recently been added to these diagnostic tools.[20,21] Myositis-specific antibodies are useful tools for predicting specific clinical features (e.g., anti-Jo-1 antibody may be associated with interstitial lung disease, Raynaud's, and mechanic's hands).[19] Classic cutaneous features of dermatomyositis include the heliotrope rash, Gottron's papules, the V-sign, and the shawl sign.[18] The heliotrope rash is often accompanied by edema of the eyelids. Gottron's lesions tend to be flat-topped papules or patches over dorsal articular surfaces. Malignancy may precede, coincide with, or postdate the diagnosis of dermatomyositis. Histological findings of the involved skin in dermatomyositis include vacuolar basal layer change, necrotic keratinocytes, vascular dilatation, and superficial/sparse perivascular infiltrate. This histology may be indistinguishable from SLE (systemic lupus erythematosus).

Immunopathological studies suggest a role for complement-mediated injury of vessels in dermatomyositis. Interstitial lung disease (ILD) in IIM may present as an acute onset syndrome, as a chronic slowly progressive syndrome, or as an asymptomatic abnormal chest X ray[17] Anti-tRNA-synthestase antibodies are the strongest predictors for development of ILD, but they should not be solely relied upon for diagnostic purposes. Pulmonary function tests (PFTs) and high-resolution CT (HRCT) appear to be the most useful means for detecting ILD in IIM. PFTs typically show restrictive ventilatory defects with decreased total lung capacity and decreased carbon dioxide diffusion (DLCO). HRCT can discriminate between fibrotic and inflammatory disease. The most common HRCT findings are irregular linear opacities with areas of consolidation and ground glass attenuation.

Histological features of the muscle in dermatomyositis include inflammatory infiltrates that are predominantly perivascular and/or perifascicular. This is in contradistinction to polymyositis, where infiltrates are seen mostly within fascicles (endomysial inflammation). Perifascicular atrophy is another distinguishing feature limited to dermatomyositis. Prednisone, methotrexate, azathioprine, cyclosporine, and high-dose monthly intravenous immunoglobulins are the most significant drugs for the treatment of these conditions.

Conflicts of Interest

The authors declare no conflicts of interest.

References

1. Kuroda, R., A. Usas, S. Kubo, *et al.* 2006. Cartilage repair using bone morphogenetic protein 4 and muscle-derived stem cells. *Arthritis Rheum.* **54:** 387–389.
2. Embry Flory, J.J., A.J. Fosang & W. Knudson. 2006. The accumulation of intracellular ITEGE and DIPEN neoepitopes in bovine articular chondrocytes is mediated by CD44 internalization of hyaluronan. *Arthritis Rheum.* **54:** 443–454.
3. Singh, R., D.B. Robinson & H.S. El-Gabalawy. 2005. Emerging biologic therapies in rheumatoid arthritis: Cell targets and cytokines. *Curr. Opin. Rheumatol.* **17:** 274–279.
4. Sarzi-Puttini, P. & F. Atzeni. 2004. New developments in our understanding of DISH (diffuse idiopathic

skeletal hyperostosis). *Curr. Opin. Rheumatol.* **16:** 287–292.

5. Svendsen, S.W., J. Gelineck, S.E. Mathiassen, *et al.* 2004. Work above shoulder level and degenerative alterations of the rotator cuff tendons. A magnetic resonance imaging study. *Arthritis Rheum.* **50:** 3314–3322.

6. Hanlon, C.D. 2004. Treatment complications from biological agents. *Curr. Opin. Rheumatol.* **16:** 393–398.

7. von Andrian, U.H. & C.R. Mackay. 2000. T-cell function and migration. Two sides of the same coin. *N. Engl. J. Med.* **343:** 1020–1034.

8. Walport, M.J. 2001. Complement. *N. Engl. J. Med.* **344:** 1058–1066.

9. Imperato, A.K., S. Smiles & S.B. Abramson. 2004. Long-term risks associated with biological response modifiers used in rheumatic diseases. *Curr. Opin. Rheumatol.* **16:** 199–205.

10. van der Helm-van Mil, A.H.M., K.N. Verpoort, S. le Cessie, *et al.* 2007. The HLA-DRB1 shared epitope alleles differ in the interaction with smoking and predisposition to antibodies to cyclic citrullinated peptide. *Arthritis Rheum.* **56:** 425–432.

11. Kloppenberg, M. 2007. Hand osteoarthritis: An increasing need for treatment and rehabilitation. *Curr. Opin. Rheumatol.* **19:** 179–183.

12. Kaltwasser, J.P., P. Nash, D. Gladman, *et al.* 2004. Efficacy and safety of Leflunomide in the treatment of psoriatic arthritis and psoriasis: A multinational, double-blind, randomized, placebo-controlled clinical trial. *Arthritis Rheum.* **50:** 1939–1950.

13. Healy, P.J., C. Groves, M. Chandramohan & P.S. Helliwell. 2008. MRI changes in psoriatic dactylitis: Extent of pathology, relationship to tenderness and correlation with clinical indices. *Rheumatology (Oxford)* **47:** 561–562.

14. Liu, Y., D. Cortinovis & M.A. Stone. 2004. Recent advances in the treatment of the spondyloarthropathies. *Curr. Opin. Rheumatol.* **16:** 357–365.

15. Rosenthal, A.K. 2007. Update in calcium deposition diseases. *Curr. Opin. Rheumatol.* **19:** 158–162.

16. Cheng, X.G., Y.H. You, W. Liu, *et al.* 2004. MRI features of pigmented villonodular synovitis (PVNS). *Clin. Rheumatol.* **23:** 31–34.

17. Fathi, M. & I.E. Lundberg. 2005. Interstitial lung disease in polymyositis and dermatomyositis. *Curr. Opin. Rheumatol.* **17:** 701–706.

18. Santmyire-Rosenberger, B. & E. Dugan. 2003. Skin involvement in dermatomyositis. *Curr. Opin. Rheumatol.* **15:** 714–722.

19. Levine, S.M., A. Rosen & L.A. Casciola-Rosen. 2003. Anti-aminoacyl tRNA synthetase immune responses: Insights into the pathogenesis of the idiopathic inflammatory myopathies. *Curr. Opin. Rheumatol.* **15:** 708–713.

20. Adams, E.M., C.K. Chow, A. Premkumar & P.H. Plotz. 1995. The idiopathic inflammatory myopathies: Spectrum of MR imaging findings. *Radiographics* **15:** 563–574.

21. Stiglbauer, R., W. Graninger, L. Prayer, *et al.* 1993. Polymyositis: MRI-appearance at 1.5 T and correlation to clinical findings. *Clin. Radiol.* **48:** 244–248.

Overview of Imaging in Inflammatory Arthritis

James D. Katz, Geeta Nayyar, and Erinn Noeth

Departments of Medicine and Radiology, The George Washington University, Washington, DC, USA

Whether magnetic resonance imaging (MRI) or ultrasound (US) are chosen for the purposes of musculoskeletal interrogation depends upon a variety of factors ranging from the anatomy targeted to cost considerations and the time of acquisition. Newer technologies such as higher-strength MRI or 3D-US promise to help overcome some of the disadvantages of each option. Improving technical proficiency is the thrust of efforts to support more widespread application of sonographic assessment in various clinical arenas. Finally, these technologies offer the opportunity to diagnose inflammatory conditions at early stages of their disease progression.

Key words: MRI; arthritis; myositis

Overview of Imaging in Musculoskeletal Conditions

The principal target of disease activity in rheumatoid arthritis (RA) is the lining of the synovial joints. As a general rule, the plain radiographic appearance of RA reflects the pathologic changes associated with soft tissue swelling, thickening of the affected joint capsule, and osteoporosis. As the disease progresses, there is destruction of the articular cartilage with narrowing of the joint space. Juxta-articular erosions of bone are associated with hypertrophied synovium. Ultimately the disease may result in destruction and even subluxation of joints.

In the hands and wrists, RA is usually bilateral and symmetrical. Involvement of the metacarpophalangeal (MCP) and proximal interphalangeal (PIP) joints is the rule. The disease also commonly affects the carpal joints. For the assessment of early inflammatory arthritis, the small joints of the hands and feet are of primary interest.

Spinal arthritis is characteristic of the various seronegative spondyloarthropathies. Magnetic resonance imaging (MRI) may detect earlier sacroiliitis than is possible with plain radiography.[1]

High-field-strength (>1.0 T), whole-body MRI scanners, as well as medium-field (0.5–1.0 T) and low-field (<0.5 T) extremity scanners are widely available. MRI is excellent for soft tissue evaluation, especially as it relates to cases of tumor invasion and infection. MRI can be performed in multiple planes (sagittal, coronal, and axial) and bone edema is readily visualized. Evidence is accumulating that bone edema seen in MRI correlates with histological osteitis as well as the clinical symptoms associated with pain. Inflammatory tissue in the bone marrow results in increased water content, which appears as bright signal enhancement on STIR (short-tau inversion recovery) MRI sequences. In the case of the knee joint, MRI is unsurpassed in delineating meniscal pathology.[2] Similarly, inflammatory disease of the synovium is also readily imaged by MRI.[3]

Three-dimensional contrast-enhanced MRI has already proven reliable in cases of psoriatic arthritis of the hands,[4] and may eventually be useful in measuring the volume of

Address for correspondence: Dr. Geeta Nayyar, George Washington University, 1111 Army Navy Drive, Apt 1106, Arlington, VA 22202, USA. Voice: 305–794-6524. geeta.nayyar@gmail.com synovitis in RA. Another promising diagnostic procedure may be dynamic contrast-enhanced magnetic resonance imaging (DCE-MRI), but these modalities have yet to be fully developed. Furthermore, MRI is still plagued by problems with interreader and intermachine reliability. Finally, some anatomical sites remain challenges for radiological imaging. For example, the labral areas in the hip and shoulder may require special imaging sequences.[5]

High-Tesla MRI (using a 3-T magnet) may overcome some of the limitations of conventional MRI. It improves resolution while reducing data acquisition times, but at the cost of increased radiofrequency energy deposition.[6] Toward this end, quantitative imaging, such as by high-resolution MRI, promises to enable improved cartilage morphometric assessment.[7]

Within the past decade, musculoskeletal ultrasound has become an established imaging technique for the diagnosis and follow-up of patients with rheumatic diseases. Ultrasound (US) has two primary roles in musculoskeletal medicine. It can serve as an extension of the physical examination or it may be used to measure objective outcomes.[8] There are several advantages to using US as an imaging technique.

The "real-time" capability of US allows dynamic assessment of joint and tendon movements. The short scanning time necessary to evaluate each joint makes it possible to evaluate multiple joints in one clinical sitting. Other advantages are that it is noninvasive, portable, and relatively inexpensive; there is no ionizing radiation; and it is easily repeatable. All of these characteristics make it particularly useful for the monitoring of treatment. It can also be used for guiding aspiration, biopsy, and injection treatment.[8]

Ultrasound is most commonly employed to assess soft tissue disease or detect fluid collection. High-frequency US transducers enable ultrasonographic assessment of small joints. The more superficial the structure that is imaged the better the spatial resolution. Articular and periarticular fluid, as well as enthesitis, are read-

ily apprehended. It can also be used to visualize other structures, such as cartilage and bone surface, and can detect cortical defects, extensor tendon sheath thickening, synovial proliferation, and even median nerve diameter. In certain situations, US may improve the clinical accuracy of diagnosing joint effusions. Owing to the better axial and lateral resolution of US, even minute bone surface abnormalities can be depicted. Thus, destructive and/or reparative/hypertrophic changes on the bone surface can be seen before they are apparent on plain X rays or even MRIs. However, US wave frequencies cannot penetrate into bone, rendering imaging of intraosseous (and sometimes intra-articular) disease impossible. For deeply situated joints such as the hip, the limited acoustic window of the US beam poses a challenge to the reliability and validity of sonographic imaging.

Most musculoskeletal evaluation is performed using "gray scale," which means that images are produced in a black-and-white format, where each white dot in the image represents a reflected sound wave. Sound waves travel in a similar manner to light waves and therefore the denser the material is (e.g., bone cortex), the more reflective it is and the whiter it appears on the screen. Water is the least reflective body material and therefore appears as black as the sound waves travel straight through it.

Newer US techniques include color and power Doppler imaging, which provide color maps of tissues. The amount of color is related to the degree of blood flow, which may be of use in the assessment of vascular tissues and soft tissue inflammation. Doppler and power Doppler techniques offer the opportunity to evaluate synovial vascularity and potentially predict disease activity and radiographic outcome. Intravenous bubble contrast agents are being explored as potential enhancers of power Doppler sensitivity.

Data are limited regarding the particular imaging modality that is most appropriate in various clinical scenarios and only rarely have the diagnostic values of different imaging techniques been compared. Nevertheless, from a clinical standpoint, the place of US in patient management is becoming increasingly clear.

Future research on ultrasonography for joints will include development of a volumetric probe for 3D-US. Three-dimensional US imaging appears to be as reliable and accurate as the two-dimensional technique, and it may improve the imaging of smaller lesions.[9] Owing to the lack of cross-sectional orientation during the US procedure, current research efforts are focused on improving the reliability of data with respect to intra- and interreader reliability.

Two particular challenges facing the ultrasonographer are skill acquisition and standardization of technique. The precise placement of the probe over the anatomical target is just one of the skills necessary to achieve a high-quality image. Owing to the fact that the procedure itself entails dynamic/real-time imaging, static "snapshots" obtained by the operator may not fully represent the knowledge derived from the study. For example, observing the movement of a tendon or acquiring an image during muscle contraction may provide important clinical information that is difficult to capture otherwise.

Research is needed to ensure adequate skill attainment by sonographers. Generally, sonography training involves either "hands-on" courses or apprenticeship-style instruction. The American College of Radiology recommends that 500 supervised scans be adopted as a minimum standard of training. The EULAR Working Group for Musculoskeletal Ultrasound has proposed guidelines for basic training.

The production of high-quality US images is intimately linked with rigorous standardization of US techniques. In recent years, experts have published guidelines on the correct approach to imaging a variety of anatomical sites in an attempt to produce a standard for clinical practice, training, and research. As a concept, standardization is well known in the field of plain radiography. Ultrasound presents specific difficulties in relation to standardization by virtue of its dynamic nature and the dependence of the acquisition process on the operator. The advent of 3D-US should address many of these difficulties. However, since the majority of practitioners will continue to use 2D-US, these issues will remain important in the foreseeable future.

Over the last 5 years, the EULAR Working Group has been organizing basic and advanced US courses, which have been successful in terms of the number of participants and the level of satisfaction among those who have attended. Recently, a group of rheumatologists from Belfast described a series of steps they took over a 5-year period, to gain sufficient experience to achieve a basic level of competency in US. At the end of that period, they were assessed by an experienced rheumatologist-sonographer in a formal test of their ability to perform basic US examinations on normal volunteers and patients. This system has the advantage of being a "real-time" assessment of a dynamic technique, but it requires a considerable time commitment on the part of all the participants.

Perhaps a more universal means of training and assessment can be devised with the help of the latest techniques of web-based learning. These are not a substitute for mentoring by an experienced sonographer, but they could be a powerful adjunct to face-to-face learning. This approach has already been the subject of a pilot study in Italy, where trainees have the benefit of a continuous interaction with tutors by submitting their US images to a web-based tutor for comment and feedback.

As physicians have gained experience with ultrasonography, it has become natural to rely increasingly upon this technique to guide procedures and therapeutic interventions.[10] Moreover, in an emergency department setting, US has proven invaluable for rapid low-cost assessment of peripheral soft tissue injuries.[11]

MRI as an Aid in the Diagnosis of Early Inflammatory Arthritis

The focus on diagnosis of inflammatory arthritis early in the course of the disease is motivated by the advent of effective therapeutic strategies. The advantage to these strategies is that early administration affords the best treatment outcome.[12–18] When left untreated, substantial and irreversible joint damage often occurs within the first few months of rheumatoid onset,[17,19–22] so identification of RA patients in the initial stages of the disease could improve their quality of life.[14,17,21,23]

The diagnosis of RA encompasses a spectrum of disease manifestations established by the American College of Rheumatology (ACR), which includes clinical and laboratory findings in addition to the conventional radiographic signs of osseous erosions or periarticular osteopenia in the hands or wrist joints.[24] An early diagnosis is often clinically difficult because the nonspecific signs and symptoms of the disease are relatively slow to develop and often overlap with other inflammatory polyarthropathies.[25,26] As a more objective tool, conventional radiographs have played an important role in the initial evaluation of patients with polyarthritis. However, the hallmarks of RA, which include osseous marginal erosions and symmetric joint space narrowing, are often late developments on conventional radiographs. Some studies have shown a delay in radiographic findings of 6–12 months from symptom onset,[20,27] at which time these lesions may be irreversible. With its multiplanar tomography and superior soft tissue detail, MRI has been the subject of considerable attention as a more sensitive imaging modality with an important role in the early diagnosis of rheumatological disorders.

The pathogenesis of RA is not well understood, but follows a generalized inflammatory cascade. Cytokine release stimulates synovial hyperplasia and pannus formation, with the earliest involvement occurring in synovial joints and tendon sheaths. Ongoing synovitis leads to subsequent bone damage in those areas covered solely by synovium (the so-called bare areas of bone), located between the insertion of the joint capsule and the cartilage.[28] Within these areas one can see bone marrow edema and the subsequent development of osseous erosions.[28] If untreated, bone destruction and deformity ensue, often with associated secondary degenerative arthritis.

The clear advantage of MRI over conventional radiography is the ability to image the synovium. The fibrous synovial tissue of the normal joint has the signal intensity of simple joint fluid on an MRI. When inflamed, the synovium becomes thickened and hyperemic, demonstrating early and avid contrast enhancement with gadolinium-diethyltriaminepentaacetic acid (Gd-DTPA).[29] This enhancement enables the differentiation between inflamed synovial tissue and joint effusion, as the latter does not enhance.[29]

The importance of this is multifold. First, synovitis has no radiographic correlate and is often asymptomatic in its earliest stages, which renders MRI more sensitive than either radiography or a clinical examination for the detection of synovitis.[15,30–32] Second, the presence of synovitis serves as a prognostic indicator for later bone destruction, with osseous damage occurring in proportion to the degree of synovitis, but not in its absence.[15,33] This finding has led several investigators to focus on more quantitative analyses of synovial hyperplasia, using both volume measurements and rates of synovial enhancement with dynamic MRI.[29,34,35] Østergaard *et al.* demonstrated that MRI-calculated synovial membrane volumes are closely related to the rate of progression of joint destruction.[34] Third, effective suppression of synovitis has been shown to actually prevent bone damage.[15] Certainly, this last point underscores the critical role of MRI in the detection of synovitis at an early, reversible stage.

With ongoing inflammation, synovitis ultimately elicits a local edematous response in the underlying bone marrow, identified with

MRI as an increased water signal in subcortical bone. This edema tends to occur in those areas of bone that have no protective cartilage, and is best illustrated on water-sensitive MRI sequences with fat suppression. Edematous bone, sometimes referred to as "osteitis," demonstrates significant enhancement with Gd-DTPA,[29] and has been shown to correlate with clinical markers of inflammation.[36] Bone edema has been identified in patients within the first 4 weeks of symptom onset,[33] and it tends to evolve into bony erosions at the same site.[20,36–38] In fact, marrow edema at initial MRI is the factor most predictive not only of subsequent osseous erosion,[37,39] but also of functional outcome in later disease.[36,38] In summary, marrow edema represents an early and reversible finding on MRI but one that has no plain radiographic correlate.

Osseous marginal erosions are a classic radiographic finding in RA, and are found in up to 47% of rheumatoid patients within the first year of disease.[22] On MRI, erosions appear as focal defects in cortical bone, often with increased signal on water-sensitive (T2-weighted) sequences and increased enhancement with Gd-DTPA. Enhancement with intravenous contrast indicates the presence of inflamed synovium within the defect,[29,40] and may help to distinguish erosions from simple and degenerative bone cysts, which do not enhance.[20]

Multiple studies have illustrated the superiority of MRI over radiography in identifying erosions.[20,31,39–41] In a 1998 study by McQueen *et al.*, radiographically identified osseous erosions were detected in only 15% of RA patients at presentation; MRIs of those same patients demonstrated erosions in 70% at presentation.[20] Other longitudinal studies have confirmed that erosions detectable on an initial MRI are seen later on conventional radiographs in the same location.[31,37,39,42] For instance, Albers *et al.* demonstrated that conventional radiography identified 20% of MRI-detectable erosions in an RA cohort at baseline but detected 60% of those same erosions in 5 years time.[42] These data speak not only

to the delay inherent in conventional radiographic imaging, but also to its inferior sensitivity when compared with MRI. Other studies have supported the superiority of MRI in erosion detection and have further suggested that MRI better illustrates the progression of erosions over time.[31,41]

At the present time, there are few guidelines to aid the clinician in the appropriate use of MRI in the early diagnosis of inflammatory arthritis. One use of MRI in patients with early arthritis is to distinguish between RA and the other chronic inflammatory arthropathies. As with conventional radiography, MRI relies on the characteristic pattern of rheumatoid involvement to distinguish it from these other arthropathies. Bilateral symmetric arthritis of more than three joints is the hallmark of RA, with a majority of patients presenting with symmetric arthritis of multiple small wrist and hand joints (particularly the MCP and PIP joints). In addition, RA is an erosive disease that does not demonstrate the proliferative bony changes that may be seen in various other disorders. Simultaneous synovitis of the wrist and hand tendon sheaths is another distinct finding in RA, which may further differentiate this intrasynovial disease from the other entheseal-based arthropathies.[28] MRI may also have differentiating utility in large joints such as the knee[43,44] and shoulder.[45]

Some investigators have argued that MRI should be employed as a first-line modality in suspected cases of inflammatory arthritis. In a small-cohort study, Sugimoto *et al.* demonstrated a promising 94% accuracy in the detection of early RA, compared with 81 and 83% using the traditional ACR method and classification tree alone.[46,47]

In order to provide more accurate and reproducible interpretation of MRIs, several investigators have proposed scoring systems.[48–50] Some MRI-based systems score individual findings such as bony erosions, synovitis, bone edema, and tendinous involvement in various combinations,[29,36,51] whereas others actually measure the volume of erosions and the inflamed synovium.[52] However, no single grading system has as yet gained general acceptance, owing in part to the variability of joint involvement and disease activity, as well as to imaging artifacts and other pitfalls inherent to MRI.[53,54]

Another potential role for MRI in clinical practice may be in its ability to separate patients with more severe prognoses from those whose conditions may not progress as rapidly.[22,37,55] As discussed earlier, investigators have established a relationship between the level of synovial involvement on MRIs and the likelihood of progression to subsequent bone damage by using quantitative analyses of the synovium in early RA patients.[34,43,56] Other investigators have focused on the relationship between early MRI findings and more long-term functional outcomes. In a 2004 study by Benton *et al.*, initial MRI of the wrist was found to help predict function at 6-year follow-up in RA patients.[36] With such correlations, it may be possible to determine which patients would benefit from early aggressive therapy. In short, MRI offers advanced sensitivity in the diagnosis of early inflammatory arthritis, particularly RA.

Conflicts of Interest

The authors declare no conflicts of interest.

References

1. Weber, U., R.O. Kissling & J. Hodler. 2007. Advances in musculoskeletal imaging and their clinical utility in the early diagnosis of spondyloarthritis. *J. Curr. Rheumatol. Rep.* **9:** 353–360.
2. Fox, M.G. 2007. MR imaging of the meniscus: Review, current trends, and clinical implications. *Radiol. Clin. North Am.* **45:** 1033–1053.
3. Frick, M.A., D.E. Wenger & M. Adkins. 2007. MR imaging of synovial disorders of the knee: An update. *Radiol. Clin. North Am.* **45:** 1017–1031.
4. Tehranzadeh, J., O. Ashikyan, A. Anavim & J. Shin. 2008. Detailed analysis of contrast-enhanced MRI of hands and wrists in patients with psoriatic arthritis. *Skeletal Radiol.* **37:** 433–442.
5. Lee, M.J., K. Motamedi, K. Chow & L.L. Seeger. 2008. Gradient-recalled echo sequences in direct shoulder MR arthrography for evaluating the labrum. *Skeletal Radiol.* **37:** 19–25.
6. Griffin, N., I. Joubert, D.J. Lomas *et al.* 2008. High resolution imaging of the knee on 3-Tesla MRI: A pictorial review. *Clin. Anat.* 21 10.1002/ca.20632.
7. Augat, P. & F. Eckstein. 2008. Quantitative imaging of musculoskeletal tissue. *Ann. Rev. Biomed. Eng.* **10:** 369–390.
8. Wakefield, R.J., W.W. Gibbon & P. Emery. 1999. The current status of US in rheumatology. *Rheumatology* **38:** 195–201.
9. Serafin-Król, M. *et al.* 2008. Potential value of three-dimensional ultrasonography in diagnosing muscle injuries in comparison to two-dimensional examination: Preliminary results. *Orthop. Traumatol. Rehabil.* **10:** 134–143.
10. Nazarian, L.N. 2008. The top 10 reasons musculoskeletal sonography is an important complementary or alternative technique to MRI. *Am. J. Roentgen.* **190:** 1621–1626.
11. Mankad, K., E. Hoey, A.J. Grainger & D.A. Barron. 2008. Trauma musculoskeletal ultrasound. *Emerg. Radiol.* **15:** 83–89.
12. Pincus, T. 1998. Aggressive treatment of early rheumatoid arthritis to prevent joint damage. *Bull. Rheum. Dis.* **47:** 2–7.
13. Lard, L.R., H. Visser, I. Speyer, *et al.* 2001. Early versus delayed treatment in patients with recent-onset rheumatoid arthritis: Comparison of two cohorts who received different treatment strategies. *Am. J. Med.* **111:** 446–451.
14. Quinn, M.A., P.G. Conaghan, P. Emery, *et al.* 2001. The therapeutic approach of early intervention for rheumatoid arthritis: What is the evidence? *Rheumatology* **40:** 1211–1220.
15. Conaghan, P., P. O'Connor, D. McGonagle, *et al.* 2003. Elucidation of the relationship between synovitis and bone damage: A randomized MRI study of individual joints in patients with early rheumatoid arthritis. *Arthritis Rheum.* **48:** 64–71.
16. Emery, P. 2002. Evidence supporting the benefit of early intervention in rheumatoid arthritis. *J. Rheumatol.* **66**(Suppl.): 3–8.
17. Nell, V.P.K., K.P. Machold, G. Eberl, *et al.* 2004. Benefit of very early referral and very early therapy with disease modifying anti-rheumatic drugs in patients with early rheumatoid arthritis. *Rheumatology* **43:** 906–914.
18. Kary, S., J. Fritz, U. Scherer, *et al.* 2004. Do we still miss the chance of effectively treating early rheumatoid arthritis? New answers from a new study. *Rheumatology* **43:** 819–820.
19. Brook, A. & M. Corbett. 1977. Radiographic changes in early rheumatoid arthritis. *Ann. Rheum. Dis.* **36:** 71–73.

20. McQueen, F.M., N. Stewart, J. Crabbe, *et al.* 1998. Magnetic resonance imaging of the wrist in early rheumatoid arthritis reveals high prevalence of erosions at 4 months after symptom onset. *Ann. Rheum. Dis.* **57:** 350–356.

21. Fuchs, H.A., J.J. Kaye, L.F. Callahan, *et al.* 1989. Evidence of significant radiographic damage in rheumatoid arthritis within the first 2 years of disease. *J. Rheumatol.* **16:** 585–591.

22. Fex, E., K. Jonsson, U. Johnson & K. Eberhardt. 1996. Development of radiographic damage during the first 5–6 years of rheumatoid arthritis: A prospective follow-up study of a Swedish cohort. *Br. J. Rheumatol.* **35:** 1106–1115.

23. Green, M., H. Marzo-Ortega & D. McGonagle. 1999. Persistence of mild, early inflammatory arthritis. *Arthritis Rheum.* **42:** 2184–2188.

24. Arnett, F.C., S.M. Edworthy, D.A. Bloch, *et al.* 1988. The American Rheumatism Association 1987 revised criteria for the classification of rheumatoid arthritis. *Arthritis Rheum.* **31:** 315–324.

25. Emery, P. 2002. Magnetic resonance imaging: Opportunities for rheumatoid arthritis disease assessment and monitoring long-term treatment outcomes. *Arthritis Res.* **4**(Suppl. 2): S6–S10.

26. Saraux, A., J.M. Berthelot, G. Chales, *et al.* 2001. Ability of the American College of Rheumatology 1987 criteria to predict rheumatoid arthritis in patients with early arthritis and classification of these patients two years later. *Arthritis Rheum.* **44:** 2485–2491.

27. van der Heijde, D.M., M.A. van Leeuwen, P.L. van Riel, *et al.* 1992. Biannual radiographic assessments of hands and feet in a three year prospective follow-up of patients with early rheumatoid arthritis. *Arthritis Rheum.* **35:** 26–34.

28. Sommer, O.J., A. Kladosek, V. Weiler, *et al.* 2005. Rheumatoid arthritis: A practical guide to state-of-the-art imaging, image interpretation, and clinical implications. *Radiographics* **25:** 381–398.

29. Rominger, M.B., W.K. Bernreuter, P.J. Kenney, *et al.* 1993. MR imaging of the hands in early rheumatoid arthritis: Preliminary results. *Radiographics* **13:** 37–46.

30. Klarlund, M., M. Østergaard & I. Lorenzen. 1999. Finger joint synovitis in rheumatoid arthritis: Quantitative assessment by magnetic resonance imaging. *Rheumatology* **38:** 66–72.

31. Klarlund, M., M. Østergaard, K.E. Jensen, *et al.* 2000. Magnetic resonance imaging, radiography and scintigraphy of the finger joints: One year follow-up of patients with early arthritis. *Ann. Rheum. Dis.* **59:** 521–528.

32. Kraan, M.C., H. Versendaal, M. Jonker, *et al.* 1998. Asymptomatic synovitis precedes clinically manifest arthritis. *Arthritis Rheum.* **41:** 1481–1488.

33. McGonagle, D., G. Conaghan, P. O'Connor, *et al.* 2001. The relationship between synovitis and bone changes in early untreated rheumatoid arthritis: A controlled magnetic resonance imaging study. *Arthritis Rheum.* **42:** 1706–1711.

34. Østergaard, M., M. Hansen, M. Stoltenberg, *et al.* 1999. Magnetic resonance imaging: Determined synovial membrane volume as a marker of disease activity and predictor of joint destruction in rheumatoid arthritis wrists. *Arthritis Rheum.* **42:** 918–929.

35. Østergaard, M., M. Stoltenberg & P. Lougreen-Nielson. 1998. Quantification of synovitis by MRI: Correlation between dynamic and static gadolinium-enhanced magnetic resonance imaging and microscopic and macroscopic signs of synovial inflammation. *Magn. Reson. Imaging* **16:** 743–754.

36. Benton, N., N. Stewart, J. Crabbe, *et al.* 2004. MRI of the wrist in early rheumatoid arthritis can be used to predict functional outcome at 6 years. *Ann. Rheum. Dis.* **63:** 555–561.

37. McQueen, F.M., N. Benton, J. Crabbe, *et al.* 2001. What is the fate of erosions in early rheumatoid arthritis? Tracking individual lesions using x-rays and magnetic resonance imaging over the first two years of disease. *Ann. Rheum. Dis.* **60:** 859–868.

38. McQueen, F.M., N. Benton, D. Perry, *et al.* 2003. Bone edema scored on magnetic resonance imaging scans of the dominant carpus at presentation predicts radiographic joint damage of the hands and feet six years later in patients with rheumatoid arthritis. *Arthritis Rheum.* **48:** 1814–1827.

39. McQueen, F.M., N. Stewart, J. Crabbe, *et al.* 1999. Magnetic resonance imaging of the wrist in early rheumatoid arthritis reveals progression of erosions despite clinical improvement. *Ann. Rheum. Dis.* **58:** 156–163.

40. McQueen, F.M. 2000. Magnetic resonance imaging in early inflammatory arthritis: What is its role? Review. *Rheumatology* **39:** 700–706.

41. Foley-Nolan, D., J.P. Stack, M. Ryan, *et al.* 1991. Magnetic resonance imaging in the assessment of rheumatoid arthritis: A comparison with plain film radiographs. *Br. J. Rheumatol.* **30:** 101–106.

42. Albers, J.M., P. Kurki, B. Eberhardt, *et al.* 2001. Treatment strategy, disease activity, and outcome in four cohorts of patients with early rheumatoid arthritis. *Ann. Rheum. Dis.* **60:** 453–458.

43. Gaffney, K., J. Cookson, D. Blake, *et al.* 1995. Quantification of rheumatoid synovitis by magnetic resonance imaging. *Arthritis Rheum.* **38:** 1610–1617.

44. McGonagle, D., W. Gibbon, P. O'Connor, *et al.* 1998. Characteristic magnetic resonance imaging entheseal changes of knee synovitis in spondyloarthropathy. *Arthritis Rheum.* **41:** 694–700.

45. McGonagle, D., C. Pease, H. Marzo-Ortega, *et al.* 2001. Comparison of extracapsular changes by magnetic resonance imaging in patients with rheumatoid arthritis and polymyalgia rheumatica. *J. Rheumatol.* **28:** 1837–1841.

46. Sugimoto, H., A. Takeda & J. Masuyama. 1996. Early-stage rheumatoid arthritis: Diagnostic accuracy of MR imaging. *Radiology* **198:** 185–192.

47. Sugimoto, H., A. Takeda & K. Hyodoh. 2000. Early-stage rheumatoid arthritis: Prospective study of the effectiveness of MR imaging for diagnosis. *Radiology* **216:** 569–575.

48. Larsen, A., K. Dale & M. Eek. 1977. Radiographic evaluation of rheumatoid arthritis and related conditions by standard reference films. *Acta Radiol. Diagn. (Stockholm)* **18:** 481–491.

49. Edmonds, J., A. Saudan, M. Lassere & D. Scott. 1999. Introduction to reading radiographs by the Scott modification of the Larsen method. *J. Rheumatol.* **26:** 740–742.

50. Steinbrocker, O., G.H. Traeger & R.C. Batterman. 1949. Therapeutic criteria in rheumatoid arthritis. *JAMA* **140:** 659–662.

51. Østergaard, M., P. Gideon, K. Sorenson, *et al.* 1995. Scoring of synovial membrane hypertrophy and bone erosions by MR imaging in clinically active and inactive rheumatoid arthritis of the wrist. *Scand. J. Rheumatol.* **124:** 212–218.

52. Bird, P., M. Lassere, R. Shnier & J. Edmonds. 2003. Computerized measurement of magnetic resonance imaging erosion volumes in patients with rheumatoid arthritis: A comparison with existing magnetic resonance imaging scoring systems and standard clinical outcome measures. *Arthritis Rheum.* **48:** 614–624.

53. Goldbach-Mansky, R., J. Woodbum, L. Yao, *et al.* 2003. Magnetic resonance imaging in the evaluation of bone damage in rheumatoid arthritis: A more precise image or just a more expensive one? *Arthritis Rheum.* **48:** 585–589.

54. McQueen, F.M., M. Østergaard, C. Peterfly, *et al.* 2005. Pitfalls in scoring MR images of rheumatoid arthritis wrist and metacarpal joints. *Ann. Rheum. Dis.* **64:** 48–55.

55. Peterfly, C.G. 2004. MRI of the wrist in early rheumatoid arthritis. *Ann. Rheum. Dis.* **63:** 473–477.

56. Reiser, M.F., G.P. Bongartz, R. Erlemann, *et al.* 1989. Gadolinium-DTPA in rheumatoid arthritis and related diseases: First results with dynamic magnetic resonance imaging. *Skeletal Radiol.* **18:** 591–597.

Section II. Magnetic Resonance Imaging

The MRI View of Synovitis and Tenosynovitis in Inflammatory Arthritis

Implications for Diagnosis and Management

Fiona M. McQueen

Department of Molecular Medicine and Pathology, University of Auckland, Auckland, New Zealand

MRI scanning is the current gold standard modality for imaging synovitis and tenosynovitis in patients with inflammatory arthritis. Inflamed synovial membrane within the joints and investing tendon sheaths appears thickened on T1-weighted sequences and enhances postcontrast. On T2-weighted sequences, synovitis and synovial effusions typically show a high signal. Studies have shown correlations between the degree of inflammation and vascularity of synovium obtained at biopsy and postcontrast enhancement on matching dynamic MRI scans. Scoring systems have been devised that are based on quantifying synovial membrane thickening and signal intensity on static postcontrast scans and have been validated in multireader settings. Moderate to high reliability has been demonstrated with trained readers and quantification of synovitis in this way is being used increasingly as an outcome measure in clinical trials to assess response to therapy. MRI-observed synovitis is almost invariable in those with active rheumatoid arthritis, but recent studies have also demonstrated its presence in patients in clinical remission, emphasizing the sensitivity of this technique and the importance of subclinical joint inflammation. MRI-observed synovitis has been validated against other imaging modalities, including power Doppler ultrasound, and has also been investigated in normal subjects (where mild enhancement can rarely occur). Studies over 1–2 years have suggested that MRI synovial membrane volume and postcontrast enhancement on dynamic imaging can predict the development of erosions. In the long term, an overall score of inflammation incorporating synovitis, tenosynovitis, and bone edema may be a more useful MRI predictor of aggressive erosive disease.

Key words: MRI; inflammatory arthritis; rheumatoid arthritis; synovitis; tenosynovitis

Introduction

The optimal imaging modality for investigating inflammatory arthritis must be able to provide information about the extent of joint inflammation (as it affects the synovium, tenosynovium, and bone) as well as joint damage (in terms of bone erosion, cartilage loss, and tendon rupture). MRI scanning is capable of imaging all of these tissues tomographically to a high degree of resolution and defining these pathological changes, so it is an ideal tool for informed clinical decision making. Over the past 10 years a considerable body of literature has been assembled on the appropriate MRI techniques for imaging inflamed synovium and tenosynovium, as well as on how to interpret the data provided and use these for directing clinical management in the individual patient. The present chapter reviews this literature with an emphasis on its clinical applications.

Address for correspondence: Fiona McQueen, M.B.Ch.B., M.D., F.R.A.C.P., Associate Professor of Rheumatology, Department of Molecular Medicine and Pathology, University of Auckland, PO Box 92019 Auckland, New Zealand. f.mcqueen@auckland.ac.nz

MRI and Ultrasound in Diagnosis and Management: Ann. N.Y. Acad. Sci. 1154: 21–34 (2009).
doi: 10.1111/j.1749-6632.2009.04382.x © 2009 New York Academy of Sciences.

Imaging the Synovial Membrane

How does MRI allow us to see the inflamed synovium? The generation of an image by MRI scanning depends on the detection of protons that are exposed to an extremely powerful magnetic field applied in pulses. This affects the spin of the individual protons in certain ways that are recorded as variations in signal on different magnetic resonance sequences.[1] Spatial information is also obtained and transformed by computing software into an image depicting not only structure but also pathological change, particularly in terms of increased water content. High concentrations of H^+ ions (as H_2O) are contained within the cells, which traffic to sites of inflammation and are also within blood contained in new vessels formed as a result of angiogenic stimuli. Clinically, inflamed joints become swollen and tender and these parameters can be used by the examining rheumatologist to quantify disease activity. At the level of MRI, which provides an internal image of the joint at a resolution that is an order of magnitude greater than clinical examination, the synovium and tenosynovium can be seen to have become thickened because of the accumulation of cells and blood vessels, and volume can be calculated from serial three-dimensional slices.[2] This measure provides a surrogate marker for synovitis but does not distinguish actively inflamed synovium from fibrous pannus, which may still retain volume but possesses only low-grade inflammatory activity.[3]

A second method for quantifying synovitis involves identifying regions of inflammation by their increased T2-weighted (T2w) signal, associated with the accumulation of water (in cells or vessels).[4] A third method employs intravenous contrast in the form of gadolinium diethylenetriamine pentaacetic acid (Gd-DTPA), which has paramagnetic properties to produce increased signal on postcontrast T1w images[5] and can be used to produce a static image. Alternatively, a dynamic image can be built up, depicting the movement of the small contrast molecules from the vasculature to the intersti-

tium of the synovial membrane and from there into any accompanying synovial effusion. Various MRI parameters can be recorded, including the maximum signal intensity achieved after a set period of time or its rate of increase, which is linear over the first 40 to 80 s and termed either the enhancement rate (E-rate) or enhancement ratio (E-ratio) according to the method used. Figure 1 shows an example of rheumatoid synovitis in the wrist with severe tenosynovitis involving the extensor carpi ulnaris (ECU). These scans illustrate the typical MRI characteristics of rheumatoid synovitis with thickened and brightly enhancing synovium and tenosynovium seen on T1 post-GdDTPA images in the coronal and axial planes, contrasting with low signal on precontrast images.

Correlating MRI Evidence of Synovitis with Histology

It is important to know how closely the measurement of synovitis on MRI scans correlates with the degree of inflammation determined from histological examination of the synovium. Relevant studies have mostly focused on the knee, where synovial tissue can be most readily obtained. One of the first descriptions came from Konig *et al.*, who evaluated inflammation in the knees in 20 rheumatoid arthritis (RA) patients using dynamic enhanced MRI and compared these results with histological data obtained from biopsy of the synovial membrane performed arthroscopically or operatively in 12 patients.[3] Their preliminary findings revealed hyperintense signal on T2w images, correlating with "remarkable" enhancement on post-Gd-DTPA T1w images in three patients, and this appearance matched hypervascular pannus in a histological assessment. In contrast, hypointense lesions on MRI correlated with histologic evidence of fibrous pannus with a "burnt out" appearance.

A more comprehensive study followed from Gaffney *et al.*,[6] who compared the intensity of rheumatoid synovitis in the knee, measured

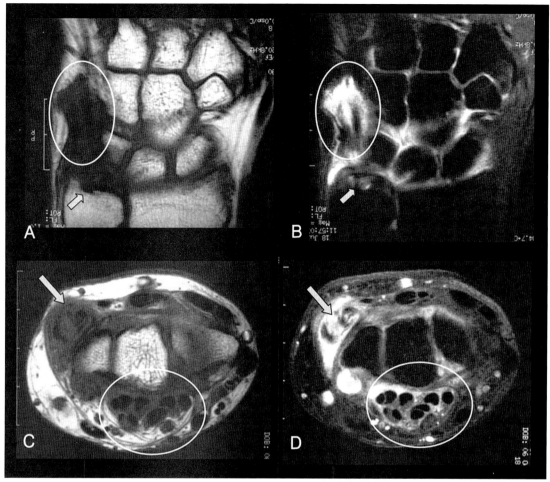

Figure 1. MRI scans from a 58-year-old woman with a 6-year history of RA: (**A**) coronal T1w image and (**B**) coronal T1w fat-saturated postcontrast image showing radiocarpal and intercarpal synovitis, extensive tenosynovitis involving the ECU (circle), and small erosions in the distal ulna (short arrow). (**C**) and (**D**) are equivalent images in an axial plane at the level of the lunate, showing a split within the ECU tendon itself (long arrow), as well as tenosynovitis involving the flexor tendon compartment (circle).

using the initial rate of enhancement on post-contrast MRI scans, with a score for inflammation calculated from multiple synovial biopsy samples taken from the suprapatellar bursa (a total of 98 examined for the group). They found a strong correlation ($r = 0.63$) between the E-rate and a composite histologic inflammatory score quantifying polymorphonuclear (PMN) cellular infiltration, hyperemia, and fibrin deposition. The same group followed up on this work in 1998 with a study specifically examining blood vessels identified immunohistochemically using an endothelial cell marker.[7] The

MRI E-rate correlated with both the numerical density of blood vessels and their fractional area, emphasizing the fact that this parameter is closely linked to vascularity (Fig. 2). Similar results were obtained by Tamai *et al.*, who compared the E-ratio with a histologic score for inflammation on synovial biopsy specimens taken from the knee in 10 patients.[8] In their study, enhancement postcontrast was greater in regions with a high degree of fibrin exudation, cellular infiltration, villous hypertrophy, vascular proliferation, and infiltration by granulation tissue but not in regions affected by fibrosis.

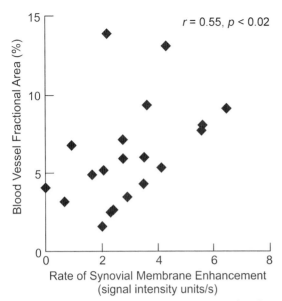

$r = 0.55, p < 0.02$

Figure 2. Graph showing the relationship between the rate of synovial membrane enhancement, from dynamic enhanced MRI scans, and blood vessel fractional area, from synovial membrane biopsy. Adapted from Gaffney *et al. Ann. Rheum. Dis.* 1998. **57:** 152–157, with permission.

Østergaard *et al.* approached the same question from a different direction in their study of 17 RA and 25 OA (osteoarthritic) knees.[9] The volume of synovial membrane was determined using a manual outlining method to determine its boundaries on consecutive slices, and this surrogate measure of synovitis was then compared with a histologic assessment of inflammation, again from biopsy specimens taken from the knee arthroscopically. A strong correlation was found between this MRI synovial volume score and a composite histologic inflammation score (Spearman's $\sigma = 0.55, p < 0.001$), as well as separately with fibrin deposition, subsynovial mononuclear, and PMN leukocyte infiltration. Synovial membrane volumes were also shown to be higher in RA than OA knees and to correlate with the erythrocyte sedimentation rate (ESR) and C-reactive protein (CRP). In a separate study, these authors compared the same histological data with synovial signal intensity (postcontrast), represented by the E-ratio. However, instead of quantifying this in a small re-

gion of interest (ROI) as in other studies, they calculated it for the entire synovium (identified by outlining) in a preselected slice. This gave a much stronger correlation with histological inflammation ($\sigma = 0.73$) than the smaller regions ($\sigma = 0.49$).[10]

Moving away from the knee, Ostendorf *et al.* examined the 2nd MCP joint of 22 RA patients using miniarthroscopy and synovial biopsy and made comparisons with MRI data relating to synovitis.[11] Arthroscopic synovial findings including hyperemia and increased vascularity, as well as villous proliferation, were found in more than 90% of patients. MRI examination revealed increased synovial membrane thickness in all but one individual and synovial enhancement postcontrast in 19 (86%). These MRI features correlated with arthroscopic synovial inflammation (hyperemia and vascularity). However, in only a small number of samples were microscopic biopsy data available and features correlating with MRI synovial thickening ranged from florid synovial proliferation and hyperemia to a more chronic appearance with subsynovial fibrosis and flattening of the lining layer.

Thus, MRI cannot give the same detailed information as histological examination when it comes to the specifics of cellular infiltration and vascularity, but it does allow synovitis to be quantified without resorting to an invasive procedure. Regional heterogeneity is the bugbear of attempting to quantify synovitis from synovial biopsies and this means the time-consuming analyses of multiple samples to obtain an estimate of the average degree of inflammation.[12] The same problem complicates the interpretation of E-MRI images, especially when the E-rate or E-ratio is calculated from small ROIs. Although the computer interpretation of the intensity of the MRI signal is highly reproducible, the placement of the ROI itself is directed by the observer's decision regarding the point of maximal enhancement within the synovial membrane and is therefore highly subjective and potentially a source of error.[13] However, if synovial membrane can be identified from postcontrast MRI scans and its overall volume assessed from consecutive slices, a "broad brush" surrogate marker for synovitis is produced, and this circumvents most of the problems associated with sampling error. This is the measure of synovitis that has been incorporated into the most widely used RA MRI scoring system (RAMRIS),[14] which is discussed more fully below.

Validation against Other Imaging Modalities

Further validation of MRI as a tool for detecting and quantifying synovitis comes from studies comparing this modality with ultrasound (US). Using B-mode and gray-scale US, synovitis appears as thickening of the synovial membrane as it invests joints, bursae, or tendon sheaths.[15] Increased blood flow can be imaged using Doppler techniques allowing quantitation of membrane thickening and color intensity.[16] Szkudlarek *et al.* compared dynamic MRI with contrast-enhanced power Doppler ultrasonography (CE PDUS) of RA MCP joints and found the rate of early synovial MRI enhancement to be highest in joints with a positive CE PDUS signal.[17] Another study found a strong relationship between the thickness of synovial membrane on postcontrast MRI scans and both the color fraction and mean resistance index (RI) from color Doppler US (both giving a measure of abnormal perfusion in inflamed synovial membrane).[18] Scheel *et al.* recently reported a prospective 7-year follow-up imaging study comparing radiography, ultrasonography, and MRI of RA finger joints and demonstrated a reduction in US synovitis from 83% of joints at baseline to 52% at follow-up, which paralleled the fall in MRI-observed synovitis from 63 to 41%.[19] Looking at a different modality, Beckers *et al.* found that MRI-observed synovial volumes in the knee were highly correlated with proton emission tomography (PET) measures of glucose metabolism, which indicated the expected link between structure and function in the inflamed synovium.[20]

Sensitivity and Specificity

Once it had been established that MRI synovitis is a reasonable indicator of true synovial inflammation, it was interesting to investigate whether these changes can occur in normal controls. This was done most comprehensively by Ejbjerg *et al.*, who studied 28 healthy individuals using contrast-enhanced MRI of the wrist and MCP joints.[21] MRI depicted low-grade changes that resembled synovitis in 9% of the MCP joints and 10% of the wrist joints, but almost half of these changes were observed in three subjects who had elevated CRP levels (and therefore could possibly have had subclinical inflammation). The changes were all at the lowest level scored (1 out of 3 on the RAMRIS scale), and dynamic MRI revealed only minimal synovial enhancement (Δ signal intensity) compared with levels in RA patients that were 30-fold higher. These results give an insight into the specificity of MRI synovitis and indicate that while low-grade enhancement can occur in normal joints, most RA joints exhibit much greater degrees of membrane thickening and enhancement, which is strongly indicative of disease.

There is now extensive literature describing MRI-defined synovitis in RA,[22] and most authors agree that it is a sensitive indicator of the presence and activity of disease. McQueen *et al.* found that 93% of a cohort of 42 RA patients had evidence of synovitis at the dominant wrist within 6 months of the onset of symptoms,[23] and Boutry *et al.* echoed these results, finding synovitis in the wrist and the MCP and MTP joints in 90, 93, and 97%, respectively, of their group with a similar disease duration.[24] Ostendorf *et al.* studied 10 RA patients who had only had symptoms for a median of 9 weeks and of these, none had synovitis in the MCP joints of the hands (although four had tenosynovitis), but all 10 had MRI synovitis in the

MTP joints of the feet, where it was often associated with tenosynovitis and bone edema.[25] These findings recall radiographic studies indicating that rheumatoid erosions develop first in the metatarsal heads (most specifically the 5th).[26] However, there has not previously been an imaging modality capable of depicting soft tissue inflammation to this degree of resolution, so MRI can provide new insights into the disease process in RA and indicate which joint areas are affected earliest.

Not surprisingly, given its ability to image the joint in three dimensions, MRI has been shown to be more sensitive than clinical examination for imaging synovitis.[27,28] Goupille *et al.* found MRI-observed synovitis in RA MCP joints 10 times more often than by clinical examination, but in only 2 of 107 joints examined was clinical synovitis diagnosed in the absence of MRI inflammation.[27] For reasons of feasibility, MRI and not histology was used as the gold standard measure of synovitis, but, as noted earlier, links between the two have been fairly conclusively demonstrated.[6,8,10]

An interesting recent development has been a growing awareness that MRI synovitis often persists in the face of clinical remission, and this has major implications for disease modifying antirheumatic drug (DMARD)-efficacy in suppressing joint damage.[28,29] Cohen *et al.* showed that radiographic damage progression occurred in 17% of patients in sustained clinical remission,[30] and, more recently, Brown *et al.* found that 96% of 107 RA patients in clinical remission had MRI synovitis (and 46% had bone edema), while 3 of 17 controls showed mild synovial thickening but none had bone edema.[28] DMARD-induced clinical remission was compared with biologically induced remission in another small study of Mexican RA patients.[29] These authors found the effect of biological therapies to be much greater from an MRI perspective, with only two MRI-inflamed joints detected out of 120 assessed compared with 24 joints in patients on DMARDs alone. Clearly, the goal of complete imaging remission is harder to achieve but is increasingly becoming the target for efficacy as far as biological therapies are concerned.

Measurement of MRI Synovitis and Tenosynovitis

For MRI synovitis and tenosynovitis to be useful tools for assessing patients' responses to therapeutics, validated scoring systems have had to be devised.[14,23] The most widely accepted is now the RAMRIS system,[14] produced as the result of an international collaboration under the Outcome Measures for Rheumatoid Arthritis Clinical Trials (OMERACT) banner. This group extended the project to produce an atlas incorporating images for synovitis, bone edema, and bone erosion for use as a reference.[31] Reliability and sensitivity to change of this system were tested separately by four readers, who scored 10 sets of baseline and 1-year follow-up MRI scans of the wrist in a group of RA patients with early or established disease.[32] Measurement reliability for synovitis status scores was moderately high with interreader intraclass correlation coefficients (ICCs) of 0.7 and 0.78 for baseline and follow-up scores, with similar results for change in synovitis over time (ICC = 0.74). However, the minimal detectable change (MDC) for synovitis change scores was 26%, and this degree of variability must be borne in mind when interpreting study results.

A number of studies have shown MRI-observed tenosynovitis to be a prominent feature of early rheumatoid disease in both the hands[23,25] and the feet,[25] suggesting that this is an important pathological change to capture. As applies to the detection of synovitis, the incorporation of post-GdDTPA sequences seems to be significant in scoring tenosynovitis, as these are more sensitive and show greater signal change than T2 sequences alone.[33] The scoring of MRI-observed tenosynovitis was omitted from the original RAMRIS score for reasons of feasibility, but had been incorporated into an earlier system.[23] Recently, a tenosynovitis score has been developed and tested in a multireader longitudinal setting,[34] where it was found to have a similar degree of reliability to the synovitis score (interobserver ICC for change of 0.67). The median time for scoring was 7 min, so this would not make its addition to the standard RAMRIS too unwieldy. In another study, the same group found a composite MRI inflammation score encompassing synovitis, tenosynovitis, and bone edema to be the most sensitive outcome measure for detecting response to anti-TNF agents,[35] and this is likely to become a useful tool in the clinical trial setting. How soon it will filter into clinical practice to assist the clinician in detecting an early response to DMARD or biologic therapy remains to be seen, as application of RAMRIS, with or without the tenosynovitis component, is relatively complex and may be beyond the reach of the average clinician.

Predicting Prognosis

Østergaard *et al.* produced early evidence that synovial volume, measured in the wrist using a manual outlining technique, and the area-under-the-curve (AUC) for synovial volume over a 12-month period, correlated with the rate of erosive progression ($\sigma = 0.53$ and 0.69, respectively) in a cohort of 26 RA patients.[36] Given the relative difficulty of measuring synovial volume, these authors also scored synovial hypertrophy and found this to be fairly strongly related to volume at different points in time. Unfortunately, the baseline synovial hypertrophy score did not predict erosive progression, but the AUC for this measure did to a moderate degree. Extrapolation of these findings to a clinical situation is difficult, as prediction of an aggressive erosive phenotype really has to be done from baseline measurements rather than AUC estimations (which continue until the point at which the erosions are measured). However, the results can be interpreted more broadly and suggest that persistent inflammation within a joint provides an appro-

priate milieu for bone erosion to occur, emphasizing the importance of good disease control.

McQueen *et al.* also examined the predictive power of MRI synovitis and tenosynovitis in their cohort of early RA patients. They found that the baseline score for synovitis predicted the MRI erosion score at 1 year (OR = 2.1) but this was not as strong as the predictive power of bone edema (OR = 6.5) or a high composite MRI score encompassing synovitis, tenosynovitis, bone edema, and erosion (OR = 12.4).[37] Dynamic enhanced MRI evidence of synovitis at baseline (the E-rate) also predicted the MRI erosion score at 1 year, but not as strongly as the quantitative synovitis score.[38] When the same patients were reassessed at 6 years, baseline MRI synovitis scores did not predict erosions or joint space narrowing, as opposed to bone edema scores, which were predictive, but incorporating all baseline MRI measures together into a composite score with CRP and ESR yielded the best results, with a model that predicted 60% of the variability of the 6-year Sharp–van der Heijde score.[39] Tendinopathy, incorporating a score for tenosynovitis and signal change within the tendon itself, was also separately examined and the most commonly affected site was the extensor carpi ulnaris.[23,40] Tendon rupture had occurred in 11% of the group by 6 years and was predicted by high tendinopathy scores at baseline and 1 year.[40]

Others have examined the predictive power of MRI-observed synovitis with varying results. Savnik *et al.* showed that the volume of synovial membrane in the MCP joints predicted the development of bone erosions 1 year later,[41] but the opposite was reported by Haavardsholm *et al.* who found no predictive effect from baseline synovitis in their group of 84 RA patients (although bone edema was predictive).[42] Taken together, these various studies indicate that MRI observed synovitis alone is probably not a very useful tool for prediction of later erosion, and this is partly due to its frequency, as it occurs in 80–90% of patients. However, its inclusion in a composite MRI score, with tenosynovitis and, crucially, bone edema could be a very helpful addition to clinical acumen when trying to assess which patients are likely to go on to develop erosive, damaging disease. Tendon rupture is a separate form of structural damage and limited evidence suggests some prediction from baseline tendinopathy scores even out as far as 6 years, but larger studies are required to confirm this.

Imaging the Response to Therapy

The ability of MRI synovitis to act as an "imaging biomarker" for measuring patient responses to therapy was first assessed in the knee by Østergaard *et al.*, who demonstrated a 50–60% decrease in synovial membrane and effusion volumes during the first week after intra-articular steroid injection.[43] In a similar study in the wrist, the same authors found that the MRI estimate of synovial membrane volume could differentiate between the response to DMARDs alone and the slightly greater response to DMARDs plus prednisolone.[36] In a similar vein, Conaghan *et al.* investigated the response to intra-articular steroid plus methotrexate versus methotrexate alone in 40 untreated RA patients using MRI synovitis, this time scored according to the thickness of enhancing synovium (in millimeters).[44] They found a difference in the reduction of synovitis between the two treatment groups, suggesting that this is a sensitive tool for discriminating degrees of response. They also found that bone erosions were most likely to occur in joints affected by synovitis, but as in other studies only the AUC for synovitis was predictive of new erosions. Reece *et al.* used dynamic enhanced MRI scans of affected knees as their outcome measure in a 4-month trial comparing leflunomide with methotrexate.[45] Despite the fact that patient numbers in each treatment group were very small (18 and 21, respectively), a difference was demonstrated in that those on leflunomide had significantly lower initial rates of synovial enhancement than those on methotrexate. Although the results of this study were positive, the pitfalls of the measurement of synovitis from dynamic MRI scans have already been alluded to, so these findings should be interpreted with caution.

The most exciting application for MRI synovitis as an outcome measure is in the clinical trial setting, monitoring responses to biologics. Here the potential advantages of having a sensitive measure that can detect change fairly reliably and over a short period of time makes MRI assessment of synovitis very attractive, especially when compared with the much more cumbersome end point of radiographic erosions. Kalden-Nemeth *et al.* performed the first MRI-based trial investigating the effect of anti-TNF agents in 18 RA patients. They used dynamic MRI before and 4 weeks after an infusion of CA2, which would later be called infliximab (IFX).[46] Enhancing ROIs were defined (once more depending to a high degree on the observer's ability to correctly identify maximally enhancing synovium), and in this early study, MRI scans were performed at a variety of regions, including the knees, ankles, and hands. A highly significant reduction in Gd-DTPA uptake was reported in the patients receiving the anti-TNF agent, and although caveats apply to interpretation of these data, they were encouraging.

Another trial of IFX plus methotrexate (MTX) over 12 months incorporated MRI scoring to assess response.[47] This time the earliest incarnation of the RAMRIS criteria was used,[48] including a score for synovitis, by two observers. Although a significant difference between the MTX alone and MTX + IFX groups was shown, surprisingly this was quite modest, with a fall in the synovitis score in the IFX group from 5.5 to 3.4, compared with the placebo group, where a reduction from 6.2 to 5.9 was observed. However, despite a trend toward less damage in the IFX-treated patients over time, there was no significant between-group difference in the change in the Sharp score over 12 months, reinforcing the notion that MRI may offer a better way of measuring outcome.

Zikou *et al.* recently used high-field postcontrast MRI to evaluate the volume of inflammatory synovial pannus in patients pre- and post-treatment with adalimumab.[49] They found this measure of synovitis to be decreased in 86% of patients after 1 year of therapy and to correlate with the fall in other measures of inflammation, including ESR and swollen joint count. Interestingly, data have not always been positive and a Danish study of anakinra with and without MTX failed to show a significant change in the MRI synovitis score despite improvements in tender and swollen joint counts.[50] In this study, the MRI erosion score fared better as an outcome measure, demonstrating progression in erosions from baseline to 12 weeks, which could only be detected by the Sharp score over 36 weeks. The authors concluded that the evidence supported the value of MRI for accelerated assessment of structural joint damage. Evidence from large clinical trials of biologics is awaited, but the early publications suggest that MRI may sensitively detect residual synovitis that could persist even in the face of a clinical response. This returns us to the concept of imaging remission, which may be the target of future therapy.

High-Field versus Low-Field Extremity MRI

Dedicated extremity MRI (E-MRI) units are capable of detecting synovitis and tenosynovitis in RA and are being used increasingly because they offer improved patient comfort at lower cost,[51] albeit with some reduction in image clarity and a less favorable signal-to-noise ratio. Results are dependent on the type of unit being employed but Ejbjerg *et al.* showed excellent agreement between high-field (1.5 T) and low-field (0.2 T) scans for the assessment of synovitis in their 2005 study that examined the wrists and MCP joints of established RA patients.[52] High-field MRI revealed synovitis in 172 sites compared with 164 sites on low-field scans, giving sensitivity, specificity, and predictive accuracy

of low-field MRI (using high field as the gold standard) of 90, 96, and 94%. More recently an OMERACT imaging working group investigated interobserver reliability for the detection of synovitis using 0.2-T E-MRI in cross-sectional and longitudinal settings.[53] Average measures ICCs for synovitis indicated fair to moderate agreement among the three readers at a single time point (ICCs of 0.53 in MCP joints and 0.66 in the wrist) but change scores over time were more reliable (ICC for wrists and MCPs combined = 0.89).

Schirmer *et al.* recently reported another study comparing low-field and high-field MRI in RA joints and included tenosynovitis in the parameters measured.[54] Of 68 evaluations, flexor tenosynovitis was diagnosed by low-field MRI in 24 and by high-field MRI in 33 instances, with kappa values of 0.5–0.6 indicating moderate reliability; but clearly tenosynovitis is seen better using 1.5-T machines. Overall, the impression from the literature is that E-MRI units may be helpful for monitoring the response of joint inflammation to DMARD or biological DMARD therapy over time, but results must be interpreted with caution and two different readers will always be required to provide an indication of scoring variability. Whether the information gleaned will add to the standard clinical workup to the extent of altering outcomes remains controversial,[55] but technical advances and the steady improvement of image quality suggest that E-MRI will assume an increasingly important role in the management of RA as time goes on.

Using MRI to Help Diagnose Inflammatory Arthritis

The finding of erosions on MRI may help classify the patient with undifferentiated arthritis as having early RA well before the appearance of radiographic erosions.[23,56]

However, it is also interesting to examine the question of whether there are disease-specific features of MRI synovitis or tenosynovitis that could assist the clinician in differentiating among the different forms of inflammatory arthropathy. Synovitis in the wrist has been shown to have the same appearance in psoriatic arthritis (PsA) as it does in RA on enhanced dynamic MRI scans,[57] as would be expected from the similar synovial histology in these conditions.[58] However, documentation of distal interphalangeal (DIP) joint synovitis by MRI makes PsA more likely, consistent with the clinical distribution of joint disease.[59] Dactylitis is another PsA feature that is well-imaged using MRI (and not found in RA) and is usually associated with flexor tenosynovitis, plus or minus bone edema and small joint synovitis within the affected ray.[60,61]

Narvaez *et al.* sought differentiating MRI features in patients with early RA compared with a PsA cohort and also concluded that flexor tendons were more commonly involved in PsA and extensor tendons in RA.[62] Another distinguishing PsA feature was diaphyseal bone edema, but this was relatively uncommon.[62] Jevtic *et al.* first described extracapsular soft tissue edema on PsA MRI scans of the fingers as "inflamed tissue extending far beyond the joint capsule, involving neighboring structures such as thickened collateral ligaments and periarticular soft tissue."[63] This feature was further characterized in the knee in patients with PsA and other spondyloarthopathies (SpA) by McGonagle *et al.*[64] These investigators also found extracapsular changes to be more common in polymyalgia rheumatica (PMR) than in RA.[65]

There are very few MRI data on synovitis/tenosynovitis in the other connective tissue diseases but Ostendorf *et al.* investigated a small group of systemic lupus erythematosus (SLE) patients with Jaccoud's arthropathy and described edematous and proliferative tendinopathy as well as capsular swelling and synovial hypertrophy.[66] Taken together, the evidence suggests that the MRI appearances of synovitis and tenosynovitis are fairly similar across all inflammatory arthropathies, but in some instances certain features might be identified that could help direct the clinician toward making a specific diagnosis.

Summary

In summary, MRI offers a view of the inflamed synovial membrane that is unparalleled in terms of image clarity and tomographic definition. Not only are anatomical features delineated, but the pathological appearance and degree of synovial inflammation can be clearly observed as can any associated synovial effusions and articular damage. Studies have confirmed a close association between the extent of MRI observed synovitis and histological features of inflammation from synovial biopsy.[3,6–9] Owing to problems associated with ROI sampling error on dynamic scans,[13] the most reliable results come from summative or average estimations as incorporated into the RAMRIS system.[14] With a 1.5-T scanner and trained readers, this score can be highly reliable,[32] but when monitoring change over time (e.g., to measure drug efficacy), there is significant interobserver variability, emphasizing the need for two readers when measuring outcome. This caution is particularly relevant to the use of low-field dedicated extremity scanners in this context. However, MRI is capable of more comprehensive imaging with a higher degree of resolution than US, which is the only other widely used modality for detection of synovitis and tenosynovitis.

Further studies are needed regarding the place of MRI in diagnosing inflammatory arthritis, and although there are some characteristic features in RA, PsA, SLE,[23,60,62–64,67] and possibly PMR,[65] these tend to occur in the minority of patients. Regarding prognostication, short-term studies link MRI synovial membrane volume to subsequent joint erosion,[36,41] but over the longer term this association may not hold and an overall "MRI inflammation score" incorporating synovitis, tenosynovitis, and bone edema seems to be more valuable.[35] MRI outcomes have been incorporated into a number of large clinical trials of biologics now underway, and these should provide much better data on prognosis and outcome, as well as addressing the question of imaging remission. Overall, despite any misgivings clinicians may have about its relative complexity, MRI provides information about joint inflammation that represents a quantum leap forward from plain radiography. Given the constant technical advances, including the advent of 3-T and even 7-T scanners, ever-improving dedicated extremity machines, and more comprehensive scoring systems, this can only improve patient care if applied judiciously by the astute clinician.

Conflicts of Interest

The author declares no conflicts of interest.

References

1. Peterfy, C.G. 2001. Magnetic resonance imaging of the wrist in rheumatoid arthritis. *Sem. Musculoskeletal Radiol.* **5:** 275–288.
2. Østergaard, M., M. Hansen, M. Stoltenberg & I. Lorenzen. 1996. Quantitative assessment of the synovial membrane in the rheumatoid wrist: An easily obtained MRI score reflects the synovial volume. *Br. J. Rheumatol.* **35:** 965–971.
3. Konig, H., J. Sieper & K.J. Wolf. 1990. Rheumatoid arthritis: Evaluation of hypervascular and fibrous pannus with dynamic MR imaging enhanced with Gd-DTPA. *Radiology* **176:** 473–477.
4. Gilkeson, G., R. Polisson, H. Sinclair, *et al.* 1988. Early detection of carpal erosions in patients with rheumatoid arthritis: A pilot study of magnetic resonance imaging. *J. Rheumatol.* **15:** 1361–1366.
5. Beltran, J., V. Chandnani, R.A. McGhee, Jr. & S. Kursunoglu-Brahme. 1991. Gadopentetate dimeglumine-enhanced MR imaging of the musculoskeletal system. *AJR Am. J. Roentgenol.* **156:** 457–466.
6. Gaffney, K., J. Cookson, D. Blake, *et al.* 1995. Quantification of rheumatoid synovitis by magnetic resonance imaging. *Arthritis Rheum.* **38:** 1610–1617.
7. Gaffney, K., J. Cookson, S. Blades, *et al.* 1998. Quantitative assessment of the rheumatoid synovial microvascular bed by gadolinium-DTPA enhanced magnetic resonance imaging. *Ann. Rheum. Dis.* **57:** 152–157.
8. Tamai, K., M. Yamato, T. Yamaguchi & W. Ohno. 1994. Dynamic magnetic resonance imaging for the evaluation of synovitis in patients with rheumatoid arthritis. *Arthritis Rheum.* **37:** 1151–1157.
9. Østergaard, M., M. Stoltenberg, P. Lovgreen-Nielsen, *et al.* 1997. Magnetic resonance imaging-determined synovial membrane and joint effusion volumes in rheumatoid arthritis and osteoarthritis: Comparison with the macroscopic and microscopic appearance of the synovium [see comment]. *Arthritis Rheum.* **40:** 1856–1867.
10. Østergaard, M., M. Stoltenberg, P. Lovgreen-Nielsen, *et al.* 1998. Quantification of synovistis by MRI: Correlation between dynamic and static gadolinium-enhanced magnetic resonance imaging and microscopic and macroscopic signs of synovial inflammation. *Magn. Reson. Imaging* **16:** 743–754.
11. Ostendorf, B., R. Peters, P. Dann, *et al.* 2001. Magnetic resonance imaging and miniarthroscopy of metacarpophalangeal joints: Sensitive detection of morphologic changes in rheumatoid arthritis. *Arthritis Rheum.* **44:** 2492–2502.
12. Rooney, M., D. Condell, W. Quinlan, *et al.* 1988. Analysis of the histologic variation of synovitis in rheumatoid arthritis. *Arthritis Rheum.* **31:** 956–963.
13. McQueen, F.M., J. Crabbe & N. Stewart. 2004. Dynamic gadolinium-enhanced magnetic resonance imaging of the wrist in patients with rheumatoid arthritis: Comment on the article by Cimmino et al. *Arthritis Rheum.* **50:** 674–675; Author reply 675–676.
14. Østergaard, M., C. Peterfy, P. Conaghan, *et al.* 2003. OMERACT rheumatoid arthritis magnetic resonance maging studies: Core set of MRI acquisitions, joint pathology definitions, and the OMERACT RA-MRI scoring system. *J. Rheumatol.* **30:** 1385–1386.
15. Backhaus, M., T. Kamradt, D. Sandrock, *et al.* 1999. Arthritis of the finger joints: A comprehensive approach comparing conventional radiography, scintigraphy, ultrasound, and contrast-enhanced magnetic resonance imaging. *Arthritis Rheum.* **42:** 1232–1245.
16. Newman, J.S., T.J. Laing, C.J. McCarthy & R.S. Adler. 1996. Power Doppler sonography of synovitis: Assessment of therapeutic response—preliminary observations [see comment]. *Radiology* **198:** 582–584.
17. Szkudlarek, M., M. Court-Payen, C. Strandberg, *et al.* 2001. Power Doppler ultrasonography for assessment of synovitis in the metacarpophalangeal joints of patients with rheumatoid arthritis: A comparison with dynamic magnetic resonance imaging. *Arthritis Rheum.* **44:** 2018–2023.
18. Terslev, L., S. Torp-Pedersen, A. Savnik, *et al.* 2003. Doppler ultrasound and magnetic resonance imaging of synovial inflammation of the hand in rheumatoid arthritis: A comparative study. *Arthritis Rheum.* **48:** 2434–2441.

19. Scheel, A.K., K.G.A. Hermann, S. Ohrndorf, *et al.* 2006. Prospective 7 year follow up imaging study comparing radiography, ultrasonography, and magnetic resonance imaging in rheumatoid arthritis finger joints. *Ann. Rheum. Dis.* **65:** 595–600.

20. Beckers, C., X. Jeukens, C. Ribbens, *et al.* 2006. (18)F-FDG PET imaging of rheumatoid knee synovitis correlates with dynamic magnetic resonance and sonographic assessments as well as with the serum level of metalloproteinase-3. *Eur. J. Nucl. Med. Mol. Imaging* **33:** 275–280.

21. Ejbjerg, B., E. Narvestad, E. Rostrup, *et al.* 2004. Magnetic resonance imaging of wrist and finger joints in healthy subjects occasionally shows changes resembling erosions and synovitis as seen in rheumatoid arthritis. *Arthritis Rheum.* **50:** 1097–1106.

22. Østergaard, M. & B. Ejbjerg. 2004. Magnetic resonance imaging of the synovium in rheumatoid arthritis. *Sem. Musculoskeletal Radiol.* **8:** 287–299.

23. McQueen, F.M., N. Stewart, J. Crabbe, *et al.* 1998. Magnetic resonance imaging of the wrist in early rheumatoid arthritis reveals a high prevalence of erosions at four months after symptom onset. *Ann. Rheum. Dis.* **57:** 350–356.

24. Boutry, N., A. Larde, F. Lapegue, *et al.* 2003. Magnetic resonance imaging appearance of the hands and feet in patients with early rheumatoid arthritis. *J. Rheumatol.* **30:** 671–679.

25. Ostendorf, B., A. Scherer, U. Modder & M. Schneider. 2004. Diagnostic value of magnetic resonance imaging of the forefeet in early rheumatoid arthritis when findings on imaging of the metacarpophalangeal joints of the hands remain normal. *Arthritis Rheum.* **50:** 2094–2102.

26. Mottonen, T.T. 1988. Prediction of erosiveness and rate of development of new erosions in early rheumatoid arthritis. *Ann. Rheum. Dis.* **47:** 648–653.

27. Goupille, P., B. Roulot, S. Akoka, *et al.* 2001. Magnetic resonance imaging: A valuable method for the detection of synovial inflammation in rheumatoid arthritis. *J. Rheumatol.* **28:** 35–40.

28. Brown, A.K., M.A. Quinn, Z. Karim, *et al.* 2006. Presence of significant synovitis in rheumatoid arthritis patients with disease-modifying antirheumatic drug-induced clinical remission: Evidence from an imaging study may explain structural progression. *Arthritis Rheum.* **54:** 3761–3773.

29. Martinez-Martinez, M.U., E. Cuevas-Orta, G. Reyes-Vaca, *et al.* 2007. Magnetic resonance imaging in patients with rheumatoid arthritis with complete remission treated with disease-modifying antirheumatic drugs or anti-tumour necrosis factor alpha agents. *Ann. Rheum. Dis.* **66:** 134–135.

30. Cohen, G., L. Gossec, M. Dougados, *et al.* 2007. Radiological damage in patients with rheumatoid arthritis on sustained remission. *Ann. Rheum. Dis.* **66:** 358–363.

31. Østergaard, M., J. Edmonds, F. McQueen, *et al.* 2005. An introduction to the EULAR-OMERACT rheumatoid arthritis MRI reference image atlas. *Ann. Rheum. Dis.* **64**(Suppl. 1): i3–i7.

32. Haavardsholm, E.A., M. Østergaard, B.J. Ejbjerg, *et al.* 2005. Reliability and sensitivity to change of the OMERACT rheumatoid arthritis magnetic resonance imaging score in a multireader, longitudinal setting. *Arthritis Rheum.* **52:** 3860–3867.

33. Tehranzadeh, J., O. Ashikyan, A. Anavim & S. Tramma. 2006. Enhanced MR imaging of tenosynovitis of hand and wrist in inflammatory arthritis. *Skeletal Radiol.* **35:** 814–822.

34. Haavardsholm, E.A., M. Østergaard, B.J. Ejbjerg, *et al.* 2007. Introduction of a novel magnetic resonance imaging tenosynovitis score for rheumatoid arthritis: Reliability in a multireader longitudinal study. *Ann. Rheum. Dis.* **66:** 1216–1220.

35. Haavardsholm, E., M. Østergaard, A. Schildvold & T. Kvien. 2006. MRI findings reflecting inflammation is more responsive than clinical measures of disease activity when monitoring anti-TNF alpha treatment in RA patients. *Arthritis Rheum.* **54**(Suppl.): S800.

36. Østergaard, M., M. Hansen, M. Stoltenberg, *et al.* 1999. Magnetic resonance imaging-determined synovial membrane volume as a marker of disease activity and a predictor of progressive joint destruction in the wrists of patients with rheumatoid arthritis [see comment]. *Arthritis Rheum.* **42:** 918–929.

37. McQueen, F.M., N. Stewart, J. Crabbe, *et al.* 1999. Magnetic resonance imaging of the wrist in early rheumatoid arthritis reveals progression of erosions despite clinical improvement. *Ann. Rheum. Dis.* **58:** 156–163.

38. Huang, J., N. Stewart, J. Crabbe, *et al.* 2000. A 1-year follow-up study of dynamic magnetic resonance imaging in early rheumatoid arthritis reveals synovitis to be increased in shared epitope-positive patients and predictive of erosions at 1 year. *Rheumatology* **39:** 407–416.

39. McQueen, F.M., N. Benton, D. Perry, *et al.* 2003. Bone edema scored on magnetic resonance imaging scans of the dominant carpus at presentation predicts radiographic joint damage of the hands and feet six years later in patients with rheumatoid arthritis. *Arthritis Rheum.* **48:** 1814–1827.

40. McQueen, F., V. Beckley, J. Crabbe, *et al.* 2005. Magnetic resonance imaging evidence of tendinopathy in early rheumatoid arthritis predicts tendon rupture at six years. *Arthritis Rheum.* **52:** 744–751.

41. Savnik, A., H. Malmskov, H.S. Thomsen, *et al.* 2002. MRI of the wrist and finger joints in inflammatory joint diseases at 1-year interval: MRI features

to predict bone erosions. *Eur. Radiol.* **12:** 1203–1210.

42. Haavardsholm, E.A., P. Bøyesen, M. Østergaard, *et al.* 2007. MRI-detected bone marrow edema is a predictor of subsequent radiographic progression in early rheumatoid arthritis. *Ann. Rheum. Dis.* [DOI: 10.1136/ard.2007.071977]

43. Østergaard, M., M. Stoltenberg, P. Gideon, *et al.* 1996. Changes in synovial membrane and joint effusion volumes after intraarticular methylprednisolone. Quantitative assessment of inflammatory and destructive changes in arthritis by MRI. *J. Rheumatol.* **23:** 1151–1161.

44. Conaghan, P.G., P. O'Connor, D. McGonagle, *et al.* 2003. Elucidation of the relationship between synovitis and bone damage: A randomized magnetic resonance imaging study of individual joints in patients with early rheumatoid arthritis. *Arthritis Rheum.* **48:** 64–71.

45. Reece, R.J., M.C. Kraan, A. Radjenovic, *et al.* 2002. Comparative assessment of leflunomide and methotrexate for the treatment of rheumatoid arthritis, by dynamic enhanced magnetic resonance imaging [see comment]. *Arthritis Rheum.* **46:** 366–372.

46. Kalden-Nemeth, D., J. Grebmeier, C. Antoni, *et al.* 1997. NMR monitoring of rheumatoid arthritis patients receiving anti-TNF-alpha monoclonal antibody therapy. *Rheumatol. Int.* **16:** 249–255.

47. Quinn, M.A., P.G. Conaghan, P.J. O'Connor, *et al.* 2005. Very early treatment with infliximab in addition to methotrexate in early, poor-prognosis rheumatoid arthritis reduces magnetic resonance imaging evidence of synovitis and damage, with sustained benefit after infliximab withdrawal: Results from a twelve-month randomized, double-blind, placebo-controlled trial. *Arthritis Rheum.* **52:** 27–35.

48. Conaghan, P., J. Edmonds, P. Emery, *et al.* 2001. Magnetic resonance imaging in rheumatoid arthritis: Summary of OMERACT activities, current status, and plans. *J. Rheumatol.* **28:** 1158–1162.

49. Zikou, A.K., M.I. Argyropoulou, P.V. Voulgari, *et al.* 2006. Magnetic resonance imaging quantification of hand synovitis in patients with rheumatoid arthritis treated with adalimumab. *J. Rheumatol.* **33:** 219–223.

50. Østergaard, M., A. Duer, H. Nielsen, *et al.* 2005. Magnetic resonance imaging for accelerated assessment of drug effect and prediction of subsequent radiographic progression in rheumatoid arthritis: A study of patients receiving combined anakinra and methotrexate treatment. *Ann. Rheum. Dis.* **64:** 1503–1506.

51. Lindegaard, H.M., J. Vallo, K. Horslev-Petersen, *et al.* 2006. Low-cost, low-field dedicated extremity magnetic resonance imaging in early rheumatoid arthritis: A 1-year follow-up study. *Ann. Rheum. Dis.* **65:** 1208–1212.

52. Ejbjerg, B.J., E. Narvestad, S. Jacobsen, *et al.* 2005. Optimised, low cost, low field dedicated extremity MRI is highly specific and sensitive for synovitis and bone erosions in rheumatoid arthritis wrist and finger joints: Comparison with conventional high field MRI and radiography. *Ann. Rheum. Dis.* **64:** 1280–1287.

53. Bird, P., B. Ejbjerg, M. Lassere, *et al.* 2007. A multi-reader reliability study comparing conventional high-field magnetic resonance imaging with extremity low-field MRI in rheumatoid arthritis. *J. Rheumatol.* **34:** 854–856.

54. Schirmer, C., A.K. Scheel, C.E. Althoff, *et al.* 2007. Diagnostic quality and scoring of synovitis, tenosynovitis and erosions in low-field MRI of patients with rheumatoid arthritis: A comparison with conventional MRI. *Ann. Rheum. Dis.* **66:** 522–529.

55. American College of Rheumatology. 2006. Extremity magnetic resonance imaging in rheumatoid arthritis: report of the American College of Rheumatology Extremity Magnetic Resonance Imaging Task Force. [see comment]. *Arthritis Rheum.* **54:** 1034–1047.

56. Østergaard, M., A. Duer & K. Horslev-Petersen. 2005. Can magnetic resonance imaging differentiate undifferentiated arthritis? *Arthritis Res. Ther.* **7:** 243–245.

57. Cimmino, M.A., M. Parodi, S. Innocenti, *et al.* 2005. Dynamic magnetic resonance of the wrist in psoriatic arthritis reveals imaging patterns similar to those of rheumatoid arthritis. *Arthritis Res. Ther.* **7:** R725–R731.

58. van Kuijk, A.W.R., P. Reinders-Blankert, T.J.M. Smeets, *et al.* 2006. Detailed analysis of the cell infiltrate and the expression of mediators of synovial inflammation and joint destruction in the synovium of patients with psoriatic arthritis: Implications for treatment. *Ann. Rheum. Dis.* **65:** 1551–1557.

59. McQueen, F., M. Lassere, P. Bird, *et al.* 2007. Developing a magnetic resonance imaging scoring system for peripheral psoriatic arthritis. *J. Rheumatol.* **34:** 859–861.

60. Olivieri, I., L. Barozzi, L. Favaro, *et al.* 1996. Dactylitis in patients with seronegative spondylarthropathy. Assessment by ultrasonography and magnetic resonance imaging. *Arthritis Rheum.* **39:** 1524–1528.

61. Healy, P.J. & P.S. Helliwell. 2006. Dactylitis: Pathogenesis and clinical considerations. *Curr. Rheumatol. Rep.* **8:** 338–341.

62. Narváez, J., J.A. Narváez, J.M. Nolla & J. Valverde. 2007. Comparative study of MR imaging findings in wrist and hands in early psoriatic arthritis and rheumatoid arthritis. *Arthritis Rheum.* **56:** S281.

63. Jevtic, V., I. Watt, B. Rozman, *et al.* 1995. Distinctive radiological features of small hand joints

in rheumatoid arthritis and seronegative spondyloarthritis demonstrated by contrast-enhanced (Gd-DTPA) magnetic resonance imaging. *Skeletal Radiol.* **24:** 351–355.

64. McGonagle, D., W. Gibbon, P. O'Connor, *et al.* 1998. Characteristic magnetic resonance imaging entheseal changes of knee synovitis in spondylarthropathy [see comment]. *Arthritis Rheum.* **41:** 694–700.

65. Marzo-Ortega, H., L.A. Rhodes, A.L. Tan, *et al.* 2007. Evidence for a different anatomic basis for joint disease localization in polymyalgia rheumatica in comparison with rheumatoid arthritis. *Arthritis Rheum.* **56:** 3496–33501.

66. Ostendorf, B., A. Scherer, C. Specker, *et al.* 2003. Jaccoud's arthropathy in systemic lupus erythematosus: Differentiation of deforming and erosive patterns by magnetic resonance imaging. *Arthritis Rheum.* **48:** 157–165.

67. McQueen, F., M. Lassere & M. Østergaard. 2006. Magnetic resonance imaging in psoriatic arthritis: A review of the literature. *Arthritis Res. Ther.* **8:** 207.

Bone Marrow Edema

Georg Schett

*Department of Internal Medicine 3, University of Erlangen-Nuremberg,
Erlangen, Germany*

A bone marrow edema pattern on MRI has a similar signal quality as an inflamed synovium and may, in fact, reflect true inflammatory infiltrates rather than a pure accumulation of extracellular fluid. Bone lesions near sites of rheumatoid arthritis–related inflammation are heavily vascularized, contributing to the high water content and enhanced visibility on MRI. However, even without erosive change, periarticular bone marrow lesions may be seen. This chapter describes the nature of bone marrow lesions detected by MRI in patients with inflammatory arthritis.

Key words: bone marrow edema; magnetic resonance imaging; rheumatoid arthritis

Arthritis has always been considered to be a disease that affects the joint space and its neighboring structures, particularly the articular cartilage and the synovial membrane. All forms of inflammatory arthritis as well as osteoarthritis are characterized by impairment of the normal function of the joint, which is a smooth and painless gliding of the articular surfaces. Joint disease clinically manifests as pain, swelling, and stiffness, which indicates that the pathophysiological process directly involves those structures that are important for normal motion of the joint. Inflammatory arthritis and, to a lesser extent, osteoarthritis are characterized by profound changes in the synovial membrane, leading to an influx of immune and inflammatory cells as well as to increased vascularity. Damage to the surface of the articular cartilage associated with proteoglycan loss, damage of the collagen backbone of cartilage, and erosions all are closely associated with the synovial pathology. There are differences associated with the respective impact of each of these processes in joint pathology. It is evident that rheumatoid arthritis (RA), for instance, is driven by synovial inflammation, whereas osteoarthritis (OA), for example, is presumably driven by cartilage damage.

These concepts include anatomic structures that are in direct contact with the joint space but traditionally have not considered other tissue compartments that are closely connected to the joint. In this regard, the bone marrow compartment is of particular interest since a very thin layer of bone separates it from the joint cavity. The bone marrow cavity harbors fat cells (adipocytes, white marrow), a dense trabecular network of bone, which provides stability, as well as the hematopoietic system with stem cells and the cells differentiating into the three primary hematopoietic lineages (red marrow). The bone marrow compartment has not received much attention in arthritis research since its direct assessment is difficult. Unlike the synovium, the bone marrow is not accessible by physical examination. Similarly, synovial biopsy and synovectomy do not invade this compartment. Therefore other avenues must be pursued in order to provide insight into bone marrow changes.

MRI has dramatically changed the situation as it can depict changes of tissue composition irrespective of whether the tissue is "hidden" by bone or not. It is generally known that an MRI can show inflammatory alteration of the

Address for correspondence: Georg Schett, Department of Internal Medicine 3, University of Erlangen-Nuremberg, Krankenhausstrasse 12 Erlangen Germany 91080. georg.schett@uk-erlangen.de

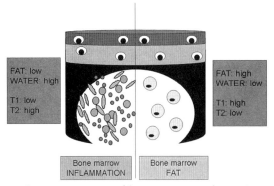

Figure 1. Basics of bone marrow edema. Normal peripheral bone marrow is filled by adipocytes and is a fat-rich compartment (*right*). Bone marrow edema is characterized by an accumulation of immune cells and microvessels in the bone marrow replacing the marrow adipocytes. This leads to an increase in water content and a decrease in fat content (*left*).

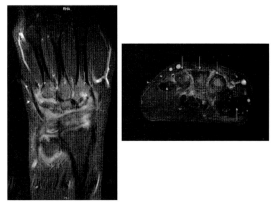

Figure 2. MRI image of bone marrow edema. Coronal (*left*) and transversal (*right*) section of a T1 weighted, fat-saturated contrast-enhanced MRI of the wrist joint in a patient with active RA. Orange arrows show bone marrow edema at the bases of the metacarpals II to IV. In the transversal section, the unaffected metacarpals II to IV (dark, blue arrows) show a signal clearly different from the one found in the metacarpals II to IV. (Color figure can be seen in the online version.)

synovial membrane in patients with RA and other forms of inflammatory arthropathy, and that it is an excellent technique for viewing inflammatory changes in the synovial membrane (synovitis) and tendons (tenosynovitis). Details concerning this aspect of MRI are addressed elsewhere in this book. However, MRI of joints affected by inflammatory arthritis also shows that morphological changes extend to sites beyond the articular space. In particular, bone marrow changes associated with arthritis are of increasing interest.

Normal bone marrow is a fat-rich tissue, particularly at peripheral sites, where hematopoiesis is not prominent. As a fat-rich tissue, it has a characteristic signal pattern on MRI scans, appearing as a bright signal on T1-weighted images and as a dark signal on T2-weighted images. Changes in this pattern are a consequence of replacement of fatty tissue by more water-rich material (Fig. 1). These lesions have been named "bone marrow edema," a term that has arisen from imaging studies and which describes an altered signal pattern (decreased T1 signal and increased T2 signal) of a specific part of the bone marrow, where fat is replaced by water.[1] Moreover, bone marrow edema is clearly visible in a contrast-enhanced

MRI, where it appears as a bright lesion (Fig. 2). However, one cannot distinguish bone marrow edema from true edema, since the increase in water content is relative, in part because fatty tissue retracts and is replaced by nonfat tissue. Indeed bone marrow edema has a signal quality similar to that of inflamed synovium and may in fact reflect true inflammatory infiltrates rather than a pure accumulation of extracellular fluid. Instruments to describe the severity of bone marrow edema have been developed such as the rheumatoid arthritis MRI scoring (RAMRIS) system of T2-weighted images,[2,3] which has been recognized as reliable and sensitive.[4]

Changes in bone marrow are common in RA patients. Sixty-eight percent of patients with established RA have bone marrow lesions, and these lesions affect a higher percent of bones in established disease than in early disease.[5] The presence of bone marrow edema is more likely in patients with high inflammatory disease activity (as measured by C-reactive protein), a high level of pain, and antibodies against citrullinated proteins.[6,7] Even in early RA, bone

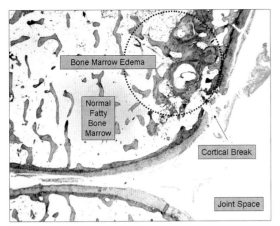

Figure 3. Histological section through a joint with bone marrow edema. A proximal PIP joint of a patient with RA showing accumulation of immune cells and blood vessels at the site of MRI signs of bone marrow edema. Note the replacement of fat by an inflammatory infiltrate.

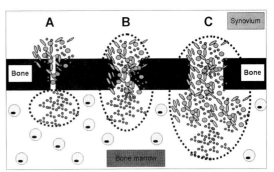

Figure 4. Generation of bone marrow edema. (**A**) Small bone marrow lesion consisting of lymphocyte aggregates, which is connected to inflammatory synovial tissue by small cortical bone channels. This may lead to the impression of isolated bone marrow edema with no bone erosion. (**B**) Bone erosion with resorption of cortical bone and widening of bone marrow edema. This image would reflect MRI bone erosion, which is the sum of inflammatory tissue within the bone marrow as well as within cortical bone. (**C**) More severe bone erosion with widening of the cortical break and extensive marrow edema.

marrow lesions may be seen in the affected joints, sometimes within the first months after the onset of the disease.[8] Interestingly, bone marrow edema is not found in patients with pure arthralgia, that is, without signs of inflammatory joint disease. However, these lesions can be present in RA patients in clinical remission, suggesting that subclinical inflammation may still add to further damage in such cases. A recent study from Leeds has shown that among 107 RA patients in clinical remission, 96% had MRI-based evidence for residual synovitis and 46% had bone marrow edema.[9]

Studies addressing the nature of MRI-based bone marrow edema are scarce, as it is difficult to examine the bone marrow adjacent to inflamed joints in humans directly. From a handful of histopathologic studies on material derived from joint replacement surgery it is known that juxta-articular bone marrow does show signs of inflammation[10–12] (Fig. 3). Bone marrow fat is replaced by immune cells, particularly T and B lymphocytes, which form aggregates in the bone marrow and are associated with the accumulation of blood vessels. In fact, this exactly reflects the increased water content observed in bone marrow edema.

Specifically, the fat is replaced by a vascularized, cell-rich inflammatory tissue. Importantly, bone marrow edema is not exclusive to RA: MRI of patients with spondylarthropathies reveals extensive changes in the bone marrow of vertebral bodies, the pelvis along the sacroiliac joints, and in bone marrow compartments close to peripheral joints. Moreover, these lesions are also found in joints affected by OA, suggesting that the formation of inflammatory infiltrates in the bone marrow might be a common finding in diseased joints. Other conditions that involve bone marrow edema are transient osteoporosis of the hip[13,14] and osteonecrosis.[15]

The mechanisms that lead to the generation of bone marrow infiltrates in arthritis are as yet poorly understood.[16] Recent studies comparing MRIs of joints in patients with RA with sequential sections of the same joints after joint replacement surgery have clearly shown that the bone marrow changes observed on the MRI scans are based on inflammatory infiltrates.[6,17] How these infiltrates form is still a matter of speculation (Fig. 4). There are two potential scenarios: (1) Bone marrow infiltrates could represent primary lesions, which then entail articular changes, or (2) bone marrow lesions are formed as a consequence of arthritis. It is difficult to determine which of these scenarios is the more likely; moreover, it might differ among the various kinds of diseases.

In RA, for instance, synovial pathology is very prominent and may indeed represent a primary event, which is then followed by bone marrow pathology. In OA, however, the mechanism may be different and the main inflammatory changes may be localized first in the bone marrow and then in the synovium. At least, the emergence of bone marrow lesions around diseased joints suggests communication between the synovium and the bone marrow. In RA, resorption of mineralized tissue beneath the articular cartilage is a major contributor to joint pathology and leads to a break in cortical bone, allowing direct communication between the synovial tissue and the bone marrow. These penetration sites are characterized by inflammatory infiltrates in the neighboring bone marrow, which are based either on the formation of lymphocytic aggregates or on the invasion of synovial tissue into the marrow space. In both cases these lesions are heavily vascularized, which contributes to a high water content and their visibility on MRI scans.

Classical bone erosions are thus a major factor in the involvement of the bone marrow in RA. Bone marrow lesions, however, are found early in the disease, even before overt bone erosions have been formed. How can this be explained? In fact, bone erosions may not be a *conditio sine qua non* for communication between the synovium and the bone marrow. Cortical bone is crossed by a number of channels, which allows blood vessels to enter into the marrow space and thus represents pathways for inflammatory tissue to cross the cortical barrier before creating a large break in the cortical bone. Widening of cortical bone channels has been observed in histopathologic examination of joints of RA patients. Thus, inflammatory tissue may reach the bone marrow and create inflammatory lesions well before true

cortical breaks form. This can be visualized on MRI scans and sometimes even on plain radiographs.

As bone marrow edema reflects true inflammation, it is likely that such lesions specifically affect the arthritic process. First, these lesions may precipitate trabecular bone loss. In fact, loss of periarticular trabecular bone is a well-known and early feature in RA patients. It is also known as periarticular osteoporosis, owing to its appearance on plain radiographs. Periarticular osteoporosis has so far been considered as a kind of paracrine effect of inflammatory tissue leading to cytokine-induced bone resorption. However, the fact that bone marrow edema is located at these sites and reflects inflammatory tissue in the bone marrow suggests that trabecular bone loss is indeed a direct consequence of the accumulation of immune cells and increased formation of osteoclasts. Moreover, bone marrow edema may also affect the formation of bone erosions. This postulate is supported by the high correlation between MRIs showing bone marrow edema and MRIs indicating bone erosions.[18] It is known that the sites of bone marrow edema predict the later formation of bone erosion.[19]

In a Norwegian cohort of patients ($N = 84$) with early arthritis, bone marrow edema (RAMRIS score for BME > 2) predicted the progression of radiographic bone erosions as well as MRI bone erosions in the wrist joint after 1 year. Similar results were obtained in a Finnish cohort of 27 patients with early arthritis, where the BME at baseline was the best predictor among other MRI-based variables (e.g., synovitis score) and laboratory parameters (e.g., C-reactive protein) for the MRI bone erosions in the wrist joint after 2 years.[20] Moreover, these bone marrow lesions also preceded radiographic bone erosions in RA.[21] These observations suggest that bone marrow edema could contribute to the formation of cortical bone erosions. This is conceivable as inflammatory tissue in the bone marrow that has the potential to create osteoclasts from mononuclear precursors also has the ability to degrade cortical bone. The observation that bone marrow edema can be found before overt bone erosion does not necessarily exclude the possibility that synovial inflammatory tissue has made use of small cortical bone channels to pass the bone barrier and create inflammatory sites in the marrow. The MRI characteristics of bone erosions support the close relationship between bone erosion and bone marrow lesions. MRI bone erosions, in fact, do not reflect only the site where cortical bone has been broken, but also depict the intramedullar inflammatory tissue close to the penetration site.

The presence of bone marrow edema in diseases such as RA reveals that inflammatory joint diseases are not exclusive to the synovial membrane but also extend to the neighboring bone marrow. The tethering of bone marrow edema and bone erosions indicates that these inflammatory lesions directly contribute to the disease process of RA and are relevant to progressive structural damage. The detection of bone marrow edema by MRI can therefore be considered a valuable tool for defining the severity and extent of inflammatory processes in chronic joint disease.

Acknowledgment

MRI images were kindly provided by Prof. Michael Uder, Radiology Department, University of Erlangen-Nuremberg, Erlangen, Germany.

Conflicts of Interest

The authors declare no conflicts of interest.

References

1. Wilson, A.J., W.A. Murphy, D.C. Hardy & W.G. Totty. 1988. Transient osteoporosis: Transient bone marrow edema? *Radiology* **167:** 757–760.
2. Østergaard, M., C. Peterfy, P. Conaghan, *et al.* 2003. OMERACT Rheumatoid arthritis magnetic resonance imaging studies: Core set of MRI acquisitions, joint pathology definitions, and the OMERACT RA-MRI scoring system. *J. Rheumatol.* **30:** 1385–1386.
3. Conaghan, P., P. Bird, B. Ejbjerg, *et al.* 2005. The EULAR–OMERACT rheumatoid arthritis MRI reference image atlas: The metacarpophalangeal joints. *Ann. Rheum. Dis.* **64:** i11–i21.
4. Haavardsholm, E.A., M. Østergaard, B.J. Ejbjerg, *et al.* 2005. Reliability and sensitivity to change of the OMERACT rheumatoid arthritis magnetic resonance imaging score in a multireader, longitudinal setting. *Arthritis Rheum.* **52:** 3860–3867.
5. Savnik, A., H. Malmskov, H.S. Thomsen, *et al.* 2001. Magnetic resonance imaging of the wrist and finger joints in patients with inflammatory joint diseases. *J. Rheumatol.* **28:** 2193–2200.
6. F.M. McQueen, A. Gao, M. Østergaard, *et al.* 2007. High-grade MRI bone oedema is common within the surgical field in rheumatoid arthritis patients undergoing joint replacement and is associated with osteitis in subchondral bone. *Ann. Rheum. Dis.* **66:** 1581–1587.
7. Tamai, M., A. Kawakami, M. Uetani, *et al.* 2006. The presence of anti-cyclic citrullinated peptide antibody is associated with magnetic resonance imaging detection of bone marrow oedema in early stage rheumatoid arthritis. *Ann. Rheum. Dis.* **65:** 133–134.
8. McQueen, F.M., N. Stewart, J. Crabbe, *et al.* 1998. Magnetic resonance imaging of the wrist in early rheumatoid arthritis reveals a high prevalence of erosions at four months after symptom onset. *Ann. Rheum. Dis.* **57:** 350–356.
9. Brown, A.K., M.A. Quinn, Z. Karim, *et al.* 2006. Presence of significant synovitis in rheumatoid arthritis patients with disease-modifying antirheumatic drug-induced clinical remission: Evidence from an imaging study may explain structural progression. *Arthritis Rheum.* **54:** 3761–3773.
10. Jimenez-Boj, E., K. Redlich, B. Turk, *et al.* 2005. Interaction between synovial inflammatory tissue and bone marrow in rheumatoid arthritis. *J. Immunol.* **175:** 2579–2588.
11. Appel, H., C. Loddenkemper, Z. Grozdanovic, *et al.* 2006. Correlation of histopathological findings and magnetic resonance imaging in the spine of patients with ankylosing spondylitis. *Arthritis Res. Ther.* **22:** R143.
12. Zanetti, M., E. Bruder, J. Romero & J. Hodler. 2000. Bone marrow edema pattern in osteoarthritic knees: Correlation between MR imaging and histologic findings. *Radiology* **215:** 835–840.
13. Curtiss, P.H. & W.E. Kincaid. 1959. Transitory demineralization of the hip in pregnancy. *J. Bone Joint Surg. (Am)* **41:** 1327–1333.
14. Haynes, C.W., W.F. Conway & W.W. Daniel. 1993. MR imaging of bone marrow edema pattern:

Transient osteoporosis, transient osteoporosis, transient bone marrow edema syndrome, or osteonecrosis. *Radiographics* **13:** 1001–1011.

15. Turner, D.A., A.C. Templeton, P.M. Selzer, *et al.* 1989. Femoral capital osteonecrosis: MR finding of diffuse marrow abnormalities without focal lesions. *Radiology* **171:** 135–140.

16. McQueen, F.M. & B. Ostendorf. 2006. What is MRI bone oedema in rheumatoid arthritis and why does it matter? *Arthritis Res. Ther.* **8:** 222.

17. Jimenez-Boj, E., I. Nöbauer-Huhmann, B. Hanslik-Schnabel, *et al.* 2007. Bone erosions and bone marrow edema as defined by magnetic resonance imaging reflect true bone marrow inflammation in rheumatoid arthritis. *Arthritis Rheum.* **56:** 1118–1124.

18. McQueen, F.M., N. Stewart, J. Crabbe, *et al.* 1999. Magnetic resonance imaging of the wrist in early rheumatoid arthritis reveals progression of erosions despite clinical improvement. *Ann. Rheum. Dis.* **58:** 156–163.

19. Haavardsholm, E.A., P. Bøyesen, M. Østergaard, *et al.* 2007. MRI findings in 84 early rheumatoid arthritis patients: Bone marrow oedema predicts erosive progression. *Ann. Rheum. Dis.* **67:** 794–800.

20. Palosaari, K., J. Vuotila, R. Takalo, *et al.* 2006. Bone oedema predicts erosive progression on wrist MRI in early RA–a 2-yr observational MRI and NC scintigraphy study. *Rheumatology (Oxford)* **45:** 1542–1548.

21. McQueen, F.M., N. Benton, D. Perry, *et al.* 2003. Bone edema scored on magnetic resonance imaging scans of the dominant carpus at presentation predicts radiographic joint damage of the hands and feet six years later in patients with rheumatoid arthritis. *Arthritis Rheum.* **48:** 1814–1827.

MRI for Assessing Erosion and Joint Space Narrowing in Inflammatory Arthropathies

Mahnaz Momeni and Kathleen Brindle

Rheumatology Division and Department of Radiology, The George Washington University, Washington DC, USA

The superior soft tissue contrast and multiplanar capability of magnetic resonance imaging has contributed to earlier diagnosis and implementation of effective treatment for a variety of arthropathies. Owing to overlapping clinical signs and symptoms, MRI plays a role in delineating the features and stages of these conditions. With the advent of disease-modifying therapies, it is important to diagnose inflammatory arthropathy as early as possible. In this chapter, we discuss the pathophysiology of bone erosion and joint space narrowing, as well as the role of MRI in the imaging of the seropositive and seronegative inflammatory arthropathies.

Key words: erosion; joint space narrowing; magnetic resonance imaging

Introduction

On the basis of epidemiological data,[1] rheumatoid arthritis affects 1% of the population. The disease demonstrates slow progression in some patients, whereas it rapidly destroys joint spaces and periarticular bone in others. The peak onset of symptoms is between the fourth and the sixth decades; however, juvenile rheumatoid arthritis is also well known. Before the development of MRI, clinicians had to rely on clinical examination, presenting symptoms, and radiographs to diagnose this disease. Unfortunately, radiographs demonstrate only the late changes owing to rheumatoid arthritis. MRI is able to detect early synovial changes before the development of erosions. Recent research also suggests that bone marrow edema detected by MRI may, in fact, be predictive of erosions.[2] Early diagnosis is of high priority in the initial workup of patients with suspected rheumatoid arthritis. Confirmation of the diagnosis allows clinicians to start disease-modifying therapy early, before severe secondary disability has occurred. Assessment of the severity of the disease on the baseline scans of individual patients may allow clinicians to tailor their drug regimens appropriately.

Pathophysiology for Joint Space Narrowing and Bone Erosion in Rheumatoid Arthritis

The chronic inflammatory arthritides are often associated with localized and generalized bone loss. Localized bone loss manifests as periarticular osteopenia and subchondral bone erosions and constitutes an important feature in diagnosing and directing treatment in rheumatoid arthritis (RA), psoriatic arthritis (PsA), and juvenile idiopathic arthritis. MRI has now revealed that erosions occur early in these diseases. Furthermore, erosions tend to correlate with ongoing disease activity and joint destruction. Early intervention to alter the natural progression of joint destruction has been shown to substantially improve functional status. The revelation that erosions reflect ongoing disease activity and are thus associated with an unfavorable prognosis led to increased the efforts

Address for correspondence: Dr. Mahnaz Momeni, Assistant Professor of Medicine, George Washington University, Rheumatology Division, 2150 Pennsylvania Ave NW 3-416 Washington DC, USA 20037. voice: 202-741-2488. mmomeni@mfa.gwu.edu

MRI and Ultrasound in Diagnosis and Management: Ann. N.Y. Acad. Sci. 1154: 41–51 (2009).
doi: 10.1111/j.1749-6632.2009.04384.x © 2009 New York Academy of Sciences.

to identify the underlying mechanisms behind this pathologic process. Success of the antitumor necrosis factor- (anti-TNF-) therapy in retarding and, in some cases, possibly reversing early focal bone loss has been encouraging.

Osteoclasts (OCLs), cells that are uniquely capable of bone degradation, are consistently detected at erosion sites in all animal models of destructive arthritis as well as human RA.[2] Synovial inflammation generates tumor necrosis factor (TNF)-alpha, macrophage colony-stimulating factor (M-CSF), and receptor activator of nuclear factor-κB ligand (RANKL)—cytokines that fuel osteoclastogenesis and arthritic bone destruction. The targeted removal of OCLs by TNF blockers, RANKL antagonism, or genetic manipulation in animal models potently blocks this bone destruction.[3–6]

Role of Osteoclasts in Bone Erosion

Osteoclasts are multinucleated cells derived from the mononuclear cell precursors of the monocyte/macrophage lineage that resorbs bone matrix. Bone destruction in RA is mainly attributable to the abnormal activation of OCLs. Bone is a dynamic tissue that is constantly remodeled by bone-resorbing osteoclasts and bone-forming osteoblasts. Dysfunction or imbalance in these cells is seen in RA. The discovery of RANK ligand highlighted the central role of OCLs in the pathogenesis of bone destruction in RA.[7]

OPG

The discovery of osteoprotegerin (OPG) in 1997 was a major advance in the field of bone biology. OPG is released in soluble form by stromal cells/osteoblasts. In addition to bone, OPG mRNA is expressed by a number of other tissues, including lung, heart, kidney, liver, stomach, intestine, thyroid gland, brain, and spinal cord. OPG inhibits the differentiation and activity of osteoclasts by acting as a decoy receptor for the receptor activator of nuclear factor κB

ligand (RANKL), thereby downregulating the RANKL signaling through receptor activator of nuclear factor κB (RANK). In this manner it inhibits osteoclast differentiation, suppresses mature osteoclast activation, and induces OCL apoptosis.

RANK

RANK is a transmembrane protein that belongs to the tumor necrosis factor receptor (TNFR) superfamily. It is expressed primarily in the cells of the monocytes/macrophage lineage, including osteoclastic precursors, B and T cells, dendritic cells, and fibroblasts. RANK is also present on the surface of mature osteoclasts.

RANKL

The discovery of OPG was soon followed by the identification of its ligand, initially termed "osteoprotegerin ligand" (OPG-L), which turned out to be identical with two previously described members of the TNF superfamily. RANKL is a 317 amino acid peptide that also belongs to the TNF-superfamily. It exists in two forms, soluble and membrane bound. RANKL has been detected in synovial fibroblasts, osteoblasts, and activated T cells from peripheral blood as well as tissue near the pannus–bone interface. TNF-α induces RANKL and M-CSF in stromal cells and also stimulates osteoclast precursor cells to synergize with RANKL signaling.[8,9] It is also reported that anti-TNF drugs induce apoptosis in synovial macrophages, suggesting a complex action mechanism.

Bone Erosion Provides Further Evidence of a Link between Immune System Activation and Bone Resorption

Once the function of OPG/RANK/RANKL in bone remodeling was recognized, it was hypothesized that RANKL may be of major pathophysiological importance in the bone and joint destruction observed in inflammatory arthritides such as RA. Studies by Goldring and Gravallese[45], provided initial insights into the role of RANKL in the pathogenesis of focal bone erosions. Other studies have provided compelling evidence that both activated T cells from the RA synovium and synovial fibroblasts produce RANKL. Indeed it is now assumed that activated T cells, which play a central role in the pathogenesis of RA, may contribute to the osteoclast-mediated bone resorption via RANKL expression. Although the role of RANKL in other inflammatory diseases is not yet known, Ritchlin *et al.*,[10] using immunohistochemistry, revealed striking spatial regulation of RANK, RANKL, and OPG expression in the PsA joints.

The severity of bone erosion correlated with higher circulating mononuclear OCL precursor (OcP) numbers, which revealed a novel mechanism for osteoclastogenesis in PsA.[10]

The Role of T Cells in Osteoclastogenesis

As RANKL is expressed in activated T cells, it is of vital importance to determine whether T cells have the capacity to induce osteoclast differentiation. Indeed, Kong *et al.*[11] showed that RANKL expressed on activated T cells directly induces osteoclastogenesis.

Helper T (Th) cells are divided into two main subsets according to the cytokines they produce, Th1 and Th2.[12] Th1 cells produce mainly interferon-γ and IL-2 and are involved in cellular immunity, whereas Th2 cells produce mainly IL-4, IL-5, and IL-10 and are involved in humoral immunity. Interferon-γ and IL-2 are the key cytokines produced by Th1 cells. Interferon-γ strongly inhibits osteoclastogenesis, suggesting that normal Th1 cells inhibit osteoclastogenesis and do not induce bone loss.

T cells in RA joints are defective in suppressive effect owing to the lack of interferon-γ, but they have a strong capacity to induce inflammatory cytokines, which stimulate the expression of RANKL on synovial cells. Interestingly, IL-4[13,14] and IL-10,[15] both of which are classic Th2-type cytokines, also inhibit osteoclastogenesis,[16] so the positive effect of T cells on osteoclastogenesis can only be observed under strictly limited conditions. Thus, the actual role of T cells in osteoclastogenesis is highly complex and may depend on the type of prevailing cytokines.[17] Under some conditions, T cells may not drive osteoclastogenesis, even if RANKL is expressed. In the presence of high levels of TNF, subosteoclastogenic ("permissive") amounts of RANKL may be sufficient for TNF to drive RANKL-mediated osteoclastogenesis.[18]

MRI-Observed Erosion and Joint Space Narrowing in Inflammatory Arthritis

Magnetic resonance imaging is a sensitive modality for the detection of erosions, and it does so more often and at an earlier stage than radiography.[19]

Fast spin-echo T1-weighted sequences, fat-saturated T2 fast spin-echo sequences, and postcontrast T1-weighted sequences with fat saturation are performed in axial, coronal, and sagittal orthogonal planes. If fat-saturated T2-weighted sequences are not available, a short-tau inversion recovery (STIR) sequence can be obtained. Good fat saturation and contrast enhancement are important for the evaluation of bone marrow edema and synovial hyperemia, respectively.

In many cases, bone erosions are seen on MRI scans when radiographs do not indicate abnormalities (Fig. 1).[20] In one recent study, for example, only 41% of the erosions seen on MRIs were subsequently detected on radiographs (Fig. 2).[21] Only focal lesions that demonstrate contrast enhancement are eligible to be classified as erosions. Before the development of contrast-enhanced MRI, the term erosion was applied to juxta-articular lesions in patients who demonstrated distribution of

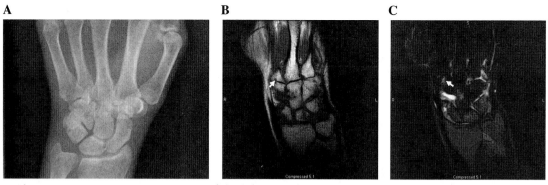

Figure 1. Postero-anterior (PA) view of the left wrist of a 43-year-old woman with rheumatoid arthritis: (**A**) The bone mineralization is normal and no joint space narrowing or erosive changes is seen in the wrist. Coronal T1- (**B**) and coronal T2-weighted fast spin-echo fat-saturated (**C**) MRI scans of the left wrist were performed approximately 1 month later. There is proliferative synovitis with a high T2 signal in the joints on T2-weighted images (white arrow in **C**) and bone marrow edema with scattered erosions (white arrow in **B**) are present throughout the wrist. The most visible erosion on these images is at the base of the 2nd metacarpal.

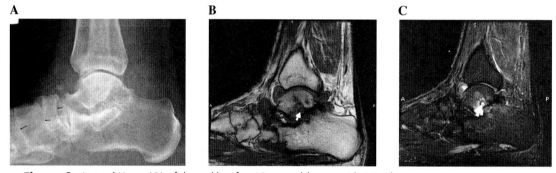

Figure 2. Lateral X ray (**A**) of the ankle of a 62-year-old man with RA. There is joint space narrowing at multiple joints (black arrows) with relative sparing of the tibiotalar joint, but there is soft tissue prominence at the tibiotalar joint, suggesting an effusion or synovitis. Erosions are not seen clearly on the X ray but are obvious on the ankle MRI performed approximately 1½ years earlier. Sagittal T1 (**B**) and sagittal STIR (**C**) MRI scans were performed. Synovial proliferation in the ankle is intermediate in signal on the T1-weighted images and bright on the STIR images. There is a large erosion (white arrow in **B**) at the posterior subtalar joint with surrounding bone marrow edema (white arrow in **C**). These findings are bright on the STIR images. Multiple erosions in other joints were also visible on the MRI.

the lesions in a pattern characteristic of RA. With the advent of contrast-enhanced MRI, the definition of the term erosion became more precise. According to the outcome measures in rheumatoid arthritis clinical trials scoring system (OMERACT),[22] erosion is defined as a sharply marginated bone lesion with correct juxta-articular localization and typical signal characteristics. According to OMERACT, to be labeled erosion the cortical break should be seen in at least two planes.

Focal lesions that show increased T2 signal without contrast enhancement can represent subchondral cysts. Such a distinction becomes particularly important in cases where RA has to be differentiated from degenerative OA (osteoarthritis). MRI allows for early detection of erosions and correct classification of osseous lesions as erosive in cases where abnormality is located far from the joint. In some cases, even large erosions are occult on radiographs but are clearly demonstrated on MRIs (Fig. 3).[23]

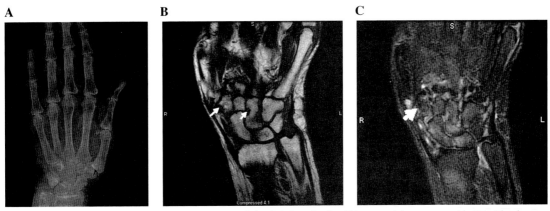

Figure 3. Postero-anterior (PA) (**A**) views of the left hand of a 76-year-old woman with RA. The bones are diffusely osteopenic. Some erosions show in the PA view at the 1ˢᵗ CMC joint. Coronal T1 (**B**) and coronal T2-weighted fast spin-echo with fat saturation (**C**) images of the left wrist of the same woman. The MRIs better demonstrate findings of RA with multiple low-signal erosions (white arrows in **B**) seen in the wrist on the T1-weighted images. Proliferative synovitis is seen as a bright signal within the joint spaces on the T2-weighted images. Bone marrow edema is also seen on the T2 images as a bright signal within the bone.

Erosions detectable by MRI are likely to progress to radiograph-detectable erosions in patients with high baseline disease activity. Moreover, before the advent of MRI, it was not possible to evaluate osseous structures for the presence of bone marrow edema. Increased T2 signal on MRIs results from increased water content in the bone marrow, which is probably related to an inflammatory response. Bone marrow edema is a strong predictor of future erosions. Bone marrow edema has been shown to be associated with a sixfold increase in risk of developing erosions at the same site at 1 year of follow-up.[24] A more recent study also demonstrated that bone marrow edema predicts erosive progression in early RA during the first 2 years of the disease.

Contrast-Enhanced Imaging in Rheumatoid Arthritis

Whereas T2-weighted imaging allows for detection of edematous tissues and joint effusions, administration of intravenous contrast enables detection of inflamed hypervascular tissues. Intravenous contrast can be used to differentiate inflamed synovium from adjacent bone marrow edema and joint effusion (Figs. 4 and 5). Several factors contribute to good contrast between the inflamed synovium and adjacent tissues, including the amount of injected contrast, the amount of joint effusion, and the vascularity of the adjacent tissues.[25,26]

If a significant amount of time is allowed to pass between contrast injection and the acquisition of the magnetic resonance images, contrast will diffuse into the joint. This phenomenon has been studied in healthy volunteers, and there is no reason to think that the same process would not occur in patients with inflammatory arthritis. If the images are not acquired in a timely fashion, it may not be possible to differentiate between synovium and joint fluid. Hence, accurate timing of the scan is very important when imaging patients with suspected RA. In the wrist, the peak steady state of contrast enhancement is reached at 60 to 120 s.[27] The initial period of 10 min after administration of contrast has been suggested as the optimal time for imaging of the knee joint, but other reports counter that the optimal timing may be as early as 5 to 6 min after administration.[28,29]

The use of contrast-enhanced MRI in evaluation of RA is supported by several studies. Moreover, it has been shown to detect

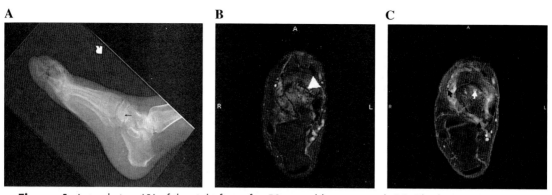

Figure 4. Lateral view (**A**) of the right foot of a 53-year-old woman with RA. The bones are osteopenic and there is joint space narrowing at the talonavicular joint (black arrows) without evidence of erosions. Axial T2 fast spin-echo images with fat saturation (**B**) and axial T1-weighted images with fat saturation and gadolinium contrast administration (**C**) were taken of the right ankle/hindfoot. Erosions are easily visualized at the talonavicular joint as focal areas of bright T2 signal (white arrowhead in **B**), and they enhance after contrast administration (white arrow in **C**). There is also enhancing rheumatoid pannus (black arrow in **C**).

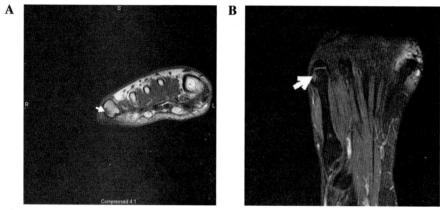

Figure 5. MRI was performed on a woman with a diagnosis of RA and pain in her 3rd through 5th toes. Coronal T1 (**A**) and axial T1-weighted images with fat saturation and gadolinium contrast administration (**B**) were taken. These images reveal an erosion at the lateral aspect of the 5th metatarsal head that is low signal on the T1-weighted images and enhances after gadolinium administration (white arrows).

more periarticular bone abnormalities than T2-weighted imaging. Figure 6 illustrates an example of erosions that are better depicted on a contrast-enhanced image than on T2-weighted fat-saturated image.

MRI as a Follow-Up Tool

With the advent of disease-modifying therapy, MRI became an important tool for the evaluation of patient responses to therapy. As the disease is now being treated early, before significant bone and joint destruction has occurred, MRI can be used to evaluate the response of synovium to therapy and accurately document the stability or progression of erosions. Tam *et al.*,[46] for example, used dynamic contrast-enhanced MRI to document changes in synovitis severity, volume of the synovium, and synovial perfusion indices after patients were treated with a combination of methotrexate and infliximab. Quantification of hand synovitis by measuring the volume of enhanced inflammatory tissue has also been used to evaluate the effectiveness of new medications in

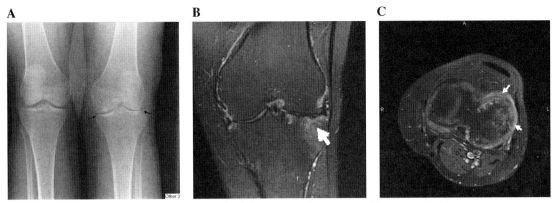

Figure 6. Antero-posterior (AP) view of both knees (**A**) of a 46-year-old woman. Although the joint spaces are maintained in the right knee, there is diffuse joint space narrowing in the left knee with erosive changes (black arrows) and no significant osteophyte formation. Despite the asymmetry, the findings in the left knee are compatible with RA. The findings are confirmed on MRIs of the knee. Coronal T2 fast spin-echo images with fat saturation (**B**) and axial T1-weighted images with fat saturation after the intravenous administration of gadolinium contrast (**C**) were taken. Erosive changes with edema, both bright on the T2-weighted images, are greatest at the lateral compartment of the knee, where they involve predominantly the tibial plateau. The erosions enhance after contrast administration.

the treatment of refractory arthritis.[30,31] Other researchers have used MRI to evaluate bone marrow edema and the progression or development of erosions to compare a new drug regimen with a placebo.

MRI can also be used to predict functional outcome in patients with early inflammatory arthritis. Benton *et al.*[32] demonstrated that MRI of patients with early RA can predict functional outcome at 6 years of follow-up. Another report based on the same cohort also demonstrated that areas of bone marrow edema at baseline evolved into erosions at follow-up. Evidence of tendinopathy on MRIs in early RA can also predict tendon rupture at 6 years.

MRI in Psoriatic Arthritis

Magnetic resonance imaging has advanced our understanding of many types of arthritis, with respect to both inflammatory processes and articular damage. Psoriatic arthritis (PsA) has been the subject of less research scrutiny than RA in many areas, including imaging, but this is likely to change because there is an increasing use of MRI outcome measures in clinical trials of new therapeutic agents such as biologics.[33]

Although the work conducted by Ritchlin and co-workers[34] recently focused attention on activated osteoclasts in PsA and raised the possibility that a disorder of bone remodeling may underlie this disease, evidence from MRI studies conducted thus far suggests that PsA erosions are rather similar to those of RA. There are differences in terms of distribution, but the erosions themselves consist of a break in cortical bone overlying a region of altered signal intensity with definite margins, as described in RA (Fig. 7). Furthermore, as those in RA, PsA erosions can be large and are frequently not visualized in conventional radiography. The study conducted by Savnik and co-workers[35] in patients with inflammatory arthritis suggested that MRI erosions in PsA patients did not progress over time to the same extent as those in patients with early RA, raising the possibility that PsA bone disease may sometimes be less aggressive. Backhaus and colleagues[36] included 15 PsA patients in their study of MRI, ultrasound, and scintigraphy of the finger joints, nine of whom were described as having MRI-observed erosions. Some of these erosions were

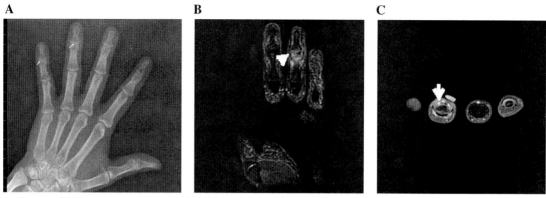

Figure 7. Postero-anterior view (**A**) of the left hand in a 50-year-old man. There is mild juxta-articular osteopenia and soft tissue swelling at the 4th DIP joint. The joints of the 4th and 5th fingers appear narrowed but on MRI only the 4th DIP joint is abnormal. Coronal STIR image (**B**) and axial T1-weighted image with fat saturation after gadolinium contrast administration (**C**) in the same patient. Imaging is focused on the 4th finger. On the STIR image there is bone marrow edema with a high signal in the distal aspect of the middle phalanx in the 4th DIP joint. A bright signal is also seen along the periosteum. (white arrow in **B**) Contrast-enhanced T1-weighted image demonstrates synovial enhancement (white arrow in **C**). The DIP joint and periosteal involvement is suggestive of PsA.

"nonenhancing" following contrast injection, suggesting that they might contain fibrous tissue rather than inflammatory pannus and therefore be relatively "inactive," but there was no clear description of these lesions.

As in RA, the histopathological correlate of MRI-observed bone edema has not been defined in PsA, but Bollow and co-workers[37] found some evidence of osteitis in subcortical bone in their biopsy study of sacroiliac joints in spondyloarthropathy patients (including two with PsA). Bone edema has been described in PsA, reactive arthritis, ankylosing spondylitis, and RA and is recognized as an ill-defined area in the subcortical bone with increased signal on STIR, T2-weighted with fat saturation (FS), and postcontrast T1-weighted with FS sequences.

Savnik and colleagues[38] found MRI-observed bone edema in PsA patients included in their cohort with early inflammatory arthritis, and noted that the total number of bones affected did not change over 1 year (compared with the RA patients, in whom it increased). They found examples in PsA of bone edema involving distal, middle, and proximal phalanges of the fingers as well as carpal bones, radius, and

ulna, and found that in various cases it either appeared or disappeared between the baseline and 1 year MRI examinations. Bone edema was a strong predictor of bone erosions in their RA group (as was described elsewhere[39]), but this was not specifically demonstrated in PsA joints, and further studies are needed to clarify this point.

In their series comparing MRIs of the hand in 28 PsA and 18 RA patients, Giovagnoni and co-workers[40] also noted signal changes in subchondral bone (bone edema) in 43% of their patients, associated with pronounced periarticular edema of the soft tissues, spreading to the subcutis, and suggested that this might constitute a "psoriatic pattern" on an MRI.

Comparing MRI Findings in Rheumatoid Arthritis and Psoriatic Arthritis

In RA and PsA, the finger joints are usually the first joints affected. Although the diagnosis is based primarily on clinical findings, it is sometimes difficult even for a trained rheumatologist to differentiate between them. This is especially true in cases of PsA *sine psoriase*. Radiographic changes in PsA are specific and differ from those in RA, but a conventional radiograph may also be normal in acute arthritis. A study done by Schoellnast and Hannes[41] compared MRI findings of the wrist and the hand in patients with PsA and RA. Using contrast-enhanced MRI, they found that erosions were statistically more frequent in patients with RA and that periostitis was statistically seen more frequently in patients with PsA. No statistically significant difference was found in the frequency of synovitis, bone marrow edema, bone cysts, or tenosynovitis between the two groups. The radiocarpal joint, the midcarpal joints, the carpometacarpal joints, and the metacarpophalangeal joints were significantly affected more frequently in patients with RA than in patients with PsA, whereas the proximal interphalangeal joints were significantly more frequently affected in patients with PsA ($p < 0.05$).

Offidani *et al.* showed that joints were frequently affected in patients with psoriasis but without clinically evident arthritis,. They reported periarticular effusion and synovitis/intra-articular effusion as the two most frequent findings (36 and 44%, respectively).[41]

Pitfalls

Several pitfalls should be considered during interpretation of MRI studies in the context of RA. Partial volume artifacts can mimic erosive changes, synovitis, and tenosynovitis. Insertion sites of interosseous ligaments can mimic erosions.[42] Close proximity of anatomical structures in the wrist can lead to confusion among bone marrow edema, synovitis, and tenosynovitis on fluid-sensitive sequences. Furthermore, bone edema, erosions, and tenosynovitis have been reported in healthy volunteers.[43] Small amounts of fluid are commonly identified in the extensor tendons, particularly extensor carpi radialis brevis and longus.[44] The cause of this finding is unknown and, in some cases, it may be confused with tenosynovitis. In-homogeneous fat suppression may mimic bone marrow edema. In some cases, bone marrow edema may be found surrounding focal erosions. In others, a small focal area of edema may mimic a focal erosion, especially on images obtained without contrast. Differentiation between an erosion and edema would be difficult in such cases. Focal bone changes, such as the development of small bone islands, can also mimic erosions on T1-weighted images. However, evaluation of all available sequences, including fat-suppressed contrast-enhanced T1-weighted images, should solve most challenging cases.

Conclusions

Magnetic resonance imaging is an excellent modality for evaluation of patients with early inflammatory arthritis. In addition to demonstrating excellent sensitivity for detection of erosions, MRI can show even earlier changes, such as synovitis and tenosynovitis. Secondary manifestations of RA, such as carpal tunnel syndrome, can also be well evaluated by means of MRI. Fat-suppressed and contrast-enhanced sequences are an important part of the MRI protocols for evaluation of RA. In addition to early detection, MRI can also be used to evaluate the effectiveness of therapies.

Conflicts of Interest

The authors declare no conflicts of interest.

References

1. Goldring, S. 2003. Osteoporosis and rheumatic diseases. In *Primer of the Metabolic Bone Diseases and Disorders of Mineral Metabolism*. 5th ed.: 379–382. Lippincott Williams & Wilkins. Philadelphia.
2. Gough, A.K., J. Lilley, S. Eyre, *et al.* 1994. Generalised bone loss in patients with early rheumatoid arthritis. *Lancet* **344:** 23–27.
3. Redlich, K., S. Hayer, A. Maier, *et al.* 2002. Tumor necrosis factor alpha-mediated joint destruction

is inhibited by targeting osteoclasts with osteoprote-gerin. *Arthritis Rheum.* **46:** 785–792.

4. Redlich, K., S. Hayer, R. Ricci, *et al*. 2002. Osteoclasts are essential for TNF-alpha-mediated joint destruction. *J. Clin. Invest.* **110:** 1419–1427.

5. Schett, G., K. Redlich, S. Hayer, *et al*. 2003. Osteoprotegerin protects against generalized bone loss in tumor necrosis factor-transgenic mice. *Arthritis Rheum.* **48:** 2042–2051.

6. Zwerina, J., S. Hayer, M. Tohidast-Akrad, *et al*. 2004. Single and combined inhibition of tumor necrosis factor, interleukin-1, and RANKL pathways in tumor necrosis factor-induced arthritis: Effects on synovial inflammation, bone erosion, and cartilage destruction. *Arthritis Rheum.* **50:** 277–290.

7. Anandarajah, A.P. 2006. Anti-RANKL therapy for inflammatory bone disorder: Mechanism and potential clinical applications. *J. Cell. Biochem.* **97:** 226–232.

8. Takayanagi, H., S. Kim, K. Matsuo, *et al*. 2002. RANKL maintains bone homeostasis through c-Fos-dependent induction of interferon-beta. *Nature* **416:** 744–749.

9. Wyzga, N., S. Varghese, S. Wikel, *et al*. 2004. Effects of activated T cells on osteoclastogenesis depend on how they are activated. *Bone* **35:** 614–620.

10. Ritchlin, C.T., S.A. Haas-Smith, P. Li, *et al*. 2003. Mechanisms of TNF-alpha- and RANKL-mediated osteoclastogenesis and bone resorption in psoriatic arthritis. *J. Clin. Invest.* **111:** 821–831.

11. Kong, Y.Y., U. Feige, I. Sarosi, *et al*. 1999. Activated T cells regulate bone loss and joint destruction in adjuvant arthritis through osteoprotegerin ligand. *Nature* **402:** 304–309.

12. Sato, K. & H. Takayanagi. 2006. Osteoclasts, rheumatoid arthritis, and osteoimmunology. *Curr. Opin. Rheumatol.* **18:** 419–426.

13. Kasono, K., K. Sato, Y. Sato, *et al*. 1993. Inhibitory effect of interleukin-4 on osteoclast-like cell formation in mouse bone marrow culture. *Bone Miner.* **21:** 179–188.

14. Abu-Amer, Y. 2001. IL-4 abrogates osteoclastogenesis through STAT6-dependent inhibition of NF-κB. *J. Clin. Invest.* **107:** 1375–1385.

15. Hong, M.H., H. Williams, C.H. Jin, *et al*. 2000. The inhibitory effect of interleukin-10 on mouse osteoclast formation involves novel tyrosine-phosphorylated proteins. *J. Bone Miner. Res.* **15:** 911–918.

16. Takahashi, N., G.R. Mundy & G.D. Roodman. 1986. Recombinant human interferon-γ inhibits formation of human osteoclast-like cells. *J. Immunol.* **137:** 3544–3549.

17. Nanes, M.S. 2003. Tumor necrosis factor-α: Molecular and cellular mechanisms in skeletal pathology. *Gene* **321:** 1–15.

18. Catrina, A.I., C. Trollmo, E. af Klint, *et al*. 2005. Evidence that anti-tumor necrosis factor therapy with both etanercept and infliximab induces apoptosis in macrophages, but not lymphocytes, in rheumatoid arthritis joints: Extended report. *Arthritis Rheum.* **52:** 61–72.

19. Klarlund, M., M. Østergaard & K.E. Jensen. 2000. Magnetic resonance imaging, radiography, and scintigraphy of the finger joints. *Ann. Rheum. Dis.* **59:** 521–528.

20. Scheel, A.K. & K.G. Hermann. 2006. Prospective 7 year follow up imaging study comparing radiography, ultrasonography, and magnetic resonance imaging in rheumatoid arthritis finger joints. *Ann. Rheum. Dis.* **65:** 595–600.

21. Ashikyan, O. 2007. The role of magnetic resonance imaging in the early diagnosis of rheumatoid arthritis. *Top. Magn. Reson. Imaging* **18:** 169–176.

22. Østergaard, M. & C. Peterfy. 2003. OMERACT rheumatoid arthritis magnetic in resonance imaging studies. *J. Rheumatol.* **30:** 1385–1386.

23. Tehranzadeh, J., O. Ashikyan, J. Dascalos & C. Dennehey. 2004. MRI of large intraosseous lesions in patients with inflammatory arthritis. *AJR Am. J. Roentgenol.* **183:** 1453–1456.

24. McQueen, F.M. & N. Benton. 2001. What is the fate of erosions in early rheumatoid arthritis? *Ann. Rheum. Dis.* **60:** 859–868.

25. Oliver, C. & S. Speake. 1996. Advantages of an increased dose of MRI contrast agent for enhancing inflammatory synovium. *Clin. Radiol.* **51:** 487–493.

26. Konig, H., J. Sieper & K.J. Wolf. 1990. Rheumatoid arthritis: Evaluation of hypervascular and fibrous pannus with dynamic MR imaging enhanced with Gd-DTPA. *Radiology* **176:** 473–477.

27. Cimmino, M.A., S. Innocenti, F. Livrone, *et al*. 2003. Dynamic gadolinium-enhanced magnetic resonance imaging of the wrist in patients with rheumatoid arthritis can discriminate active from inactive disease. *Arthritis Rheum.* **48:** 1207–1213.

28. Yamato, M., K. Tamai, T. Yamaguchi, *et al*. 1993. MRI of the knee in rheumatoid arthritis: Gd-DTPA perfusion dynamics. *J. Comput. Assist. Tomogr.* **17:** 781–785.

29. Sugimoto, H., A. Takeda & K. Hyodoh. 2001. MR imaging for evaluation of early rheumatoid arthritis. *Sem. Musculoskeletal Radiol.* **5:** 159–165.

30. Zikou, A.K., M.I. Argyropoulou, P.V. Voulgari, *et al*. 2006. Magnetic resonance imaging quantification of hand synovitis in patients with rheumatoid arthritis treated with adalimumab. *J. Rheumatol.* **33:** 219–223.

31. Argyropoulou, M.I., A. Glatzouni, P.V. Voulgari, *et al*. 2005. Magnetic resonance imaging quantification of hand synovitis in patients with rheumatoid arthritis treated with infliximab. *Joint Bone Spine* **72:** 557–561.

32. Benton, N., N. Stewart, J. Crabbe, *et al*. 2004. MRI of the wrist in early rheumatoid arthritis can be used to predict functional outcome at 6 years. *Ann. Rheum. Dis.* **63:** 555–561.

33. McQueen, F., M. Lassere & M. Østergaard. 2006. Magnetic resonance imaging in psoriatic arthritis: A review of the literature. *Arthritis Res. Ther.* **8:** 207.

34. Ritchlin, C.T., S.A. Haas-Smith, P. Li, D.G. Hicks & E.M. Schwartz. 2003. Mechanisms of TNFα and RANKL-mediated osteoclastogenesis and bone resorption in psoriatic arthritis. *J. Clin. Invest.* **111:** 821–831.

35. Savnik, A., H. Malmskov & H.S. Thomsen. 2002. MRI of the wrist and finger joints in inflammatory joint diseases at 1-year interval: MR features to predict bone erosions. *Eur. Radiol.* **12:** 1203–1210.

36. Backhaus, M., T. Kamradt & D. Sandrock. 1999. Arthritis of the finger joints. A comprehensive approach comparing conventional radiography, scintigraphy, ultrasound and contrast-enhanced MRI. *Arthritis Rheum.* **42:** 1232–1234.

37. Bollow, M., T. Fischer, H. Reißhauer & M. Backhaus. 2000. Quantitative analyses of sacroiliac biopsies in spondyloarthropathies: T cells and macrophages predominate in early and active sacroiliitis–cellularity correlates with the degree of enhancement detected by magnetic resonance imaging. *Ann. Rheum. Dis.* **59:** 135–140.

38. Savnik, A., H. Malmskov & H.S. Thomsen. 2001. Magnetic resonance imaging of the wrist and finger joints in patients with inflammatory joint diseases. *J. Rheumatol.* **28:** 2193–2200.

39. McQueen, F.M., N. Benton, D. Perry & J. Crabbe. 2003. Bone oedema scored on magnetic resonance scans of the dominant carpus at presentation predicts radiographic joint damage at the hands and feet six years later in patients with rheumatoid arthritis. *Arthritis Rheum.* **48:** 1814–1827.

40. Giovagnoni, A., W. Grassi & F. Terilli. 1995. MRI of the hand in psoriatic and rheumatical arthritis. *Eur. Radiol.* **5:** 590–595.

41. Offidani, A., A. Cellini, G. Valeri & A. Giovagnoni. 1998. Subclinical joint involvement in psoriasis: Magnetic resonance imaging and X-ray findings. *Acta Derm. Venereol.* **78:** 463–465.

42. McQueen, F., M. Østergaard, C. Peterfy, *et al*. 2005. Pitfalls in scoring MR images of rheumatoid arthritis wrist and metacarpophalangeal joints. *Ann. Rheum. Dis.* **64**(Suppl. 1): i48–i55.

43. Parodi, M., E. Silvestri, G. Garlaschi, *et al*. 2006. How normal are the hands of normal controls? A study with dedicated magnetic resonance imaging. *Clin. Exp. Rheumatol.* **24:** 134–141.

44. Timins, M.E., S.E. O'Connell, S.J. Erickson, *et al*. 1996. MR imaging of the wrist: Normal findings that may simulate disease. *Radiographics* **16:** 987–995.

45. Goldring, S.R. & E.M. Gravallese. 2004. Bisphosphonates: Environmental protection for the joint? *Arthritis Rheum.* **50:** 2044—2047.

46. Tam, L.-S., J.F. Griffith, A.B. Yu, *et al*. 2007. Rapid improvement in rheumatoid arthritis patients on combination of methotrexate and infliximab: Clinical and magnetic resonance imaging evaluation. *Clin. Rheumatol.* **26:** 941–946.

MRI in Juvenile Idiopathic Arthritis and Juvenile Dermatomyositis

Janet Mary McCrae Gardner-Medwin,[a] Greg Irwin,[b] and Karl Johnson[c]

[a] *Senior Lecturer in Paediatric Rheumatology, University of Glasgow, Royal Hospital for Sick Children, Glasgow, Scotland, UK*

[b] *Consultant Paediatric Radiologist, Department of Radiology, Royal Hospital for Sick Children, Glasgow, Scotland, UK*

[c] *Consultant Paediatric Radiologist, Department of Paediatric Radiology, Birmingham Children's Hospital, Birmingham, UK*

The use of MRI in the assessment of the musculoskeletal system in children has important differences from its use in adults. Growth in children has significant impact on the epiphysis and growth plate, which are important structures in the growing child, and there are radiological features that differ from those in adults: disease may alter structures during a period of growth; the pathologies themselves are a distinct group of diseases at variance with adult arthritis and myositis, with a different spectrum of differential diagnoses; and many technical issues are different when imaging a child. These are important considerations in choosing the appropriate imaging. MRI is a powerful and valuable imaging technique in pediatric musculoskeletal pathologies, with considerable potential for future developments to enhance its role in diagnosis, management, and therapeutic intervention for these children.

Key words: joints; arthritis; inflammation; juvenile idiopathic arthritis (JIA); juvenile dermatomyositis (JDM); children; magnetic resonance imaging; muscle

Introduction

Advances and improvements in musculoskeletal imaging have dramatically improved the service that radiologists can now offer the pediatric rheumatologist. Such imaging assists in the initial diagnosis of juvenile idiopathic arthritis to detect any disease complications at an early stage and helps facilitate optimum management. It also has a growing role in the diagnosis and management of inflammatory muscle disease, particularly juvenile dermatomyositis. Consideration has to be given to the child's age and stage of development, the symptoms under investigation, and the clinical question being considered.

Nomenclature and Classification

Juvenile Idiopathic Arthritis

Juvenile idiopathic arthritis (JIA), which affects an estimated 1 in 1000 children,[1] is a heterogeneous group of arthropathies unified by their onset in childhood. The classification of JIA was significantly revised by the Classification Task Force in Childhood Rheumatic Disease of the International League for Rheumatology (ILAR) meeting in Durban in 1997,[2] and was updated in Edmonton in 2004,[3] with the aim of advancing knowledge toward etiological and pathogenic homogeneity.[4] The classification was also designed to unite the criteria

Address for correspondence: Janet Gardner-Medwin, Senior Lecturer in Paediatric, Rheumatology, Department of Child Health, University of Glasgow, Royal Hospital for Sick Children, Yorkhill, Glasgow G38SJ, U.K. jgm4w@clinmed.gla.ac.uk

MRI and Ultrasound in Diagnosis and Management: Ann. N.Y. Acad. Sci. 1154: 52–83 (2009).
doi: 10.1111/j.1749-6632.2009.04498.x © 2009 New York Academy of Sciences.

of the American College of Rheumatology for juvenile rheumatoid arthritis (JRA)[5] and European League of Associations for Rheumatology (EULAR) for juvenile chronic arthritis (JCA).[6] It is important to note the term JRA does not include juvenile spondyloarthropathy and psoriatic arthropathy. Table 1 clarifies the difference between the classifications. Radiological differentiation among the subgroups has not yet been established, in contrast to significant work in the adult field, which suggests that exploration of this area in JIA would be fruitful.

Juvenile Dermatomyositis

Juvenile dermatomyositis (JDM) is an uncommon disorder of childhood with heterogeneous clinical features, so a diagnosis may be significantly delayed. It is characterized by a painful proximal myopathy, typically of the pelvic and shoulder girdles, but may affect a limited muscle group. The characteristic rash, with purple discoloration over the eyelids (heliotrope rash), and erythematous patchy skin on extensor surfaces (Gottron's papules) can be atypical. The range of severity contrasts between children with mild weakness responsive to short-term steroids and those significantly affected with respiratory failure and aggressive vasculitis when the prognosis is poor.

The classification criteria for JDM remain those of Bohan and Peter.[7] While the clinical features are still valid and indeed continue to be recognized as key features of dermatomyositis by clinicians,[8] the criteria are outdated. Electromyography (EMG) has now all but been replaced by MRI in clinical practice, and revision of these criteria to include MRI or ultrasound (US) are now required. Biopsy is no longer consistently performed in all centers. When the clinical picture, particularly the characteristic rash, and muscle MRI appearances are in keeping, these may be considered sufficient for a diagnosis. Clinicians with access to MRI rate it very highly, of equal value to muscle biopsy, in diagnostic value, replacing EMG and muscle biopsy.[8] With the MRI appearances of JDMs,

which are typically bilateral, and symmetrical muscle edema, in the presence of a characteristic rash, biopsy may not be needed.

Magnetic Resonance Imaging

Over the past decade the increasing use of MRI and the advances in more functional MRI techniques have improved the assessment of joint disease in JIA. These advances have allowed the radiologist to be more proactive in managing the disease. MRI is superior for detecting both inflammatory changes in the joint and damage to the cartilage than ultrasonography or plain radiography. It can accurately evaluate the later manifestations of JIA, including erosions, loss of joint space, cartilage damage, and ligamentous involvement.[9-12] Recent advances show that a quantitative assessment of synovial hypertrophy may be possible.[13] There are practical disadvantages of MRI, particularly in pediatric practice, but these can be largely overcome by the use of the technique in designated pediatric units. The availability of MRI varies worldwide. With pediatric MRI, it is important that suitable sedation or general anesthetic facilities are available to allow compliance in children of all ages. Each MRI examination may take between 30 and 60 min, which may cause some children distress. Appropriate distraction techniques and suitable rewards should be available.

Technical Aspects of Imaging

Patient Preparation

As with any aspect of pediatric imaging it is important that insofar as possible the child be fully informed as to the process. In the younger or uncooperative child, sedation or general anesthesia may be required. Often, in JIA, contrast enhancement is used, so either prior venous cannulation or the application of local anesthetic cream is useful.

Coil selection is important and the basic principle of having an increased signal-to-noise

Table 1. The New Classification of Juvenile Arthritis, Clinical Features, and Comparison to Old Classifications and Adult Disease (RF = rheumatoid factor)

Characteristic	JIA	Clinical features[3]	JRA (USA)[5]	JCA (Europe)[6]	Adult equivalent
Age at onset	<16 years		<16 years	<16 years	
Minimum duration of arthritis	6 weeks		6 weeks	3 months	
Subtypes	Systemic arthritis	Systemic manifestations often precede arthritis: Evening spikes of fever dipping to subnormal in the mornings; evanescent salmon-colored rash on the trunk, axillae, and inner thighs most marked at the height of the fever; lymphadenopathy, splenomegaly, serositis, and pallor. An aggressive polyarticular arthritis can develop associated with a worse prognosis.	Systemic onset JRA	Systemic onset JCA	Adult Still's disease
	Oligoarthritis Persistent	Arthritis in up to four joints. Continues to involve fewer than four joints throughout the disease course.	Pauciarticular JRA	Pauciarticular JCA	-
	Extended	Affects more than four joints after the first 6 months, and associated with a worse prognosis than persistent oligoarthritis.			
	Polyarthritis (RF-negative)	Affects five or more joints in first 6 months of disease. Test for RF is repeatedly negative.	Polyarticular JRA (RF does not alter classification)	Polyarticular JCA	-
	Polyarthritis (RF-positive)	Affects five or more joints in first 6 months of disease. Tests for RF are positive on two occasions at least 2 months apart.		Juvenile rheumatoid arthritis (JRA)	Rheumatoid arthritis
	Enthesitis-related arthritis	Boys older than 6 years of age, HLA B27 positive, or family history of HLA B27 associated disease. Asymmetrical large-joint arthritis of the lower limbs, enthesitis in the feet, knees, and pelvic girdle. Lumbosacral spine and sacroiliac involvement rare in childhood, but may develop ankylosing spondylitis as older teenagers/adults.	Excluded	Juvenile spondyloarthropathies (including juvenile ankylosing spondylitis, juvenile psoriatic arthritis, Reiter's syndrome, and arthropathies of inflammatory bowel disease.)	Ankylosing spondylitis

Continued

Table 1. *Continued*

Characteristic	JIA	Clinical features[3]	JRA (USA)[5]	JCA (Europe)[6]	Adult equivalent
Psoriatic arthritis		Arthritis and psoriasis may occur together. In the absence of psoriasis a family history, or nail features of psoriasis such as nail pitting may be found. The asymmetrical arthritis typical involves large and small joints or a dactylitis).	Excluded		Psoriatic arthritis
Other		Arthritis that either does not fulfill criteria for any category or fulfills criteria for more than one category. It is hoped new disease groups will emerge from this category.	–	–	–

ratio and a small field of view should be adhered to.[14] An improved signal-to-noise ratio can be achieved by the use of phased-array or send–receive coils. Manufacturers now produce a wide variety of coils for numerous anatomical areas, including the temporomandibular and the shoulder and knee joints, and these should be used whenever possible. In the young small child wrap-around coils are often useful.[12]

Choice of Sequences

The choice of imaging sequences and whether standard spin-echo or fast spin-echo techniques are used is very much dependent on the radiologist's own preference and experience, as well as the routine practice in the particular institution. Although it is not appropriate to dictate the sequences to be used, it is important that the radiologist be aware of the pathological processes and clinical issues that have to be adequately imaged in JIA.[14,15]

MRI Features in Juvenile Idiopathic Arthritis

MRI is a powerful tool for imaging the structures in and around the synovial joint.

Imaging Synovium

Inflamed synovium may occur in any inflammatory process that affects the joint. The presence of inflamed synovium is a nonspecific feature and the diagnosis of JIA should be related to the clinical features of the disease. Other causes of inflamed synovium include joint hemorrhage, periarticular tumors, ischemic damage to the epiphysis (including Perthes disease[11]), and trauma.

Within the normal joint there is a thin rim of synovial tissue lining the articular surfaces. This normal synovium produces a small amount of fluid to lubricate the joint and also provides nutrients to the underlying relatively hypovascular cartilage. Normal physiological synovium is of low signal intensity on both T1-weighted and T2-weighted images and is seen as a thin smooth rim over the cartilage, no more than

2 mm thick, with no focal areas of irregularity or nodularity. A normal synovium will show some enhancement following gadolinium administration.[16–18]

The abnormal inflamed synovium seen in JIA is, in contrast, thickened and irregular and may have a wavy outline. It is low-to-intermediate signal intensity on T1-w images and high signal intensity on T2-w sequences. The signal intensity of inflamed synovium may be similar to that of any associated joint effusion on both T1-w and T2-w standard spin-echo sequences. The use of fast spin-echo and very heavily T2-w sequences improves the discrimination between joint fluid and synovium.[10,11,18–20] Both remain high signal but there is more contrast between them. The optimum method for differentiating inflamed synovium from joint effusion is by the use of gadolinium-enhanced T1-w sequences. The use of fat saturation reduces the signal from the adjacent fatty marrow and highlights the contrast enhancement.

Alternatively, the use of pre- and postcontrast medium administration subtraction techniques improves synovium detection (Figs. 1, 2, and 3).[9,11] Inflamed synovium shows rapid enhancement after an IV injection of gadolinium and it is this rapid enhancement that helps differentiate active hypervascular synovium from fibrous inactive synovium. Fibrous synovium enhances either heterogeneously or poorly.[10] There are some reports that indicate that the rate of uptake by synovium could be of use in assessing the degree of inflammatory response within a joint.[20,21] When performing postgadolinium administration sequences it is important that the sequences be performed within minutes of the injection of contrast medium, as synovial tissue has no tight junction or basement membrane and gadolinium compounds diffuse into the joint space and gradually increase the signal intensity of the adjacent fluid.[22] This is not usually a problem when imaging a single joint, but may cause difficulties if more than two joints are to be imaged during the same appointment. If more than one joint

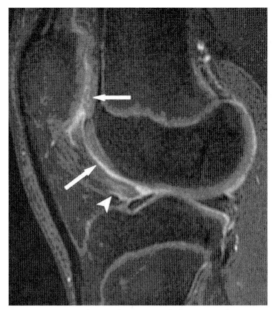

Figure 1. Sagittal, postgadolinium administration, T1-w fat-saturated image of the knee of a child with JIA. The high signal intensity around the infrapatellar fat pad (arrow) and the small area around the distal femur (arrow) indicate enhancing synovium. The synovium has a slightly irregular outline and is marginally thickened, particularly around the menisci. There is some slight irregularity of the infrapatellar fat pad (arrowhead). These appearances are borderline abnormal. This patient went on to develop more severe changes with a clinically significant joint effusion and elevated blood inflammatory markers within 3 months of the MRI examination.

is being imaged the postgadolinium administration sequences on all the joints should be done consecutively. In children a standard dose of 0.1 mmol/kg of gadolinium is sufficient; it has been shown that higher doses provide only limited additional benefit in determining the degree of synovial inflammation.[23]

In a number of studies, predominantly in adults, contrast-enhanced T1-w sequences have been used to evaluate the severity of the inflammatory arthritis,[20] and this technique is now being used in children.[13] These studies have quantified the number of joints involved, measured synovial volume, and also looked at the rate of uptake of gadolinium within the synovium.[21,24,25] In current clinical practice the presence or absence of inflamed synovium is

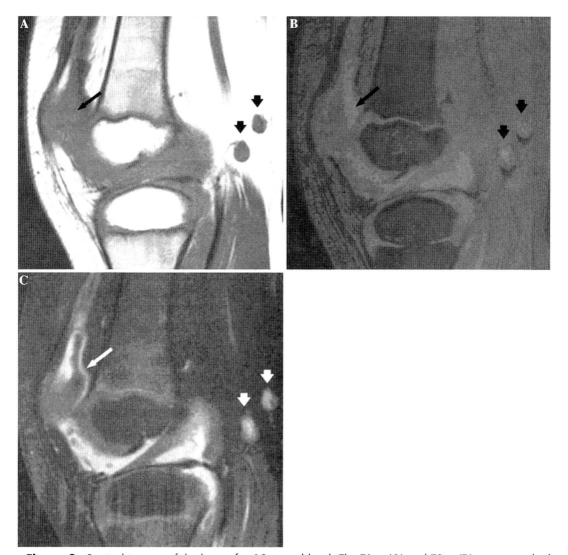

Figure 2. Sagittal images of the knee of a 13-year-old girl. The T1-w (**A**) and T2-w (**B**) sequences both demonstrate a joint effusion (arrow) and lymph nodes (arrowheads). On both sequences it is difficult to differentiate effusion from synovial hypertrophy. The gadolinium-enhanced T1-w sequence (**C**) shows marked enhancement of synovium (arrow) within the knee joint. Differentiation of fluid and synovium is much easier. The lymph nodes also enhance (arrowheads).

often all that is required by the rheumatologists, but this may change with further advancements in drug therapy. If a better measurement of disease activity is required, then synovial volumes can be determined, but this is not typically part of routine practice, as it is particularly time consuming in both sequence selection and postprocessing. The use of dynamic contrast-enhanced measurements is still not generally standard practice.[21] If these new

techniques are to be utilized in routine clinical practice proper reliability testing has to be done to assess their validity.

Imaging Cartilage

In simple terms there are three types of cartilage in a child's skeleton: growth, epiphyseal, and articular. The amount of growth cartilage present obviously depends upon the age of the child. The epiphysis of the young infant is

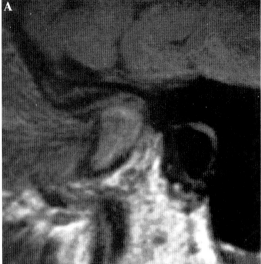

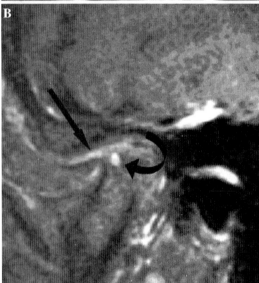

Figure 3. T1-w images of the temporomandibular joint (**A**) before and (**B**) after gadolinium administration. The contrast-enhanced image has been fat saturated to show enhancement of the temporomandibular joint anteriorly (arrow) and a small enhancing nodule within the ramus of the mandible (curved arrow).

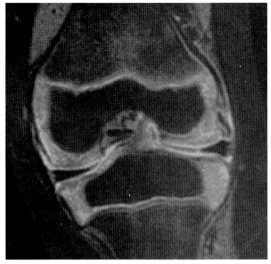

Figure 4. Coronal, proton-density fast-spin echo image of the knee of a 4-year-old boy. At the distal end of the femur the central ossified epiphysis is of low signal intensity, similar to that of the proximal femur. This epiphysis is surrounded by high-to-intermediate signal density growth cartilage. Along the joint margins the articular cartilage is of slightly high signal intensity, as is the physis.

typically composed entirely of cartilage. Discrimination between epiphyseal and articular cartilage is important and is best achieved with T2-w and proton-density-weighted sequences, particularly fast spin-echo sequences.[26] On T2-w images, physeal cartilage is of very high signal intensity, whereas the epiphyseal cartilage is of high, but slightly lower intensity. The use of fat-saturated techniques reduces the marrow signal from adjacent bone and may improve the imaging of the cartilage (Fig. 4).[9,10,26,27] On T1-w, all types of hyaline cartilage are of intermediate signal intensity. With water-sensitive sequences [STIR (short tau inversion recovery) and T2-w], epiphyseal cartilage is of relatively low signal intensity and this can distinguish it from the growth plate (physis), which is of relatively high signal. With intermediate weighted sequences (proton density), the cartilage is of relatively increased signal intensity, but with less contrast between epiphyseal and physeal.

With gradient recalled echo imaging (GRE), all forms of hyaline cartilage are of relatively high and uniform signal intensity. The use of volume acquisitions allows multiplanar reformatting and better evaluation of cartilage damage and detection of erosions. The use of fat-saturated techniques reduces marrow signal and improves the imaging of cartilage.[28]

The use of T1-w spoiled gradient-echo volume acquisition sequences [spoiled gradient-recalled acquisition at steady state (SPGR) or fast low-angle shot (FLASH); depending on the machine manufacturer] allows images to be analyzed using multiplanar reformatting with very thin slices. There is good resolution of cartilage, which is of high signal, with any defects appearing as low signal change. These sequences enable the detection of subtle cystic irregularities and focal defects with relatively high sensitivity.[26–29]

Cartilage Volume

Volume acquisition also potentially allows volume and surface area measurements of the cartilage, which may be of value in assessing long-term therapeutic response. Although these sequences are very useful, they may involve a considerably longer imaging time, which can cause problems, particularly when scanning the younger child, who may not be very compliant. The use of parallel imaging techniques and improved MRI technology has reduced scan times and these volume sequences are being used more routinely in clinical practice.

There is currently ongoing work that is looking at the T2 relaxation times of cartilage. These specialized T2-mapping sequences allow an assessment of the biochemical and biophysical changes in the extracellular cartilage and provide information about very early degenerative damage prior to any erosive damage being seen by more conventional imaging.[30,31]

Marrow Edema

Marrow edema and soft-tissue edema are best appreciated on STIR images; however, T2-w fat-saturated images also provide relatively good contrast. Contrast-enhanced, T1-w fat-saturated sequences detect areas of inflammation within joints.[10]

Applications of Magnetic Resonance Imaging

There are no clearly defined imaging protocols for JIA. The choice of imaging modality and its timing are very much patient-dependent and are a function of the clinical problem and the resources available.

In simple terms, children fall into two broad categories: (1) those who present with a relatively acute swollen joint (or joints) and in whom no firm diagnosis has been made, and (2) those in whom the diagnosis of JIA is established, but there has been an alteration of clinical symptoms or there are questions about the effects of current treatment.

Diagnosis and Differential Diagnoses

For the previously well child who presents with an acute joint problem and has been fully assessed by an experienced pediatric rheumatologist, often only a radiograph of the involved joint is necessary. This radiograph is important in excluding other causes of joint swelling, such as trauma, osteoid tumors, and dysplasias. It is important to note that a radiograph is not helpful in positively making a diagnosis of JIA early in the disease, as radiographic features such as soft tissue swelling are nonspecific and are identifiable clinically, whereas other radiographic features such as joint space narrowing and erosions only appear well after onset of the disease. In some cases, if the rheumatologist is confident of the diagnosis of JIA, there may be no request for imaging at all. If confirmation of the presence of an effusion is needed, then both US and MRI have been shown to be more sensitive in their detection than clinical examination[10,16,32,33] and plain radiographs.

Clinical features that might indicate resorting to early MRI are: (1) monoarthritis that behaves atypically, with intermittent swelling sometimes related to trauma; (2) persistent swelling resistant to therapeutic intervention, where the differential diagnoses of other intra-articular pathology such as

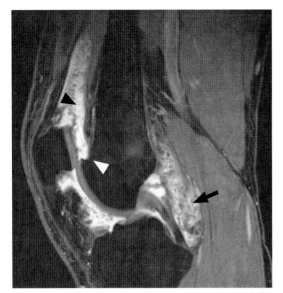

Figure 5. Sagittal T1 fat-saturated MRI of the knee postcontrast shows features of lipoma arborescens in a 17-year-old boy. There is villous lipomatous proliferation of enhancing synovium (black arrows), and an erosion at the articular margin (white arrowhead).

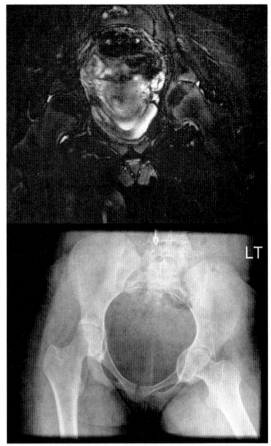

Figure 6. Idiopathic chondrolysis of the hip: MRI and radiographic features.

hemangioma, pigmented villonodular synovitis (PVNS), or lipoma arborescens (Fig. 5) are possibilities; (3) an atypical history such as atypical pain (night pain or prompt response to anti-inflammatories)[34]; or (4) history that is suggestive of JIA and clinical examination is unable to identify synovitis, often in the absence of other features such as raised acute phase response and MRI can confirm or refute this. Imaging can be helpful in common benign pediatric presentations such as synovial (Baker's) cysts when there are atypical features (Fig. 7).[35]

Idiopathic chondrolysis of the hip may present with pain and restricted range of hip movement and mimic synovitis of the hip (Fig. 6). MRI can clearly identify the loss of cartilage in the absence of inflammation or infection typical of this condition early in the disease and is of value monitoring the disease progression.[36,12] In very early cases of idiopathic chondrolysis, abnormal high and low signals, respectively, on T2-w and T1-w sequences may be seen as an unusual rectangular configuration in the femoral epiphysis and acetabulum, which along with some synovial hypertrophy may be the earliest MRI-observed features of the disease.[37]

Owing to its sensitivity to bone and soft tissue edema and abscesses, MRI can be helpful in the diagnosis of intra-articular infection, such as early tuberculosis[38] or other osteoarticular infections.[39] Isolated hip involvement is an unusual presentation of JIA, with the exception of enthesitis-related arthritis, so imaging of the hip to exclude the differential diagnoses is important. The hip is a difficult joint to assess clinically, and its evaluation by US or MRI is valuable in guiding therapy and identifying the extent of disease involvement[40]; the latter is often underassessed or missed clinically, particularly in patients of long standing or those with prior significant hip damage, with

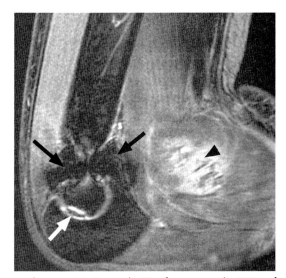

Figure 7. Sagittal T1 fat-saturated MRI of the elbow postcontrast in a 16-year-old boy with hemophilic arthropathy. There is extensive hemosiderin deposition, shown here as dark areas around the distal humerus (black arrows). There is fragmentation of the articular surface (white arrow), and a hemophilic pseudotumor in the flexor muscles of the forearm (black arrowhead).

important implications for outcome.[41] Arthritis of the temporomandibular joint (TMJ), a common feature of JIA, is also notoriously difficult to assess clinically and has a poor outcome.[42] MRI is also valuable in confirming or refuting the presence of active synovitis,[42–44] but imaging the TMJ requires a specific magnetic resonance coil not readily available in all centers.

Juxta-articular pathology can result in a small effusion mistaken for JIA, so awareness of osteomyelitis, including chronic recurrent multifocal osteomyelitis,[39,45] marrow infiltration in acute lymphoblastic leukemia, or neuroblastoma are important considerations. Although not the investigative technique of choice, MRI can identify marrow infiltration or contribute to the differentiation of tumor and infection.

In children newly diagnosed as suffering from an oligoarthritis JIA, there are preliminary studies that suggest that MRI of clinically asymptomatic joints will detect early synovitis. Follow-up on these cases appears to indicate that children who had positive findings on their MRIs are at increased risk of disease extension and conversely a negative MRI examination at presentation appears to foretell a good prognosis. This work suggests that MRI will play an increasing role in the evaluation of patients with newly diagnosed JIA and those in whom there are equivocal clinical findings.[36]

Alternatively, the request for imaging an acutely swollen joint in a previously well child may be from a clinician who is less experienced in dealing with childhood arthropathies. In this circumstance, radiology has to confirm any joint pathology and provide a differential diagnosis. Again, radiographs are important in excluding bony lesions as a cause of the swelling, but have limited value in confirming the diagnosis of JIA. Sonography and MRI are more sensitive than clinical examination in detecting synovial hypertrophy and joint effusions.[10,11]

In the acute case, the knee has been the joint most frequently studied with MRI, a consequence of it being one of the most commonly affected joints in JIA and being relatively easy to image.[9,11,46] The early MRI-observed features of JIA in the knee joint are irregularity of the infrapatellar fat pad, lymphadenopathy, and joint effusion. If these features are present within the knee, then it is important that gadolinium chelate be administered to confirm the presence and then fully delineate the degree of synovial hypertrophy. If contrast-enhanced sequences are not obtained, then the presence of synovial hypertrophy may not be fully appreciated and the diagnosis of JIA delayed. The radiologist has an important role in suggesting the diagnosis of JIA, as the clinician may not be fully aware of that possibility.

Regardless of the type of referral, in patients in whom there is an acutely swollen joint, the diagnosis of sepsis must always be excluded, and if sepsis is suspected prompt joint aspiration and/or lavage is mandatory. Infection within a joint can be severely destructive, but early appropriate treatment is curative. Care must be taken in excluding sepsis in the child who has received antibiotics for whatever reason, as the diagnostic features may be minimized. Specific

Table 2. Bohan and Peter Diagnostic Criteria for JDM[7]

A diagnosis of JDM requires:
The presence of the typical rash AND three of the following:
- Elevated serum levels of muscle-derived enzymes
- Electromyographic evidence of inflammatory myopathy
- Positive muscle biopsy
- Proximal muscle weakness

Table 3. The Differential Diagnosis of Arthritis in Children

Inflammatory
Juvenile idiopathic arthritis.
Inflammatory disease: inflammatory bowel disease, sarcoid, cystic fibrosis, autoimmune hepatitis.
Hematological malignancies: leukemia, lymphoma.
Malignancy: neuroblastoma.
Reactive: poststreptococcal, rheumatic fever, postenteric, postviral.
Infection: septic arthritis,[39] osteomyelitis,[39] discitis, tuberculosis,[38] lyme arthritis.
Irritable hip.
Systemic disease: systemic lupus erythematosus, vasculitis (Kawasaki disease, Henoch–Schönlein purpura, rarer systemic vasculitides), juvenile dermatomyositis, scleroderma.
Down's arthritis.

Mechanical
Synovial cysts (Baker's cysts).[35]
Osgood–Schlatter's disease, and other eponymous osteochondritides.
Chondromalacia patellae.
Scheuermann's disease.
Hypermobility, pes planus.
Growing pains (nocturnal idiopathic pain syndrome).
Inherited: skeletal dysplasias, congenital dislocation of the hip.
Collagen disorders: e.g., Ehlers–Danlos, Marfan's, Stickler's syndrome.
Storage disorders, e.g., mucopolysaccharidoses /lipidoses.
Avascular necrosis and other degenerative disorders: Perthes, slipped upper femoral epiphysis, idiopathic chondrolysis,[50] spondylolysis and listhesis.
Trauma: accidental and nonaccidental injury.
Hematological: hemophilia and hemoglobinopathy (sickle predominantly).
Metabolic: rickets, hypophosphatemic rickets, hypo/hyperthyroidism, diabetes, purine metabolism.
Tumors of cartilage bone or muscle: Benign: osteoid osteoma,[34] pigmented villonodular synovitis,[51] hemangioma, lipoma arborescens,[52] Malignant: synovial sarcoma, osteosarcoma, rhabdomyosarcoma.

Psychological
Idiopathic pain syndromes:
Local: e.g., reflex sympathetic dystrophy
Generalized, e.g., fibromyalgia.

differential diagnostic considerations that must be keep in mind include osteomyelitis, chronic recurrent multifocal osteomyelitis, and features of tuberculosis.[38,39,45]

In the hand the differential diagnoses in children may be wide, and MRI is a valuable scanning modality for ruling in a diagnosis, as well as for the exclusion of neoplasia, congenital malformation, infection, other inflammatory process, or trauma.[47] MRI is useful in delineating and assessing disease activity in the hands, including identifying clinically and radiographically silent lesions, soft tissue features, loss of cartilage, and erosions. Gadolinium contrast can identify areas with and without synovial enhancement. There has been some exploration of quantitative use of this technique in children with JIA.[48] The delineation of the extent of extra-articular involvement can aid a more specific diagnosis (e.g., psoriatic arthritis).[49]

Table 3 outlines the breadth of the differential diagnoses to be considered and includes specific comments on a number of differential diagnoses where MRI can be helpful.[29]

Marrow Infiltrative Diseases

In all children presenting with an oligo- or a polyarthritis it is important to consider malignancy.[53] Neuroblastoma and acute lymphoblastic leukemia (ALL) both present with effusions that mimic JIA, usually with tenderness that is typically not over the joint line as in JIA, but rather over the metaphyses, reflecting marrow infiltration. If the child is still compensating, the blood count may fail to reflect the marrow infiltration when peripheral cell counts remain within the normal ranges. Circulating leukemic blasts identified on the blood film are less common in children with a musculoskeletal presentation, and MRI of the "abnormal"

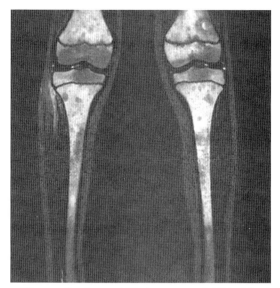

Figure 8. Coronal T2 fat-saturated MRI of both knees and upper tibias shows widespread abnormal bright signal secondary to leukemic infiltration in a 10-year-old girl.

marrow signal can be critical in making an early diagnosis (Fig. 8).

Infection

Septic arthritis is a critical differential diagnosis and should be excluded in any single inflamed joint in both established JIA, particularly in the immunosuppressed patient, or in a new presentation. In cases associated with the most common organisms (*Staphylococcus, Streptococcus,* and *Haemophilus*), the child may be systemically unwell and febrile, with a painful joint giving a pseudoparalysis guiding the diagnosis, but a more indolent presentation should always be considered and infection excluded by joint aspiration. More likely to be mistaken for JIA is the more indolent presentation of tuberculosis or osteomyelitis when there is a sympathetic effusion in the adjacent joint. Where multiple sites of osteomyelitis are identified, chronic recurrent multifocal osteomyelitis (CRMO) and the syndrome of synovitis, acne, pustulosis, hyperostosis, and osteitis (SAPHO) should be considered. Discitis is a diagnosis often overlooked clinically, particularly in the younger child, and should be considered in the child with a limp

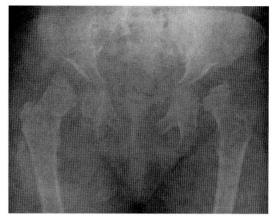

Figure 9. Mucopolysaccharidoses.

or back pain, especially one with a clear history of a preceding infective intercurrent illness.[54] Imaging of muscle may bring to light a pyomyositis[55] rather than inflammatory muscle disease.

Often the wrong diagnostic label of JIA is attributed to children with apparently widespread arthritis. Increasing the clinical awareness of confounding conditions is therefore important. Although not the diagnostic test of choice MRI may be performed and can highlight these misdiagnoses. Mucopolysaccharidosis or lipidosis are typical, with examples of imaging features given below (Fig. 9).

Back Pain

Low-back pain[52] is a common adolescent presentation, and it has been shown that MRI can identify a significant proportion of abnormalities in young teenagers, whether symptomatic or not.[53] Isolated back pain from JIA, excluding enthesitis-related arthritis, is less common, and a number of differential diagnoses should also be considered clinically, with appropriate use of MRI.[52] MRI is a useful scanning modality for both sacroiliac and lumbar spine involvement in JIA, both of which are involved in enthesitis-related arthritis, including cases associated with inflammatory bowel disease. It identifies change in advance of radiographic observations, demonstrating bone marrow edema at the sacroiliac joints sooner, and thus facilitates earlier therapy.

Monitoring Disease Progression and Response to Therapeutic Interventions

In a child with a known diagnosis of long-standing JIA, separate imaging issues are encountered. The imaging approach should be patient-centered, so the radiologist and pediatric rheumatologist should have regular multidisciplinary meetings to discuss the imaging findings on each patient and plan further investigations as appropriate.

Routine radiographs of children's joints regardless of their symptoms at each clinic visit are not indicated, as these are poor predictors of how the underlying disease is being controlled and new features are relatively slow to develop.[9,54,55] Once the diagnosis of JIA is confirmed, radiographs are only indicated when there has been a change in the child's symptoms or alteration in their management. When there has been an acute change in symptoms, radiographs may demonstrate signs of a traumatic injury, intra-articular loose bodies, or joint subluxation.

If there are concerns about an acute inflammatory reaction in a joint with underlying chronic changes, both US and MRI can identify those joints with a significant effusion that may be amenable to aspiration or intra-articular steroid injection, with MRI being the more sensitive modality for detecting inflamed synovium.[9–11,28,31,56] However, there has to be some caution in attributing all the synovial hypertrophy that is seen in a chronically affected joint to the autoimmune process, as synovial hypertrophy can be caused by the underlying degenerative process. In some cases, correlation with biochemical and hematological markers of joint inflammation will be needed.

Guiding Therapeutic Interventions

Ultrasound and radiographic imaging have the primary roles in guiding needle placement for intra-articular joint injections. Computed tomography (CT) may have a role in specific joints such as the sacroiliac joints. MRI may have an increasing role in supporting joint replacement or reconstruction, providing detailed three-dimensional images of the joints, and may also have a role in TMJ reconstruction.[57]

Radiological Features

Soft Tissue Swelling and Joint Effusions

Periarticular soft tissue swelling is one of the most common early features of JIA and typically the diagnosis is made clinically. On radiographs the detection is easier in the small joints of the hand and feet, where it is usually seen as fusiform swelling around the digits. In enthesitis-related disease the soft tissue swelling can be eccentric and irregular.[54,55] Sonography and MRI are more sensitive in delineating the swelling and any associated effusions.[10] A complication in some cases of JIA is that the child may develop persisting lymphoedema, typically of the lower limb, with soft tissue swelling extending beyond the joint.[58]

Periostitis

Periosteal new bone formation is a relatively frequent manifestation of JIA, occurring in any long bone, but is most common in the periarticular region of phalanges, metacarpals, and metatarsals. Periostitis can occur at any time during the disease process and is believed to be a consequence of inflammation of the joint capsule and the adjacent tendon insertions. The relative ease with which the periosteum can be elevated and new bone formed in children is probably a factor in its increased incidence in JIA compared with adult rheumatoid disease. In some cases the changes within the digits can be marked, causing enlargement and squaring of the bone. Diffuse swelling of the fingers or toes with associated periosteal new bone

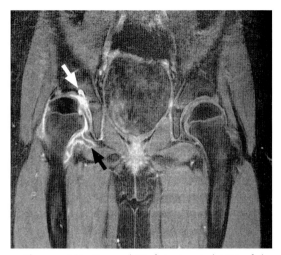

Figure 10. Coronal T1 fat-saturated MRI of the hips (postcontrast) in a 9-year-old girl with JIA. An erosion into the ileal component of the acetabulum is shown (white arrow). The black arrow indicates enhancing synovium around an effusion.

formation is a classic feature of psoriatic arthropathy, often with the bone changes preceding any dermatological features.[55,59-61]

Erosions

Erosions represent one of the endpoints of the disease process in JIA and indicate destruction of both bone and cartilage (Fig. 10). Erosions often occur at the insertion site of the intraosseous ligaments and at the sites of synovial reflection, as these areas have relatively less overlying protective cartilage, but they can occur at any point along the entire articular surface of the bone.[55,59-61]

Radiographs cannot detect any defect in either the articular or growth cartilage and so are relatively insensitive to early joint damage. They also tend to underestimate the total burden of erosive change within bone, as they are relatively insensitive to trabecular bone loss (as opposed to cortical loss), which is the largest part of the erosion. In the young child there is a generalized loss of joint space, reflecting cartilage loss, prior to bony changes, seen most commonly within the wrist joint, causing crowding of the carpal bones.[55,61] With US, erosions

are defined as a cortical defect or break that is greater than 2 mm in width with an irregular floor and acoustic enhancement within the adjacent marrow, seen in both the longitudinal and the transverse planes.[62] Sonography is superior to radiography in detecting cortical erosions in US-accessible areas, but is less reliable in detecting intramedullary lesions and those within the center of larger joints, where there is acoustic shadowing from overlying bone.[10,28,62]

MRI is the most sensitive detector of erosive changes, and it can clearly delineate between cartilage and bone defects.[9,10,28] Erosions are seen as well-circumscribed lesions that are hypointense on T1-w and hyperintense on T2-w images and they often show marked enhancement following gadolinium administration.[9-11,63]

MRI is able to demonstrate ill-defined areas of marrow edema and periarticular bone, which enhance with gadolinium administration. These abnormal areas appear prior to any radiographically observed abnormality and it is believed that they represent areas of osteitis, which are probable predictors of erosive damage. Hence MRI is able to detect inflammatory changes in the bone prior to the appearance of erosions, which may be useful in the development of disease-modifying therapies.[64,65] Postgadolinium administration sequences are the most sensitive way of quantifying the amount of erosive damage within a joint (Fig. 11).[9]

Growth Disturbances

In view of the immaturity of the pediatric skeleton, growth disturbances are a unique feature of JIA as compared to the adult inflammatory disorders. The cause of any growth disturbances is variable and may be localized or generalized. The effects of disease chronicity, prolonged steroid therapy, and immobilization result in generalized growth retardation. Any soft tissue and periarticular inflammation, epiphyseal destruction, or joint subluxation

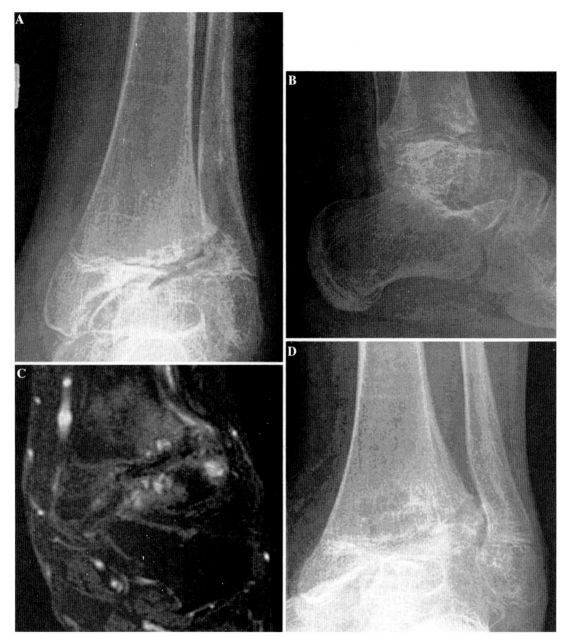

Figure 11. Serial images of a 14-year-old child with severe JIA: (A, B) Axial proton density (**A**) and lateral (**B**) radiographs of the ankle demonstrate erosive changes and sclerosis along the articular margins of the ankle joint. There is deformity of the ankle joint. (**C**) A coronal T1-w post-gadolinium administration fat-saturated image of the same ankle performed within 1 week of (**A**) and (**B**) shows marked enhancement in the bone and small enhanced cystic areas within the distal tibia. The corresponding areas appear normal on the initial radiographs (**D**).

that occurs can be associated with muscle spasms, which can create abnormal mechanical stresses on the bone that influence osseous development.[66]

Within the axial skeleton the localized inflammatory hyperemia around joints can initially cause accelerated growth, which causes epiphyseal enlargement and early bone maturation. Around the knee this epiphyseal enlargement causes widening of the intercondylar notch and squaring of the lower pole of the patella, which are classic radiographic signs of JIA, but which can also occur in hemophilia.[55,61] The initial growth acceleration that occurs in the early phase of the disease causes a relative increase in the length of the affected limb. Within the hands and feet there is earlier ossification of the growth centers of the carpal and tarsal bones, which results in a discrepancy between the child's estimated bone age and chronological age. In more long-standing disease, accelerated bone maturation promotes premature fusion of the epiphyseal physis, which ultimately leads to reduced growth and shorter limbs. If the physeal fusion is asymmetrical there will be a limb length discrepancy. The younger the child at the time of disease onset, the worse the degree of any deformity.[67]

In a significant number of children the mandible is affected by growth abnormalities. There is underdevelopment of the jaw (micrognathia) with limitation of bite, which can be a significant disability. Radiographic abnormalities include shortening of the body and ramus, flattening of the condyles, and widening of the intercondylar notch. Antegonial notching, which is a concave abnormality on the under surface of the body of the mandible, is a recognized but nonspecific radiographically observed feature of JIA. The notching is a consequence of mandibular hypoplasia and muscle imbalance acting in the region of the angle causing altered growth. The notching in JIA is typically short and close to the angle of the mandible (gonion), whereas in some congenital disorders, including Treacher–Collins syndrome, campomelic dwarfism, and neurofibromatosis, the concavity is more obtuse.[68–70] Any mandibular growth changes may or may not be associated with TMJ disease.[40] The use of dedicated TMJ coils has significantly improved the quality of MRI in this area and the use of open- and closed-mouth images helps detect any abnormal joint motion and intra-articular disc defects.

Joint Deformities

Joint subluxation, dislocation, and flexion/extension defects can occur in any joint, but are more commonly seen in the hands and feet. Any of the pathological changes seen in JIA, including erosions, ankylosis, large effusions, synovial proliferation, ligament disruption, and muscle imbalances can contribute to these deformities and, more importantly, cause loss of function. In more long-standing disease there can be new bone and osteophyte formation around the joint margins, which can cause pressure effects on adjacent structures and limit joint movement.[59–61,55]

A variety of finger abnormalities occur, which include Boutonniere deformity (flexion at the proximal interphalangeal joint and hyperextension at the distal interphalangeal joint), swan neck deformity (hyperextension at the proximal interphalangeal joint with flexion at the distal interphalangeal joint), and flexion deformity (flexion at both the proximal and distal interphalangeal joints). These changes are more common in the polyarticular subtype, particular the rheumatoid-positive group, and although they may be bilateral, they are frequently not symmetrical.[71] Similar changes are also seen in the feet.

In the wrist joint there is abnormal radial deviation, in contrast to early adult disease (though radial deviation may be a late feature of adult wrist rheumatoid arthritis). Subluxation and dislocation can also occur in the carpal bones, with the hamate being particularly affected. MRI demonstrates the degree of subluxation and identifies any localized mass of synovial tissue, which along with ligament laxity, is often responsible for causing this subluxation.[9,59,60]

Valgus or varus deformity can occur at the elbow or knee joint as a consequence of either asymmetrical epiphyseal overgrowth or significant erosive changes. Owing to this malalignment, abnormal mechanical stresses are placed on all the joints in the involved limb, which compounds any deformity. Enlargement of the femoral and humeral heads, together with loss

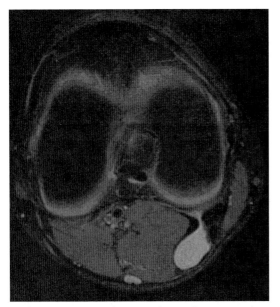

Figure 12. Axial proton density fat-saturated sequence of the knee of a 13-year-old boy showing popliteal cysts extending around the gastrocnemius muscle.

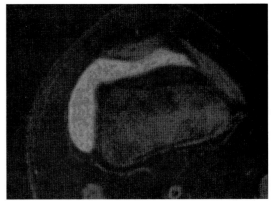

Figure 13. Axial proton density fat-saturated image of a 13-year-old girl. There is an effusion within the knee joint, which contains numerous small rice bodies. These bodies are the small low signal intensity flecks within the relatively high signal intensity fluid.

of joint space and remodeling of the acetabulum or glenoid may cause, respectively, hip and shoulder joint subluxation. The generalized osteopenia and weakened bone around the hip joint can also cause acetabular protrusion, poor iliac bone development, and coxa vara,[72–74] which is more common in the older child with more significant weight bearing. It has been suggested that in JIA the protrusion is more cephalic than that seen in adult disease. Osteonecrosis of the femoral head can occur in JIA, which may be a consequence of either JIA or joint injections.

Bursitis and Synovial Cyst Formation

Both US and MRI are more sensitive in the detection of synovial cysts and bursae than either clinical examination or radiography. The unexpected discovery of a synovial cyst is usually an isolated finding. On postgadolinium administration MRI sequences there is enhancement around the wall of the cyst. The cyst may arise from the joint capsule or the tendon sheath (Fig. 12).[75–77]

Soft Tissue Calcification

The presence of soft tissue calcification around a joint is not an uncommon finding in JIA and is typically related to joints that have had intra-articular injection of steroid. Calcification usually occurs within 2–12 months of the injection.[78]

Rice Bodies

Rice bodies are believed to result from either synovial proliferation and degeneration or synovial microinfarcts, which result in small pieces (bodies) of synovium becoming detached and falling into the joint space. These small, detached bodies vary in consistency, size, and shape and can contain coarse collagenous fibers, fibrin, or elastin. Macroscopically resembling tiny grains of rice, they may also occur in patients with other types of joint disease, such as tuberculous arthritis, agammaglobulinemia, and hypogammaglobulinemia.

On US imaging there is a joint effusion of heterogeneous echogenicity. On MRI the fluid still has high signal intensity on T2-w sequences, but there are numerous, small inhomogeneous floating bodies of low signal intensity within it (Fig. 13).[79–81]

Ankylosis

The initial osteoporosis, soft tissue swelling, and synovial hypertrophy may cause joint space widening. In more chronic disease, particularly in children who are RhF-positive, there is a gradual loss of joint space due to cartilage damage and bone erosions, which in the more severe cases may lead to bony ankylosis. This is most frequently seen in the wrist joint and in the facet joints of the cervical spine.[9,59,60,55,80] In some cases it is possible that a pseudarthrosis may develop to compensate for the loss of function that occurs with the ankylosis.[82]

Ligament/Tendon Abnormalities

Enthesitis

Enthesitis is an important pathological process in enthesitis-related arthritis (ERA) and in adult onset disease it is recognized as a key feature of psoriatic arthritis (PsA).[83,84] There is a lack of published information on the radiology of enthesitis in JIA despite its recognition in clinical practice by both clinicians and radiologists.

Inflammation around the sites of tendon and ligament insertion (enthesitis) can cause periosteal changes in the bone. The amount of new bone formation can be significant and result in either bony spurs or prominent osteophytes.[55,59,61] On MRI this enthesitis is seen as high signal at the site of tendon insertion on STIR sequences with further signal changes also being seen in the adjacent muscle; there may be an associated bursitis. These areas typically show enhancement following gadolinium administration. MRI can demonstrate fluid and inflamed synovium around the tendon sheaths and may identify subclinical tendon rupture (Fig. 14).[11,85]

Enthesitis-related arthritis (with and without inflammatory bowel disease) is clearly associated with enthesitis. Reiter's syndrome in children also has enthesitis as a prominent feature. Less clear in the pediatric literature is the presence of enthesitis in PsA, despite the fact that

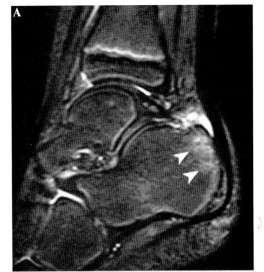

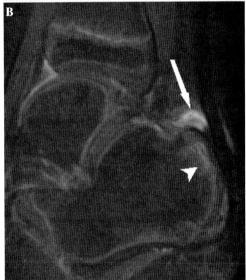

Figure 14. MRI of the foot and ankle of a 7-year-old girl with Achilles enthesitis. (**A**) Sagittal STIR image of the ankle. There is bone marrow edema around the insertion of the Achilles tendon into the calcaneum (arrowheads) with further soft tissue edema around the posterior aspect of the foot. Sagittal postgadolinium administration fat-saturated sequence shows enhancement within the bone marrow at the site of the Achilles insertion (arrowhead) and in the surrounding soft tissues (arrow).

it is clearly recognized as a feature in adult onset psoriatic disease.[47,83-85] Enthesitis is inflammation at the point of insertion of a tendon, ligament, or articular cartilage into bone. Typically, plantar fasciitis, Achilles tendon insertion, or insertion points around the patella are most commonly described in children with ERA, but many sites, including the pelvis and a number of upper limb sites, can be involved. Although peripheral enthesitis is seen in all forms of spondyloarthropathy, it is a particularly prominent feature of ERA in JIA.[21,27,29–31] Axial skeletal spondylitis occurs in about half of the cases of ERA, and mostly from the teenage years well into adult life.[86]

Work in adult ankylosing spondyloarthropathy[87,88] and psoriatic arthropathy[89] has recognized the importance of identifying enthesitis and extra-articular features on MRI in supporting the diagnosis and guiding therapy,[87] although Eshed *et al.* used an example of enthesitis in a 15-year old boy with ERA, and showed that these features are found in children as well as adults.[92] Imaging uses different techniques, such as dynamic contrast-enhanced imaging and diffusion-weighted imaging, which may work better with the younger patient[87,90] No such work has been published on JIA, but clinicians recognize the importance of enthesitis as a justification for earlier introduction of anti-TNF or other biologics in place of traditional therapies such as methotrexate.[91]

Dactilitis, along with inflammation of the joints and associated tendon sheaths giving a "sausage" toe/finger, is typical in PsA. MRI has allowed development of the concept of enthesitis to include fibrocartilage.[93–96] With teenagers it is important clinically to not confuse enthesitis of the patellar ligament with the traction apophysitis of Osgood–Schlatter or Sindig–Larsen–Johannsen disease.[97] Both US[98–102] and MRI have a role to play in the imaging of enthesitis. MRI has demonstrated the frequency of enthesitis in spondyloarthropathies, and through it we have learned that this process can be extensive, involving soft tissues and bone marrow.[92,103–105] MRI identifies diffuse bone edema next to the point of enthesis, surrounding soft tissue edema and increased ligament and bursa signal intensity after gadolinium contrast, which may be a common feature in a number of pathologies.[104,105]

In addition, the structures of the enthesis have a low water content and so have a low signal on conventional MRI, resulting in some limitations to the technique. Initial use suggested that US might be as valuable as MRI in identifying enthesitis.[106]

Ligament Abnormalities

Within joints, synovial hypertrophy causes damage and atrophy of intraosseous ligaments. In the knee, which has been the most actively studied, the cruciate ligaments can be either mildly or severely atrophic and synovial proliferation extending over the meniscal surfaces is believed to result in meniscal hypoplasia and degradation, which may precede a tear. These findings in the knee joint are more common in children who have had poorly controlled JIA for at least 4 to 5 years, but they can also occur in children with a disease duration of less than 1 year.[11] Around the wrist, ligament laxity can cause horizontal and radial deviation.

Axial Skeleton

Involvement of the cervical spine is more common in polyarticular (RhF-positive and RhF-negative) subtypes, whereas lumbar spine and sacroiliac disease are more often seen in the enthesitis-related group (particularly in children who are HLA-B27 histocompatibility antigen-positive) or associated with inflammatory bowel disease.

In the cervical spine there is hypoplasia and squaring of the vertebral bodies with synovial proliferation around the facet joints. The intervertebral disc space can become narrowed and irregular. In more severe long-standing disease, ankylosis of the apophyseal and facet joints occurs, causing significant immobility. Erosions can be seen around the odontoid process, and the synovial proliferation around the C1–C2 articulation can lead to ligament laxity and instability. Lateral radiographs may indicate widening of the gap between the posterior edge of the anterior arch of the atlas and the anterior surface of the odontoid. This gap may

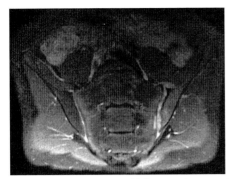

Figure 15. A 12-year-old boy with sacroiliitis. Oblique-coronal, T1-w fat-saturated images of the joints. There is widening and enhancement within the left sacroiliac joint and enhancement in the surrounding bone. There is minor enhancement around the right sacroiliac joint.

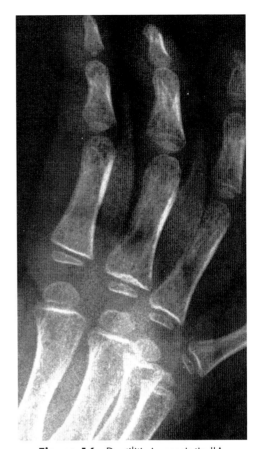

Figure 16. Dactilitis in psoriatic JIA.

show a dynamic change with flexion/extension views.[9,107]

In the lumbar spine there is more often sclerosis of the vertebral corners, loss of disc height, squaring of the anterior vertebral surface, syndesmophyte formation, and bony ankylosis. Compression fractures can occur at any level of the spine, but are particularly prevalent in the lumbar and thoracic regions if there has been long-term steroid use.

Sacroiliac disease can be difficult to detect clinically and radiographs are relatively poor at evaluating this joint. There may be joint space widening, marginal irregularity, and sclerosis that can eventually lead to ankylosis. Any of these features may be unilateral, bilateral, or symmetrical. Such findings can be slow to develop and correlate poorly with clinical function.[108–110]

MRI can demonstrate periarticular marrow edema and show enhancement within the joint space and surrounding bone, reflecting an osteitis. It is more sensitive than clinical evaluation in detecting sacroiliac disease and better at discriminating between active disease and chronic changes (Fig. 15).[109,110]

Psoriatic Arthritis

The classification of JIA[2,3] continues to exclude patients from the diagnosis of PsA if they have clinical enthesitis or lumbosacral involvement, in contrast to the diagnostic criteria in adult PsA.[85] MRI and US are recognized as being of value in identifying and defining enthesitis and other features.[85,47,111] Nevertheless, they remain research tools, with growing importance as outcome measures in clinical trials, particularly of the biologic agents.[112] Features of PsA such as synovitis and erosions are not distinguishable from rheumatoid arthritis, but other characteristics are clearly of value in identifying the seronegative group (Fig. 16). Specifically, MRI may define inflamed tissue extending beyond the joint capsule and involving structures such as ligaments and soft tissues. It may highlight involvement of sites such as distal interphalangeal (DIP) joints and entheseal insertions or find bone edema with enthesitis. MRI-observed features of enthesitis are defined[89] and increasingly well-characterized in adult spondyloarthropathies (Fig. 15).[84] Moreover, subclinical sacroiliitis has been identified on MRI in 38% of adult patients with PsA.[113] Among adults with severe psoriatic skin disease who did not have clinical arthritis, MRI distinguished subclinical arthritis in more than 60%.[114]

Magnetic Resonance Imaging in Juvenile Dermatomyositis

MRI is being used increasingly as a key diagnostic and monitoring tool for disease activity in juvenile dermatomyositis (JDM) and to identify focal muscle involvement for targeted biopsy (muscle involvement may be patchy).[117,118] A total of 78 out of 102 children (76%) had abnormal MRI-observed diagnostic images in a series of 151 cases of JDM in the United Kingdom[119] and a high proportion of clinicians with access to MRI indicated that they value it as a diagnostic tool.[8] In the presence of MRI-observed bilateral and symmetrical muscle edema accompanied by a characteristic rash, a biopsy may not be indicated.

Imaging Parameters

As with any other aspect of musculoskeletal MRI, maximized signal-to-noise ratio and the smallest field of view that is practical should be obtained. The choice of sequences and the area imaged will depend on the child and the clinical indication. Paradoxically, with a widespread myositis, it is important that the initial MRI include all the involved muscle groups to delineate the full extent of the disease. This may entail using a wide field of view or alternatively moving the patient within the magnet. Coronal sequences are useful to determine the extent of any lesion and axial images are helpful in determining the muscle groups and subcutaneous tissues that are involved. If infection is suspected it is important to include and evalu-

ate any adjacent joint to exclude an associated septic arthritis.

The choice of sequences will vary among institutions as will the choice between conventional spin-echo and fast spin-echo techniques. The use of a T2-w fat-suppressed sequence or STIR sequence is probably mandatory, as these are the most sensitive in assessing muscle edema. Conversely a T1-w sequence is useful for assessing fat infiltration within muscle.[120–124]

On standard T1-w spin-echo sequences, the signal intensity of muscle is significantly lower than that of fat and slightly lower than that of water. On T2-w spin-echo sequences, the signal intensity of muscle is significantly lower than that of both fat and water. On inversion recovery and fat-suppressed T2-w sequences, normal muscle intensity is lower than that of water but higher than that of fat.[117,120,125,126]

The presence of muscle inflammation results in both intracellular edema and extracellular free water, which causes prolongation of the T2 relaxation times. This leads to increased signal intensity on the T2-w and STIR sequences. The amount and distribution of this altered signal intensity reflects the underlying cause of the muscle inflammation,[120,121,126,127] which results in increased signal intensity on the T2-w and STIR sequences. Whereas water is of relatively high signal intensity on both STIR and T2 fast spin-echo sequences on the latter (with fat suppression), the signal for muscle is often lower than that for water. Consequently, it may be that T2 fat-saturated sequences may be more sensitive in detecting edema. STIR sequences have a more uniform degree of fat suppression and are often more suited to coronal imaging than T2 fast spin-echo sequences.

The routine use of gadolinium DTPA in all inflammatory conditions is not indicated, but is patient-dependent. Gadolinium-enhanced sequences are useful in assessing focal abscesses in muscle where there is rim enhancement.[124,125]

Postgadolinium DTPA fat-saturated sequences of adjacent joints are also useful in the septic child to help assess the presence of any

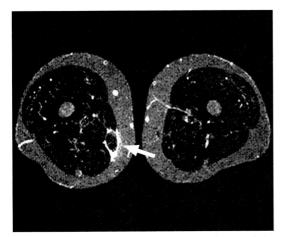

Figure 17. An axial T2 fat-saturated MRI of the thighs of an 11-year-old girl with dermatomyositis shows edema affecting only the right gracilis muscle (white arrow). A 1-year history of abnormal AST and ALT had mistakenly been interpreted as reflecting a liver rather than a muscle problem in the absence of any complaint of weakness. The diagnosis came to light when she developed a typical JDM rash. Careful clinical assessment of muscle strength identified weakness consistent with the subsequent MRI findings.

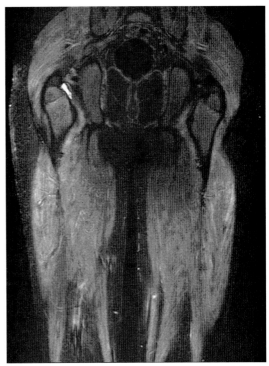

Figure 18. Coronal STIR image of a child with JDMS showing typical extensive bilateral high-signal changes affecting the muscles of the thighs and pelvis.

inflamed synovium, which reflects an associated septic arthritis.[124]

MRI is being utilized increasingly as a noninvasive guide to diagnosis and management. The MRI-observed features of the disease reflect the areas of muscle weakness and are predominantly in the proximal muscles of the upper and lower limbs. With severe disease, changes can be seen in the distal limb musculature. Typically the muscle shows widespread high signal changes on STIR and T2-w images, which are symmetrical in distribution, but not all muscle groups are affected equally (Figs. 17 and 18).[120,121,126,128–130] In JDM muscle involvement can sometimes be surprisingly focal, involving only one muscle or muscle group (Fig. 17).

Subcutaneous edema, seen as an irregular streaky high signal on STIR sequences, is a feature of early untreated disease (Fig. 20). This feature resolves relatively quickly following treatment with immunosuppressants, but where allowed to persist may be a risk fac-

tor for irreversible tissue damage. Moreover, STIR images may help to identify important pathological processes such as panniculitis.[131] Involvement of the fascia, which becomes thickened and again shows high signal change on STIR sequences, can occur. In JDMs this fascial involvement follows a distribution pattern similar to the involved muscle groups, but it is usually less noticeable than the adjacent muscle edema,[117,127,128,132] which is in contrast to eosinophilic fasciitis, where the fascial involvement is the more prominent feature and not all the adjacent muscle is involved (Fig. 19). In undifferentiated connective tissue disease (UCTD) the fascial and muscle signal intensities are similar, with a symmetrical distribution and with the muscle edema being more patchy. Both MRI and US are useful for determining the site for muscle biopsy, as the relatively patchy nature of the disease may lead to "blind" biopsies that are falsely negative.

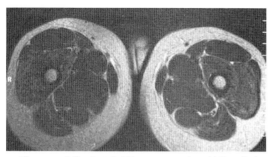

Figure 19. Axial T2-w spin-echo MRI of the thighs of a 13-year-old boy with JDMS. The distribution is bilateral and symmetrical, but involves only the vastus intermedius, vastus lateralis, and the long head of biceps femoris muscles.

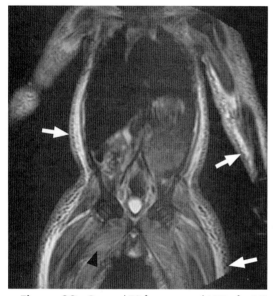

Figure 20. Coronal T2 fat-saturated MRI of a 17-month-old boy with dermatomyositis. There is extensive subcutaneous edema, seen as confluent white strands (white arrows). There is also widespread abnormal bright signal in the muscles (black arrowhead). This boy presented with profound weakness, respiratory failure, and inability to swallow. The edema had caused some initial diagnostic confusion, but is typical of JDM.

MRI is increasingly used to assess and quantify the severity of muscle disease. Presently, clinical assessment of muscle strength is dependent on patient compliance, and any loss of muscle function could be attributed to disease activity or muscle atrophy. Similarly, serum levels of muscle enzyme are partly dependent on patient muscle activity as well as disease activity,[133] and are notoriously unreliable. Most of the quantitative imaging methods rely on the fact that the more severe the disease the greater the degree of muscle inflammation; consequently there is an increase in the T2 relaxation times due to the increase in free water. The simplest method is to measure the signal values of T2-w spin-echo sequences. A refinement to this method is to calculate a ratio of the signal intensity of the muscle to the adjacent fat (the "signal intensity ratio," SIR), the assumption being that the signal intensity of fat will not change between serial studies or between patients and so acts as a "control" value. Using the SIR method, a value below 0.4 is considered normal, whereas above 0.6 is abnormal. There is obviously some overlap between normal and abnormal values.[126,127,134–136]

Signal intensity methods have inherent flaws in that they are affected by magnetic field heterogeneity, and the presence of any subcutaneous edema affects the signal intensity of the fat. More recent studies have improved the reliability of these signal intensity methods by calculating a more accurate value of the T2 relaxation time (T2 mapping).[135,136] In these studies there is very good correlation between the signal intensity value and the degree of muscle weakness, the muscle enzymes levels, and overall patient well-being. Further studies have shown that ^{32}P-spectroscopy demonstrates increased levels of phosphate in affected muscle, indicating cell inflammation and muscle breakdown.[137] Although spectroscopy shows good correlation with disease activity, this degree of functionality is less readily available on standard MRI machines, compared with T2 value measurement sequences.

In addition to assessing the acute disease and its management, radiology has a further role in imaging the longer-term complications of JDMs, which can be numerous. Muscle atrophy is a feature of more chronic disease but can also be the result of steroid therapy. It is best appreciated on T1-w sequences, as increased signal in between the muscle planes.[120,121,128,138]

Calcium deposition within muscle is another serious complication that can occur despite a normal physiological calcium/phosphate relationship. The chemical composition of calcinotic deposits has variously been described as consisting of calcium, oxalate, phosphate, uric acid, and calcium apatite.[139,140]

Calcinosis is often first detected on radiographs that are taken for a history of increasing pain or stiffness and limited mobility. Calcification is usually seen in one of two forms: nodular calcium deposits or sheetlike layers within the muscle along the length of the limb. Additionally, abnormal cystic collections filled with proteinaceous and calcium-laden fluid, known as milk of calcium collections, may occur within the muscle.[141,142] Their etiology is not fully understood, but they may be due to fracturing of calcified tissue planes, resulting in the formation of pseudobursae,[139] which then calcify around the rim, to have a more rounded or oblong appearance, as opposed to the aforementioned sheetlike calcification. On both CT and MRI, these collections show variable attenuation and signal intensity, depending on the concentration of the protein and calcium within them,[139] and minimal peripheral enhancement after contrast administration (Fig. 21).

Magnetic Resonance Imaging Compared to Other Imaging Modalities

Radiography

Conventional radiographs are the most readily available, quick, and inexpensive method of evaluating a joint. For the rheumatologist they provide an important baseline investigation and help to exclude other causes of joint pain and swelling, such as tumors, trauma, skeletal dysplasias, and infection. However, it must be remembered that radiography is unable to accurately detect damage or change to cartilage.[143]

The major drawback of radiography in JIA is that it cannot visualize synovial hyperpla-

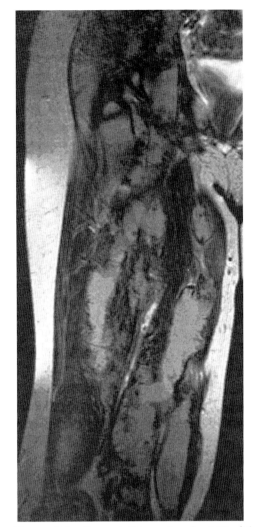

Figure 21. Coronal, T2-w spin-echo MRI of the thigh demonstrating high signal milk-of-calcium collections in a child with JDMS.

sia within a joint, so it cannot provide any relevant information about the degree of inflammatory change. The early radiographically observed changes that are visible reflect the hypervascularity and inflammatory response that accompany synovial hypertrophy, which can cause soft tissue swelling, periarticular osteopenia, and epiphyseal remodeling and widening. If the onset of JIA is relatively recent, any initial radiographs can be normal or only show minor nonspecific changes.[9,59,144]

Prolonged synovial proliferation leads to cartilage loss and bone damage, which are seen

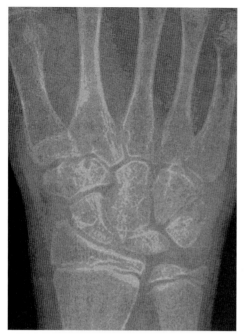

Figure 22. Radiograph of the wrist of a child with JIA. There is minor periarticular osteopenia with some metaphyseal widening. There are also some early erosive changes, particularly affecting the base of the third metacarpal and carpal bones, and some loss of joint space around the carpal bones.

radiographically as a loss of joint space and erosive changes along the joint margins (see Fig. 22). Progressive joint damage may eventually lead to bony ankylosis, with a resultant loss of function.[59,144] Radiographically observed features of chronic JIA are relatively slow to develop, their interpretation and categorization are subject to significant interobserver variability,[60,145] and they are nonspecific. A number of radiographic scoring systems for JIA have been developed, some of which have been modified from adult systems, but their use and acceptance is not agreed on universally.[144–149] In the authors' own institution the clinical assessment of function and disability of a joint is usually a more important monitor of disease progress than any radiographic changes. Radiographs are typically only obtained for children in whom there has been a significant or rapid alteration in symptoms or when surgical intervention is being considered. Radio-

graphs are important in the assessment of bone maturation and evaluating any limb length discrepancy.[150]

Sonography

Sonography is a simple, rapid, and inexpensive method of evaluating joint swelling. It is being used increasingly by rheumatologists (after suitable training) within the clinical setting.[31] The concept of the rheumatologist as a sonographer is only just beginning to impact on pediatric practice. It is a more global assessment than sonography performed by radiologists because of the integration of clinical and radiographic assessment. However, good-quality musculoskeletal US is only of value when performed with a high level of skill. Furthermore, there is a paucity of literature on musculoskeletal US in pediatric, and particularly JIA, patients.[31] There is no radiation exposure risk and in the majority of cases there is no need to sedate the child. Indeed, the older child may enjoy seeing the images and engage with the examination, particularly when it is done by a familiar clinician. Technical difficulties can occur in younger children with localized joint tenderness and pain, as they will be reluctant for the limb to be handled and moved. Moreover, in the small child, obtaining a satisfactory acoustic window to allow a proper evaluation of the internal structures of a joint can be problematic. The visualization of any intra-articular structures is significantly improved by the use of high-frequency (12–15 MHz) linear probes. The consequent loss of depth with these higher frequencies is not normally an issue when imaging on the smaller scale of a young child's joint.

Sonography is more sensitive than radiography or clinical examination in the detection of effusions, synovial thickening, and synovial cysts.[10,31] It readily distinguishes between joint fluid and inflamed synovium, the latter appearing as a thickened, irregular, and nodular relatively hyperechoic (compared to joint fluid) lining around the joint space.

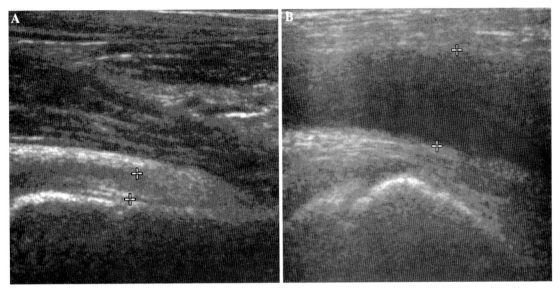

Figure 23. Sonography of a hip of a 13-year-old: (**A**) the synovium is thickened (3.5 mm) and (**B**) there is a large joint effusion.

Serial US is useful in monitoring disease activity and in evaluating any response to therapy. An increase in the size and distribution of synovium suggests active disease, whereas a reduction in the volume of joint fluid corresponds to clinical improvement. This change in fluid volume appears to occur faster than alteration in the size of the synovium.[31,32,151–153]

Color Doppler gives an indication of the degree of synovial hypertrophy and enables assessment of its vascularity. In some cases, the use of contrast enhancement has been shown to improve the detection and assessment of this vascularity.[153,154]

Normal cartilage is seen as a hypoechoic structure with a smooth outline over the bone surfaces. When there is joint inflammation there may be thickening of the cartilage, which then often has a slightly irregular outline. In chronic disease, erosions and cartilage thinning can also be detected.[10,151,32] However, in the larger joints visualization of the entire articular surface may not always be possible (Fig. 23).

Sonography is of value in assessing muscle inflammation, but is highly dependent on the skill of the operator and is being increasingly replaced by MRI, with very few centers using US or rating it as important[8] in the diagnosis or monitoring of muscle inflammation in JDM.

Bone Scintigraphy

The radionuclide bone scan can be valuable in the child with bone and soft tissue features of infection, nonaccidental injury, tumor, or inflammation, particularly where other imaging modalities have not identified a problem or are inappropriate, and a negative bone scan can help relieve concern that significant pathology has been overlooked. Scintigraphy requires high-quality images and sensitive and skilled interpretation, and is often used together with other imaging modalities to maximize the value of the technique.[155]

Novel and Exploratory Uses of Magnetic Resonance Imaging in Juvenile Dermatomyositis and Juvenile Idiopathic Arthritis

Magnetic resonance spectroscopy is a research tool with the potential to allow biochemical analysis of the severity of metabolic and vascular abnormalities in children's muscle with and without exercise, allowing exploration of the mechanism of muscle malfunction.[156] Several groups have explored the use of contrast-enhanced MRI to quantify disease activity in JIA.[157] Examination of the water content of cartilage has led to exploration of the value of assessing the quality of cartilage in children with JIA compared to controls by comparing T2 relaxation times. In children with JIA, imaging of clinically unaffected joints has suggested that subclinical MRI-observed features of arthritis may predict extension of arthritis, albeit in a small pilot study.[158] The development of a scoring system for MRIs in JIA would be valuable in advancing the utilization of MRI and in recognizing its critical role in the early and detailed assessment of inflammation and disease progression in JIA.[159]

Conflicts of Interest

The authors declare no conflicts of interest.

References

1. Andersson Garre, B. 1999. Juvenile arthritis—who gets it, where and when: A review of current data on incidence and prevalence. *Clin. Exp. Rheum* **17:** 367–377.
2. Petty, R.E., T.R. Southwood, J. Baum, *et al.* 1997. Revision of the proposed classification criteria for juvenile idiopathic arthritis: Durban. *J. Rheumatol.* **25:** 1991–1994.
3. Petty, R.E., T.R. Southwood, P. Manners, *et al.* 2004. International League of Associations for Rheumatology (ILAR) classification of juvenile idiopathic arthritis: Second revision, Edmonton, 2001. *J. Rheumatol.* **31:** 390–392.
4. Petty, R.E. & T.R. Southwood. 1998. Classification of childhood arthritis: Divide and conquer. *J. Rheumatol.* **25:** 1869–1870.
5. European League Against Rheumatism. 1977. *Bulletin 4. Nomenclature and classification of arthritis in children.* National Zeitung. Basel.
6. Cassidy, J.T., J.E. Levinson, J.C. Bass, *et al.* 1986. A study of classification criteria for a diagnosis of juvenile rheumatoid arthritis. *Arthritis Rheum.* **29:** 274.
7. Bohan, A. & J.B. Peter. 1975. Polymyositis and dermatomyositis. Parts 1 and 2. *New Engl. J. Med.* **292:** 344–347, 403–407.
8. Brown, V.E., C.A. Pilkington, B.M. Feldman & J.E. Davidson. 2006. An international consensus survey of the diagnostic criteria for juvenile dermatomyositis (JDM). *Rheumatology* **45:** 990–993.
9. Johnson, K. & J. Gardner-Medwin. 2002. Childhood arthritis: Classification and radiology. *Clin. Radiol.* **57:** 47–58.
10. Lamer, S. & G.H. Sebag. 2000. MRI and ultrasound in children with juvenile chronic arthritis. *Eur. J. Radiol.* **33:** 85–93.
11. Gylys-Morin, V.M. 1998. MR imaging of pediatric musculoskeletal inflammatory and infectious disorders. *Magn. Reson. Imaging Clin. N. Am.* **6:** 537–559.
12. Johnson, J. 2006. Imaging of juvenile idiopathic arthritis. *Pediatr. Radiol.* **36:** 743–758.
13. Graham, T.B., T. Laor & B.J. Dardzinski. 2005. Quantitative magnetic resonance imaging of the hands and wrists of children with juvenile rheumatoid arthritis. *J. Rheumatol.* **32:** 1811–1820.
14. Barnewolt, C.E. & T. Chung. 1998. Techniques, coils, pulse sequences, and contrast enhancement in pediatric musculoskeletal MR imaging. *Magn. Reson. Imaging Clin. N. Am.* **6:** 441–453.
15. Resnick, D. 1988. Common disorders of synovium lined joints: Pathogenesis, imaging abnormalities and complications. *AJR Am. J. Roentgenol.* **151:** 1079–1092.
16. Gylys-Morin, V.M., T.B. Graham, J.S. Blebea, *et al.* 2001. Knee in early juvenile rheumatoid arthritis: MR imaging findings. *Radiology* **220:** 696–706.
17. Senac, M.O., Jr., D. Deutsch, B.H. Bernstein, *et al.* 1988. MR imaging in juvenile rheumatoid arthritis. *AJR Am. J. Roentgenol.* **150:** 873–878.
18. Johnson, K., B. Wittkop, F. Haigh, *et al.* 2002. The early magnetic resonance imaging features of the knee in juvenile idiopathic arthritis. *Clin. Radiol.* **57:** 466–471.
19. Herve-Somma, C.M., G.H. Sebag, A.-M. Prieur, *et al.* 1992. Juvenile rheumatoid arthritis of the knee: MR evaluation with Gd-DOTA. *Radiology* **182:** 93–98.
20. Murray, J.G., N.T. Ridley, N. Mitchell, *et al.* 1996. Juvenile chronic arthritis of the hip: Value of contrast-enhanced MR imaging. *Clin. Radiol.* **51:** 99–102.
21. Østergaard, M. & B. Ejbjerg. 2004. Magnetic resonance imaging of the synovium in rheumatoid arthritis. *Sem. Musculoskeletal Radiol.* **8:** 287–299.
22. Østergaard, M. & M. Klarlund. 2001. Importance of timing of post-contrast MRI in rheumatoid arthritis: What happens during the first 60 minutes after IV gadolinium-DTPA? *Ann. Rheum. Dis.* **60:** 1050–1054.

23. Oliver, C. & I. Watt. 1996. Intravenous MRI contrast enhancement of inflammatory synovium: A dose study. *Br. J. Rheumatol.* **35**(Suppl. 3): 31–35.

24. Argryopoulou, M.I., S.L. Fanis, T. Xenakis, *et al*. 2002. The role of MRI in the evaluation of hip joint disease in clinical subtypes of juvenile idiopathic arthritis. *Br. J. Radiol.* **75**: 229–233.

25. Workie, D.W., B. Dardzinski, T.B. Graham, *et al*. 2004. Quantification of dynamic contrast enhanced MR-imaging of the knee in children with juvenile rheumatoid arthritis based on pharmacokinetic modelling. *Magn. Reson. Imaging* **22**: 1201–1210.

26. Jaramillo, D. & F. Shapiro. 1998. Growth cartilage: Normal appearance, variants and abnormalities. *Magn. Reson. Imaging Clin. N. Am.* **6**: 455–471.

27. Eckstein, F. & C. Glaser. 2004. Measuring cartilage morphology with quantitative magnetic resonance imaging. *Sem. Musculoskeletal Radiol.* **8**: 329–353.

28. Jaramillo, D. & T. Laor. 2008. Paediatric musculoskeletal MRI: Basic principles to optimise success. *Pediatr. Radiol.* **38**: 379–391.

29. Buchmann, R.F. & D. Jaramillo. 2004. Imaging of articular disorders in children. *Radiol. Clin. North Am.* **42**: 151–168.

30. Mosher, T.J. & B.J. Dardzinski. 2004. Cartilage MRI T2 relaxation time mapping: Overview and applications. *Sem. Musculoskeletal Radiol.* **8**: 355–368.

31. Kight, A.C., B.J. Dardzinski, T. Laor, *et al*. 2004. Magnetic resonance imaging evaluation of the effects of juvenile rheumatoid arthritis on distal femoral weight-bearing cartilage. *Arthritis Rheum.* **50**: 901–905.

32. El-Miedany, Y.M., I.H. Housny, H.M. Mansour, *et al*. 2001. Ultrasound versus MRI in the evaluation of juvenile idiopathic arthritis of the knee. *Joint Bone Spine* **68**: 222–230.

33. Eich, G.F., F. Halle, J. Hodler, *et al*. 1994. Juvenile chronic arthritis: Imaging of the knees and hips before and after intraarticular steroid injection. *Pediatr. Radiol.* **24**: 558–563.

34. Scenario, M., K. Kollo, I. Antal, *et al*. 2004. Intraarticular osteoid osteoma: clinical features, imaging results, and comparison with extraarticular localization. *J. Rheumatol.* **31**: 957–964.

35. Roth, J., I. Scheer, S. Kraft, *et al*. 2006. Uncommon synovial cysts in children. *Eur. J. Pediatr.* **165**: 178–181.

36. Johnson, K., J. Gardner-Medwin & C. Ryder. 2004. The use of MRI to predict disease progression in juvenile idiopathic arthritis. *Pediatr. Radiol.* **34**: s102–s103.

37. Laor, T. 2008. Early MRI characteristic of idiopathic chondrolyis of the hip. *Pediatr. Radiol.* **38**(Suppl. 2): s294.

38. De Backer, A.I., K.J. Mortelé, F.M. Vanhoenacker & P.M. Parizel. 2006. Imaging of extraspinal musculoskeletal tuberculosis. *Eur. J. Radiol.* **57**: 119–130.

39. Gylys-Morin, V.M. 1998. MR imaging of paedatric musculoskeletal inflammatory and infectious disorders. *Magn. Reson. Imaging Clin. N. Am.* **6**: 537–558.

40. Argyropoulou, M.I., S.L. Fanis, T. Xenakis, *et al*. 2002. The role of MRI in the evaluation of hip joint disease in clinical subtypes of juvenile idiopathic arthritis. *Br. J. Radiol.* **75**: 229–233.

41. Nistali, K., J. Babar, K. Johnson, *et al*. 2007. Clinical assessment and core outcome variables are poor predictors of hip arthritis diagnosed by MRI in juvenile idiopathic arthritis. *Rheumatology* **46**: 699–702.

42. Kuseler, A., T.K. Pederson, T. Herlin, *et al*. 1998. Contrast enhanced magnetic resonance imaging as a method to diagnose early inflammation changes in the temporomandibular joint in children with juvenile chronic arthritis. *J. Rheumatol.* **25**: 1406–1412.

43. Taylor, D.B., P. Babyn, S. Blaser, *et al*. 1993. MR evaluation of the temporomandibular joint in juvenile rheumatoid arthritis. *J. Comput. Assist. Tomogr.* **17**: 449–454.

44. Arabshahi, B., E.M. Dewitt, A.M. Cahill, *et al*. 2005. Utility of corticosteroid injection for temporomandibular arthritis in children with juvenile idiopathic arthritis. *Arthritis Rheum.* **52**: 3563–3569.

45. Robertson, L.P. & P. Hickling. 2001. Chronic recurrent multifocal osteomyelitis is a differential diagnosis of juvenile idiopathic arthritis. *Ann. Rheum. Dis.* **60**: 828–831.

46. Ramsey, S.E., R.A. Cairns, D.A. Cabral, *et al*. 1999. Knee magnetic resonance imaging in childhood chronic monarthritis. *J. Rheumatol.* **26**: 2238–2243.

47. Jimenez, R.M., D. Jaramillo & S.A. Connolly. 2005. Imaging of the pediatric hand: Soft tissue abnormalities. *Eur. J. Radiol.* **56**: 344–357.

48. Graham, T.B., T. Laor & B.J. Dardzinski. 2005. Quantitative magnetic resonance imaging of the hands and wrists of children with juvenile rheumatoid arthritis. *J. Rheumatol.* **32**: 1811–1820.

49. McQueen, F., M. Lassere, P. Bird, *et al*. 2007. Developing a magnetic resonance imaging scoring system for peripheral psoriatic arthritis. *J. Rheumatol.* **34**: 859–861.

50. Johnson, K., S.F. Haigh, S. Ehtisham, *et al*. 2003. Childhood idiopathic chondrolysis of the hip: MRI features. *Pediatr. Radiol.* **33**: 194–199.

51. Brenner, J.S. 2007. Pigmented villonodular synovitis causing painless chronic knee swelling in an adolescent. *Clin. Pediatr.* **46**: 268–271.

52. Cil, A., O. Ahmet Atay, U. Aydmgoz, *et al*. 2005. Bilateral lipoma arborescens of the knee in a child: a case report. *Knee Surg. Sports Traumatol. Arthrosc.* **13**: 463–467.

53. Jones, O.Y., C.H. Spencer, S.L. Bowyer, *et al*. 2006. A multicenter case-control study on predictive factors distinguishing childhood leukemia from juvenile rheumatoid arthritis. *Pediatrics* **117:** e840–e844.

54. Faingold, R., G. Saigal, E.M. Azouz, *et al*. 2004. Imaging of low back pain in children and adolescents. *Sem. Ultrasound CT MRI* **25:** 490–505.

55. Kjaer, P., C. Leboeuf-Yde, J.S. Sorensen & T. Bendix. 2005. An epidemiological study of MRI and low back pain in 13 year old children. *Spine* **30:** 798–806.

56. Lang, B.A., R. Schneider, B.J. Reilly, *et al*. 1995. Radiological features of systemic onset juvenile rheumatoid arthritis. *J. Rheumatol*. **22:** 168–173.

57. Martel, W., J.F. Holt & J.T. Cassidy. 1962. Roentgenologic manifestations of juvenile rheumatoid arthritis. *Am. J. Roentgenol. Radium Ther. Nucl. Med*. **88:** 400–423.

58. Hoving, J.L., R. Buchbinder, S. Hall, *et al*. 2004. A comparison of magnetic resonance imaging, sonography, and radiography of the hand in patients with early rheumatoid arthritis. *J. Rheumatol*. **31:** 663–675.

59. Kitai N, Kreiborg S, Murakami S, Bakke M, Møller E, Darvann TA, Takada K. 2002. A three-dimensional method of visualizing the temporomandibular joint based on magnetic resonance imaging in a case of juvenile chronic arthritis. *Int J Paediatr Dent*. **12:** 109–15.

60. Schmit, P., A.M. Prieur & F. Brunelle. 1999. Juvenile rheumatoid arthritis and lymphoedema: Lymphangiographic aspects. *Pediatr. Radiol*. **29:** 364–366.

61. Ansell, B.M. & P.A. Kent. 1977. Radiological changes in juvenile chronic polyarthritis. *Skeletal Radiol*. **1:** 129–144.

62. Wilkinson, R.H. & B.N. Weissman. 1988. Arthritis in children. *Radiol. Clin. North Am*. **26:** 1247–1265.

63. Reed, M.H. & D.M. Wilmot 1991. The radiology of juvenile rheumatoid arthritis: A review of the English language literature. *J. Rheumatol*. **18:** 2–22.

64. Wakefield, R.J., W.W. Gibbon, P.G. Conaghan, *et al*. 2000. The value of sonography in the detection of bone erosions in patients with rheumatoid arthritis: A comparison with conventional radiography. *Arthritis Rheum*. **43:** 2762–2770.

65. Klarlund, M., M. Østergaard, K.E. Jensen, *et al*. 2000. Magnetic resonance imaging, radiography, and scintigraphy of the finger joints: One year follow up of patients with early arthritis. *Ann. Rheum. Dis*. **59:** 521–528.

66. McQueen, F.M., N. Benton, D. Perry, *et al*. 2003. Bone edema scored on magnetic resonance imaging scans of the dominant carpus at presentation predicts radiographic joint damage of the hands and feet six years later in patients with rheumatoid arthritis. *Arthritis Rheum*. **48:** 1814–1827.

67. Østergaard, M., M. Hansen, M. Stoltenberg, *et al*. 2003. New radiographic bone erosions in the wrists of patients with rheumatoid arthritis are detectable with magnetic resonance imaging a median of two years earlier. *Arthritis Rheum*. **48:** 2128–2131.

68. Ansell, B.M. & E.G. Bywaters. 1956. Growth in Still's disease. *Ann. Rheum. Dis*. **15:** 295–319.

69. Simon, S., J. Whiffen & F. Shapiro. 1981. Leg-length discrepancies in monoarticular and pauciarticular juvenile rheumatoid arthritis. *J. Bone Joint Surg. Am*. **63:** 209–215.

70. Larheim, T.A., K. Dale & L. Tveito.1981. Radiographic abnormalities of the temporomandibular joint in children with juvenile rheumatoid arthritis. *Acta Radiol*. **22:** 277–284.

71. Larheim, T.A., H.M. Hoyeraal, A.E. Stabrun, *et al*. 1982. The temporomandibular joint in juvenile rheumatoid arthritis. *Scand. J. Rheumatol*. **11:** 5–12.

72. Ronchezel, M.V., M. Odete, O.E. Hilario, *et al*. 1995. Temporomandibular joint and mandibular growth alterations in patients with juvenile rheumatoid arthritis. *J. Rheumatol*. **22:** 1956–1961.

73. Chaplin, D., T. Pulkki, A. Saarimaa, *et al*. 1969. Wrist and finger deformities in juvenile rheumatoid arthritis. *Acta Rheumatol. Scand*. **15:** 206–223.

74. Jacqueline, F., A. Boujot & L. Canet. 1961. Involvement of the hips in juvenile rheumatoid arthritis. *Arthritis Rheum*. **4:** 500–513.

75. Hastings, D.E., E. Orsini, P. Myers, *et al*. 1994. An unusual pattern of growth disturbance of the hip in juvenile rheumatoid arthritis. *J. Rheumatol*. **21:** 744–747.

76. Harris, C.M. & J. Baum. 1988. Involvement of the hip in juvenile rheumatoid arthritis. A longitudinal study. *J. Bone Joint Surg. Am*. **70:** 821–833.

77. Iversen, J.K., H. Nelleman, A. Buus, *et al*. 1996. Synovial cysts of the hips in seronegative arthritis. *Skeletal Radiol*. **25:** 396–399.

78. Bloom, B.J., L.B. Tucker, L.C. Miller, *et al*. 1995. Bicipital synovial cysts in juvenile rheumatoid arthritis: Clinical description and sonographic correlation. *J. Rheumatol*. **22:** 1953–1955.

79. Lang, I.M., D. Hughes, J.B. Williamson, *et al*. 1997. MRI of popliteal cysts in childhood. *Pediatr. Radiol*. **27:** 130–132.

80. Gilsanz, V. & B.H. Bernstein. 1984. Joint calcification following intra-articular corticosteroid therapy. *Radiology* **151:** 647–649.

81. Chung, C., B.D. Coley & L.C. Martin. 1998. Rice bodies in juvenile rheumatoid arthritis. *AJR Am. J. Roentgenol*. **170:** 698–700.

82. Maldonado-Cocco, J.A., O. Garcia-Morteo, A.J. Spindler, *et al*. 1980. Carpal ankylosis in juvenile rheumatoid arthritis. *Arthritis Rheum.* **23:** 1251–1255.

83. Martini, G., A. Tregnaghi, T. Bordin, *et al*. 2003. Rice bodies imaging in juvenile idiopathic arthritis. *J. Rheumatol.* **30:** 2720–2721.

84. Cuomo, A., M. Pirpiris & N.Y. Otsuka. 2006. Case report: Biceps tenosynovial rice bodies. *J. Pediatr. Orthop.* **15:** 423–425.

85. Stovell, P.B., S.C. Ahuja & A.E. Inglis. 1975. Pseudarthrosis of the proximal femoral epiphysis in juvenile rheumatoid arthritis. A case report. *J. Bone Joint Surg. Am.* **57:** 860–861.

86. McGonagle, D., P.G. Conaghan & P. Emery. 1998. Classification of inflammatory arthritis by enthesitis. *Lancet* **352:** 1137–1140.

87. McGonagle, D., P.G. Conaghan & P. Emery. 1999. Psoriatic arthritis. A unified concept twenty years on. *Arthritis Rheum.* **42:** 1080–1086.

88. Gladman, D.D., P.J. Mease, V. Strand, *et al*. 2007. Consensus on a core set of domains for psoriatic arthritis. *J. Rheumatol.* **34:** 1167–1170.

89. Azouz, E.M. 2003. Arthritis in children: Conventional and advanced imaging. *Sem. Musculoskeletal Radiol.* **2:** 95–101.

90. Azouz, E.M. & C.M. Duffy. 1995. Juvenile spondyloarthropathies: Clinical manifestations and medical imaging. *Skeletal Radiol.* **24:** 399–408.

91. Gaspersic, N. *et al*. 2007. Monitoring Ank Spond therapy by dynamic contrast enhanced and diffusion weighted MRI. *Skeletal Radiol*.

92. Eshed, I. *et al*. 2008. MRI of hindfoot involvement in patients with spondyloarthritides: Comparison of low-field and high-field 'strength' units. *Eur. J. Radiol.* **65:** 140–147

93. Barozzi, L., I. Olivieri, M. De Matteis, *et al*. 1988. Seronegative spondyloarthropathies: Imaging of spondylitis, enthesitis and dactylitis. *Eur. J. Radiol.* **27:** S12–17.

94. Braun, J. *et al*. 2004. Analysing chronic spinal changes in ankylosing spondylitis: A systematic comparison of conventional x-rays with magnetic resonance imaging (MRI) using established and new scoring systems. *Ann. Rheum. Dis.* 63: 1046–1055.

95. Tse, H. *et al*. 2006. Radiologic Improvement of juvenile idiopathic arthritis-enthesitis-related arthritis following anti-tumor necrosis factor-alpha blockade with etanercept. *J. Rheumatol.* **33:** 1186–1188.

96. Jevtic, V., I. Watt, B. Rozman, *et al*. 1995. Distinctive radiological features of small hand joints in rheumatoid arthritis and seronegative spondyloarthritis demonstrated by contrast-enhanced (Gd-DTPA) magnetic resonance imaging. *Skeletal Radiol.* **24:** 351–355.

97. Benjamin, M. & D. McGonagle. 2001. The anatomical basis for disease localisation in seronegative spondyloarthropathy at entheses and related sites. *J. Anat.* **199**(Pt 5): 503–526.

98. McGonagle, D., M. Benjamin, H. Marzo-Ortega & P. Emery. 2002. Advances in the understanding of entheseal inflammation. *Curr. Rheumatol. Rep.* **4:** 500–506.

99. McGonagle, D., H. Marzo-Ortega M. Benjamin & P. Emery. 2003. Report on the Second International Enthesitis Workshop. *Arthritis Rheum.* **48:** 896–905.

100. McGonagle, D. 2003. Diagnosis and treatment of enthesitis. *Rheum. Dis. Clin. North Am.* **29:** 549–560.

101. Olivieri, I., C. Salvarani, F. Cantini, *et al*. 2002. Fast spin echo-T2-weighted sequences with fat saturation in dactylitis of spondylarthritis. No evidence of entheseal involvement of the flexor digitorum tendons. *Arthritis Rheum.* **46:** 2964–2967.

102. Lehtinen, A., M. Taavitsainen & M. Leirisalo-Repo. 1994. Sonographic analysis of enthesopathy in the lower extremities of patients with spondylarthropathy. *Clin. Exp. Rheumatol.* **12:** 143–148.

103. Balint, P.V., D. Kane, J. Hunter, *et al*. 2002. Ultrasound guided versus conventional joint and soft tissue fluid aspiration in rheumatology practice: A pilot study. *J. Rheumatol.* **29:** 2209–2213.

104. Gillet, P., P. Péré, J.Y. Jouzeau, *et al*. 1994 Enthesitis of the ligamentum teres during ankylosing spondylitis: histopathological report. *Ann Rheum Dis* **53:** 82.

105. Newman, J.S., T.J. Laing, C.J. McCarthy, *et al*. 1996. Power Doppler sonography of synovitis: Assessment of therapeutic response—preliminary observations. *Radiology* **198:** 582–584.

106. Schmidt, W.A. 2004. Doppler sonography in rheumatology. *Best Pract Res Clin Rheumatol* **18:** 827–846.

107. McGonagle, D., W. Gibbon, P. O'Connor, *et al*. 1998. Characteristic magnetic resonance imaging entheseal changes of knee synovitis in spondylarthropathy. *Arthritis Rheum.* **41:** 694–700.

108. McGonagle, D., H. Marzo-Ortega, P. O'Connor, *et al*. 2002. The role of biomechanical factors and HLA-B27 in magnetic resonance imaging-determined bone changes in plantar fascia enthesopathy. *Arthritis Rheum.* **46:** 489–493.

109. Marzo-Ortega, H., D. McGonagle, P. O'Connor & P. Emery. 2001. Efficacy of etanercept in the treatment of the entheseal pathology in resistant spondylarthropathy: A clinical and magnetic resonance imaging study. *Arthritis Rheum.* **44:** 2112–2117.

110. Kamel, M., H. Eid & R. Mansour. 2003. Ultrasound detection of heel enthesitis: A comparison with magnetic resonance imaging. *J. Rheumatol.* **30:** 774–778.

111. Thompson, G.H., M.A. Khan & R.M. Bilenker. 1982. Spontaneous atlanto-axial subluxation as a presenting manifestation of juvenile ankylosing spondylitis. *Spine* **7:** 78–79.

112. Foster, H.E., R.A. Carins, R.H. Burnell, *et al*. 1995. Atlantoaxial subluxation in children with seronegative enthesopathy and arthropathy syndrome: 2 case reports and a review of the literature. *J. Rheumatol.* **22:** 548–551.

113. Bollow, M., J. Braun, T. Biedermann, *et al*. 1998. Use of contrast-enhanced MR imaging to detect sacroiliitis in children. *Skeletal Radiol.* **27:** 606–616.

114. Bollow, M., T. Biedermann, J. Kannenberg, *et al*. 1998. Use of dynamic magnetic resonance imaging to detect sacroiliitis in HLA-B 27 positive and negative children with juvenile arthritides. *J. Rheumatol.* **25:** 556–564.

115. Muche, B., M. Bollow, R.J. Francois, *et al*. 2003. Anatomic structures in early and late stage sacroiliitis in spondyloarthritis. A detailed analysis by contrast enhanced magnetic resonance imaging. *Arthritis Rheum.* **48:** 1374–1384.

116. Marzo-Ortega, H., D. McGonagle, S. Jarrett, G. Haugeberg, E. Hensor, P. O'Connor, A.L. Tan, P.G. Conaghan, A. Greenstein & P. Emery. 2005. Infliximab in combination with methotrexate in active ankylosing spondylitis: A clinical and imaging study. *Ann. Rheum. Dis.* **64:** 1568–1575.

117. Williamson, L., J.L. Dockerty, N. Dalbeth, *et al*. 2004. Clinical assessment of sacroiliitis and HLA-B27 are poor predictors of sacroiliitis diagnoses by MRI in psoriatic arthritis. *Rheumatology* **43:** 85–88.

118. Offidani, A., A. Cellini, G. Valeri & A. Gionagnoni. 1998. Subclinical joint involvement in psoriasis: Magnetic resonance imaging and X ray findings. *Acta Derm. Venereol.* **78:** 463–465.

119. McCann, L.J., A.D. Juggins, S.M. Maillard, *et al*; Juvenile Dermatomyositis Research Group. 2006 The Juvenile Dermatomyositis National Registry and Repository (UK and Ireland)–clinical characteristics of children recruited within the first 5 yr. *Rheumatology* (Oxford) **45:** 1255–1260.

120. Walker, U.A. 2008. Imaging tools for the clinical assessment of idiopathic inflammatory myositis. *Curr Opin Rheumatol* **20:** 656–661.

121. Hernandez, R.J., D.R. Keim, D.B. Sullivan, *et al*. 1990. Magnetic resonance imaging appearance of the muscles in childhood dermatomyositis. *J. Pediatr.* **117:** 546–550.

122. Johnson, K., P.J. Davis, J.K. Foster, J.E. McDonagh, *et al*. 2006. Imaging of muscle disorders in children. *Pediatr. Radiol.* **36:** 1005–1018.

123. McCann, L.J., A.D. Juggins, S.M. Maillard, *et al*. 2006. Juvenile Dermatomyositis Research Group. The Juvenile Dermatomyositis National Registry

124. Fleckenstein, J.L. & C.D. Reimers. 1996. Inflammatory myopathies: Radiologic evaluation. *Radiol. Clin. North Am.* **34:** 427–439.

125. May, D.A., D.G. Disler, E.A. Jones, *et al*. 2000. Abnormal signal intensity in skeletal muscle at MR imaging: Patterns, pearls, and pitfalls. *Radiographics* **20:** S295–S315.

126. Bydder, G.M. & I.R. Young. 1985. MR imaging: Clinical use of the inversion recovery sequence. *J. Comput. Assist. Tomogr.* **9:** 659–675.

127. Delfaut, E.M., J. Beltran, G. Johnson, *et al*. 1999. Fat suppression in MR imaging: Techniques and pitfalls. *Radiographics* **19:** 373–382.

128. Hopkins, K.L., K.C. Li & G. Bergman. 1995. Gadolinium-DPTA-enhanced magnetic resonance of musculoskeletal infectious processes. *Skeletal Radiol.* **24:** 325–330.

129. Gylys-Morin, V.M. 1998. MR imaging of pediatric musculoskeletal inflammatory and infectious disorders. *Magn. Reson. Imaging Clin. N. Am.* **6:** 537–559.

130. Adams, E.M., C.K. Chow, A. Premkumar, *et al*. 1995. The idiopathic inflammatory myopathies: Spectrum of MR imaging findings. *Radiographics* **15:** 563–574.

131. Keim, D.R., R.J. Hernandez & D.B. Sullivan. 1991. Serial magnetic resonance imaging in juvenile dermatomyositis. *Arthritis Rheum.* **34:** 1580–1584.

132. Hernandez, R.J., D.B. Sullivan, T.L. Chenevert, *et al*. 1993. MR imaging in children with dermatomyositis: Musculoskeletal findings and correlation with clinical and laboratory findings. *AJR Am. J. Roentgenol.* **161:** 359–366.

133. Schweitzer, M.E. & J. Fort. 1995. Cost-effectiveness of MR imaging in evaluating polymyositis. *AJR Am. J. Roentgenol.* **165:** 1469–1471.

134. Pachman, L.M. & M.C. Maryjowski. 1984. Juvenile dermatomyositis and polymyositis. *Clin. Rheum. Dis.* **10:** 95–115.

135. Kimball, A.B., R.M. Summers, M. Turner, *et al*. 2000. Magnetic resonance imaging detection of occult skin and subcutaneous abnormalities in juvenile dermatomyositis. *Arthritis Rheum.* **43:** 1866–1873.

136. Kaufman, L.D., B.L. Gruber, D.P. Gerstman, *et al*. 1987. Preliminary observations on the role of magnetic resonance imaging for polymyositis and dermatomyositis. *Ann. Rheum. Dis.* **46:** 569–572.

137. Fraser, D.D., J.A. Frank, M. Dalakas, *et al*. 1991. Magnetic resonance imaging in the idiopathic inflammatory myopathies. *J. Rheumatol.* **18:** 1693–1700.

138. Chapman, S., T.R. Southwood, J. Fowler, *et al*. 1994. Rapid changes in magnetic resonance imaging of

muscle during the treatment of juvenile dermatomyositis. *Br. J. Rheumatol.* **33:** 184–186.

139. Davis, P.J.C., C. Ryder, S. Wayte, *et al.* 2003. Use of the novel magnetic resonance image technique of T2 mapping in the monitoring of juvenile dermatomyositis. *Pediatr. Rheumatol. Online Journal,* Number 4, Abstract 121.

140. Maillard, S.M., R. Jones, C. Owens, *et al.* 2004. Quantitative assessment of MRI T2 relaxation time of thigh muscles in juvenile dermatomyositis. *Rheumatology* **43:** 603–608.

141. Park, J.H., J.P. Vansant, N.G. Kumar, *et al.* 1990. Dermatomyositis: Correlative MR imaging and P-31 MR spectroscopy for quantitative characterization of inflammatory disease. *Radiology* **177:** 473–479.

142. Tymms, K.E. & J. Webb. 1985. Dermatomyositis and other connective tissue diseases: A review of 105 cases. *J. Rheumatol.* **12:** 1140–1148.

143. Brown, A.L., J.G. Murray, S.P. Robinson, *et al.* 1996. Case report: Milk of calcium complicating juvenile dermatomyositis—imaging features. *Clin. Radiol.* **51:** 147–149.

144. Mukamel, M., G. Horev & M. Mimouni. 2001. New insight into calcinosis of juvenile dermatomyositis: A study of composition and treatment. *J. Pediatr.* **138:** 763–766.

145. Samson, C., R.L. Soulen & E. Gursel, 2000. Milk of calcium fluid collections in juvenile dermatomyositis: MR characteristics. *Pediatr. Radiol.* **30:** 28–29.

146. Blane, C.E., S.J. White, E.M. Braunstein, *et al.* 1984. Patterns of calcification in childhood dermatomyositis. *AJR Am. J. Roentgenol.* **142:** 397–400.

147. Cohen, P.A., C.H. Job-Deslandre, G. Lalande, *et al.* 2000. Overview of the radiology of juvenile idiopathic arthritis (JIA). *Eur. J. Radiol.* **33:** 94–101.

148. Pettersson, H. & U. Rydolm. 1984. Radiologic classification of knee joint destruction in juvenile chronic arthritis. *Pediatr. Radiol.* **14:** 419–421.

149. Doria, A.S., C.C. de Castro, M.H. Kiss, *et al.* 2003. Inter- and intrareader variability in the interpretation of two radiographic classification systems for ju-

venile rheumatoid arthritis. *Pediatr. Radiol.* **33:** 673–681.

150. Larsen, A., K. Dale & M. Eek. 1977. Radiographic correlation of rheumatoid arthritis and related conditions by standard reference films. *Acta Radiol. Diagn. (Stockholm)* **18:** 481–491.

151. Paus, A.C. & K. Dale. 1993. Arthroscopic and radiographic examination of patients with juvenile rheumatoid arthritis before and after open synovectomy of the knee joint. A prospective study with a 5-year follow-up. *Ann. Chir. Gynaecol.* **82:** 55–61.

152. Sharp, J.T., M.D. Lidsky, L.C. Collins, *et al.* 1971. Methods of scoring the progression of radiologic changes in rheumatoid arthritis. Correlation of radiologic, clinical and laboratory abnormalities. *Arthritis Rheum.* **14:** 706–720.

153. Oen, K., M. Reed, P.N. Mallerson, *et al.* 2003. Radiologic outcome and its relationship to functional disability in juvenile rheumatoid arthritis. *J. Rheumatol.* **30:** 832–840.

154. Pyle, S. & N. Hoerr. 1962. *A Radiographic Atlas of Skeletal Development of the Foot and Ankle.* Charles C. Thomas. Springfield, IL.

155. Nadel, H.R. 2007. Bone scan update. *Sem. Nucl. Med.* **37:** 332–339.

156. Park, J.H., K.J. Niermann, N.M. Ryder, *et al.* 2000. Muscle abnormalities in juvenile dermatomyositis patients. P-31 Magnetic responance spectroscopy studies. *Arthritis Rheum.* **43:** 2359–2367.

157. Workie, D.W., B.J. Dardzinski, T.B. Graham, *et al.* 2004. Quantification of dynamic contrast-enhanced MR imaging of the knee in children with juvenile rheumatoid arthritis based on pharmacokinetic modelling. *Magn. Reson. Imaging* **22:** 1201–1210.

158. Gardner-Medwin, J.M., O.G. Killeen, C.A. Ryder, *et al.* 2006. Magnetic resonance imaging identifies features in clinically unaffected knees predicting extension of arthritis in children with monoarthritis. *J. Rheumatol.* **33:** 2337–2343.

159. Doria, A.S., P.S. Babyn & B. Feldman. 2006. A critical appraisal of radiographic scoring systems for assessment of juvenile idiopathic arthritis. *Pediatr. Radiol.* **36:** 759–772.

A Regional Approach to Foot and Ankle MRI

Michael Sean Stempel

Division of Podiatry, The George Washington University, Washington, DC, USA

This chapter presents a regional anatomic approach to MRI applications in the foot and ankle. From a clinical perspective, patients often describe their symptoms in terms of the part of the foot that hurts and when and how it hurts. Clinical questioning and physical diagnosis pursue this line as well, trying to narrow down the diagnostic possibilities. There are conditions that may blur the anatomic distinctions for forefoot, midfoot, rearfoot, and ankle; involve more than one region of the foot simultaneously; or occur in any area of the foot. The chapter also includes a separate section on the presentations of inflammatory arthritides in foot and ankle joints.

Key words: foot; ankle; metatarsalgia; heel pain; tendon injuries; plantar plate; fracture

Introduction

Bone and soft tissue anatomy is particularly complex within the foot and ankle, which together comprise 30 bones, with 6 major nerves and 11 tendons crossing the ankle joint and multiple muscular layers and compartments. All of these structures are contained within a discrete space evolved uniquely for bipedal ambulation. These factors often make the foot and ankle a challenging diagnostic puzzle and also challenge professionals charged with interpreting and clinically correlating MRI scans. The close proximity of multiple tissue planes both dorsally and plantarly and the sharp angular changes at the ankle and arch make precise positioning vital and interpretation difficult. Consistent positioning protocols, proper coil selection, knowledge of lower-extremity anatomy, detailed clinical information, and experience reading these studies are all essential for obtaining clinically applicable results.

MRI is a useful diagnostic tool in the foot and ankle precisely because of these anatomic and functional complexities. Symptoms arise from arthritides, trauma, systemic disease, and overuse syndromes. Moreover, maladaptive anatomic changes due to faulty biomechanics and poorly functioning shoe gear are often present. Though statistically less common than elsewhere in the body, the foot and ankle can be a site of soft tissue masses. Manifestations of systemic disease often present in the foot. Owing to the superior soft tissue contrast of MRI and its ability to reveal normal and abnormal anatomy in multiple planes, applications for this technology in the foot and ankle have increased over time. MRI both functions as a diagnostic tool and facilitates the planning of treatment for these conditions.

Imaging the Foot and Ankle

Intrinsic difficulties are encountered when performing MRI of the foot and ankle owing to the anatomic configuration of the foot and leg. The anatomy will be distorted if the foot is not positioned at close to 90° to the leg. If the foot is in a plantar-flexed position, axial views of the forefoot produce an oval-shaped appearance of the metatarsal instead of a circular one owing to the obliquity. If the leg is externally rotated (the relaxed position when a person lies supine), the sagittal plane views of the Achilles tendon may falsely reveal thickening,

Address for correspondence: M. S. Stempel, George Washington University, 2150 Pennsylvania Ave NW, Washington, DC 20037, USA. Voice: 202-741-2496; fax: 202-741-2490. mstempel@mfa.gwu.edu

MRI and Ultrasound in Diagnosis and Management: Ann. N.Y. Acad. Sci. 1154: 84–100 (2009).
doi: 10.1111/j.1749-6632.2009.04385.x © 2009 New York Academy of Sciences.

again owing to obliquity. Even with careful positioning of the limb, magic angle artifacts can occur when a tendon's angle is approximately $55°$ to the magnetic field. On T1 images this results in an area of increase signal intensity that does not appear on the T2 image. This artifact can also be corroborated by comparison with the corresponding perpendicular view, which reveals tendon diameter and the presence or absence of fluid within the tendon sheath. A small coil or extremity coil is used to improve spatial resolution.

Pulse sequences of the lower extremity typically include T1- and T2-weighted images in the three standard planes. When detailed clinical information is provided (and it is indicated), only the clinically relevant region of the limb is imaged. This allows narrower-width sections, thus greater anatomic detail. For example, if pathology is suspected in the forefoot, only the distal half of the foot has to be included in the field of view.

Gadolinium contrast media can be helpful when diagnosing infection, differentiating a solid versus a cystic mass, assessing a suspected Morton's neuroma, and evaluating rheumatoid arthritis.

Correlating Clinical Information, Physical Examination, and MRI Evaluation

This chapter presents a regional anatomic approach to MRI applications in the foot and ankle. From a clinical perspective, patients often describe their symptoms in terms of the part of the foot that hurts and when and how it hurts. Clinical questioning and physical diagnosis pursue this line as well, trying to narrow down the diagnostic possibilities. For example, a patient with plantar fasciitis may describe pain in the heel that is noticeable after periods of rest, or a patient with a Morton's neuroma may describe pain in the ball of the foot as feeling like a sock that is bunched beneath the toes.

Forefoot Symptoms

The forefoot is anatomically a densely packed area of the foot and is subject to dramatic weight-bearing forces during the gait cycle. There are also effects due to compression from the shoe toebox, not to mention the effect of high-heeled shoes and obesity. Each metatarsophalangeal (MTP) joint comprises a functionally unique plantar ligament plate, crossed by six tendons and bordered by several neurovascular bundles.

Patients often describe generalized symptoms in the ball of the foot, indicating a broad area of discomfort or pain in the center of the forefoot. They are often unaware that there is one area or joint that is more focally painful until asked to narrow it down, or the site is localized during a physical examination. Exceptions are pain associated with the first MTP joint, especially in the face of a hallux valgus deformity, or hammertoe contractures that rub against the shoe toebox. Key clinical symptom descriptors of forefoot pain include a feeling of a swelling or lump in the ball of the foot, shooting or radiating pain, a localized area of pain, and patterns of radiating pain especially into particular toes.

Physical examination should focus on isolating anatomic structures within the forefoot. The examination should include palpation of the MTP joint structures both dorsally and plantarly; palpation of the intermetatarsal spaces, putting the digits through their ranges of motion; and loading the joints to evaluate for subluxation. It is also useful to have the patient in a weight-bearing position to evaluate for deviation of the digits.

Inflammatory Arthritides

The forefoot is the region of the foot most commonly affected by inflammatory disease

Rheumatoid Arthritis

Inflammatory changes are present in the feet of 90% of rheumatoid patients and are also often found early in the disease process. Erosive joint changes visible on MRIs are generally comparable to those seen on plain film radiographs. Pannus has been reported to have a slightly higher signal on T1-weighted images and may be visualized better with contrast, but this level of detail is not generally clinically significant. Tendonitis or partial tears may be visualized in tendons that overlie inflamed joints.

Rheumatoid nodules are commonly located subcutaneously and can also involve joints, tendons, ligaments, and bursae. Although rheumatoid nodules in the foot represent only 1% of all nodules, they can result in significant symptoms when they are on the plantar surface or are compressed by shoes. MRI findings for rheumatoid nodules are nonspecific. T1-weighted images reveal the masses to be "isointense to muscle," and there may be intense heterogeneous enhancement on T2-weighted images.[1]

Gout and Pseudogout

Standard radiographic findings, together with clinical correlation and labs are sufficient for diagnosis of gout. MRI does not typically have a primary diagnostic role, but may reveal tophaceous changes in patients previously not known to have gout. Tophi are typically low in signal on T1 and T2.

Pigmented Villonodular Synovitis

The condition known as pigmented villonodular synovitis causes synovial hypertrophy with hemosiderin deposits resulting in a darkened appearance of the affected tissue. Tendon sheaths, bursae, and joints may be affected, and the etiology is unknown. MRI findings include joint effusions with low signal enhancement of thickened synovium on T2-weighted images. Erosive and cystic changes of adjacent bone may be present.

Morton's Neuroma/Intermetatarsal Neuroma

Clinical Presentation. An intermetatarsal neuroma, known as a Morton's neuroma, when present in its most common location between the third and fourth MTP joints, is a frequent cause of forefoot pain. The condition is more accurately described as an inflamed schwannoma, not a tumor of the nerve, as the name implies. The etiology of the perineural fibrosis, neural degeneration, and adjacent soft tissue inflammation has been attributed, but not proven, to be caused by chronic nerve entrapment, repetitive trauma, and compression by the adjacent metatarsal heads. There may also be an influence of the anatomic difference in the third intermetatarsal space innervation. Instead of being supplied by a single branch from the medial or lateral plantar nerve as in the other intermetatarsal spaces, there is a joining of a lateral branch of the medial plantar nerve and a medial branch from the lateral plantar nerve in the third intermetatarsal space. The condition is reported more often in women, with women's dress shoes and heel height taking the blame; however, this increased prevalence may be due to frequency of presenting to a physician, not frequency of occurrence.

Presenting symptoms are typically described as a burning, dull, or throbbing pain in the ball of the foot, and often as a sharp or electric radiating sensation into the third and fourth toes. Similar symptoms attributed to the second and third toes suggest a neuroma between the second and third MTP joints. This is an infrequent occurrence and has to be differentiated from a plantar plate tear, predislocation syndrome of the second MTP joint, or excessive weight-bearing loading of the second metatarsal.

MRI Findings. The appearance of an intermetatarsal neuroma on MRI is typically as a teardrop-shaped soft tissue mass between the metatarsal heads that projects inferiorly into the plantar subcutaneous fat pad. Signal intensity is intermediate on T1-weighted images and usually low on T2-weighted images owing to adjacent fibrosis.[2] Radiology literature reports findings indicating fluid within the intermetatarsal bursa when it is inflamed; however, intraoperative findings and postsurgical

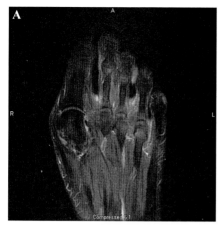 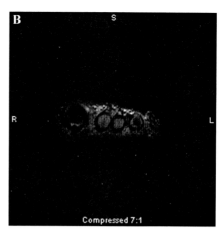

Figure 1. Morton's neuroma: An oblong low signal mass is seen between the third and fourth metatarsal heads on the coronal T2 fast spin-echo with fat-saturation images. The Morton's neuroma does not enhance significantly on the axial T1-weighted images with fat saturation after gadolinium administration, making it difficult to visualize.

pathology reports do not commonly relate the presence of a bursal structure. The use of contrast can enhance imaging of this lesion, with diffuse uptake within the mass seen when a neuroma is present (Fig. 1A, B).[3]

Plantar Plate Disruption/Lesser Metatarsophalangeal Joint Predislocation Syndrome

Clinical Presentation. This condition, only recently delineated as a clinical entity, is often not appreciated in its early stages or is misdiagnosed. Its presentation can mimic an interdigital neuroma, a plantar soft tissue mass, stress fractures, and generalized pain in the ball of the foot dubbed "metatarsalgia." Patients describe a broad area of pain involving the central portion of the ball of the foot and often the sensation, but not the presence, of a lump or swelling plantarly in this area. A change in the alignment of their toes with splaying, mild swelling, or their toe no longer touching the ground when standing may be noted.

This condition most commonly presents in the second MTP joint. The increased prevalence of presentation in this location has been attributed to factors resulting in excessive loading of the second ray during gait. Examples of these factors include restricted range of motion in the first MTP joint due to hallux rigidus, diminished propulsion due to hallux valgus, the first metatarsal functioning in a dorsiflexed position in propulsion, and an excessively long second metatarsal relative to the length of the first. Predisposing conditions may include synovitis of the MTP due to rheumatoid arthritis, spondyloarthropathies, and poorly designed or badly chosen shoes.

Clinical findings differ with progression of the condition. Initially, in the predislocation phase, there is inflammation of the MTP joint. Subtle splaying of the affected toe from the adjacent one may be observed with mild edema at the base of the toe. Dorsal subluxation of the toe with resultant lack of purchase on the ground when standing occurs when the plantar plate of the MTP becomes attenuated or ruptured near the insertion into the base of the proximal phalanx. With progression of the condition, the toe continues to sublux dorsally and ultimately often deviates medially, crossing over the hallux. The Lachman drawer test, pushing the proximal phalanx dorsally while holding the metatarsal in a fixed position, will reveal subluxation as well as pain in the plantar plate in a positive test.[4]

MRI Findings/Application. Imaging of the MTP shows the plantar plate best in the sagittal and

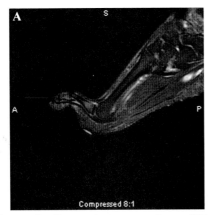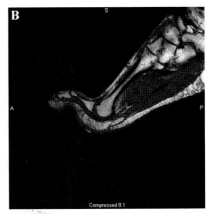

Figure 2. Plantar plate rupture: Sagittal T1 and sagittal T2 fast spin-echo with fat-saturation images of the forefoot at the level of the second MTP joint show discontinuity of the low signal plantar plate at the distal aspect of the joint.

coronal planes. T1-weighted images may reveal edema within the joint, attenuation, a tear in the plantar plate, and dorsal displacement of the digit. On T2-weighted images the normal plantar plate is a curvilinear low-signal structure. When torn, the plate appears discontinuous with an increased T2 signal at the site of the tear. T sagittal plane perspective may reveal increased signal intensity in the plantar aspect of the joint compatible with edema or disruption of the plantar plate ligament. There may also be associated tenosynovitis. Important MRI findings in the differential diagnosis of this condition include metatarsal stress fractures, intermetatarsal neuromas, and plantar or intermetatarsal soft tissue masses (Fig. 2A, B).

First MTP Joint Pain

Hallux valgus deformities and arthritic changes in the first MTP joint would rarely require the use of MRI as a primary diagnostic tool. However, significant changes may be noted within this joint incidentally when evaluating for other conditions or in the presence of various inflammatory arthritides such as rheumatoid arthritis, gout, and osteoarthritis. MRI is a useful modality for diagnosis of sesamoiditis, sesamoid fractures, and sesamoid dislocation/subluxation (turf toe).

Sesamoiditis

Clinical Presentations. Symptoms of pain in the plantar aspect of the first MTP joint can present acutely, and standard radiographs are utilized to reveal a sesamoidal fracture. However, for evaluation of long-standing pain in this region of the joint or when a fracture is not evident, MRI can assist in differentiating among osteonecrosis, stress fractures, and localized inflammation, as well as distinguishing between an acute fracture and a bipartite sesamoid.

MRI Findings/Applications. Marrow edema within a sesamoid bone may be noted by increased signal intensity on T2-weighted images and a decreased signal on T1-weighted images. Osteonecrosis is revealed by low signal intensity on both T1- and T2-weighted images. Fractures appear as a distinct linear area of low signal intensity on T1- and high or low intensity on T2-weighted images.[5]

Turf Toe

This hyperextension injury of the first MTP joint results in a sprain of the plantar ligament complex. The injury may also result in a sesamoid or phalangeal base fracture. Axial or sagittal MRIs would reveal increased signal in the plantar capsule on T2-weighted images.[6]

Bursitis: Plantar, Intermetatarsal

A bursa within the forefoot may be revealed by axial T2-weighted or STIR images. Bursae appear with high signal intensity and enhance with contrast. Typically these bursae are located plantar to the deep transverse intermetatarsal ligament and within the intermetatarsal space and are found accompanying neuromas or inflamed joints.[7]

Midfoot Symptoms

When a patient presents with a chief concern of pain in the arch or midfoot, there is, as with the forefoot, a broad range of anatomic structures that may be responsible for the symptoms. Moreover, the symptoms may have their origin in a different region of the foot. It is beneficial to have the patient try to pinpoint an area of intensity or the site of onset and try to correlate symptoms to weight bearing, gait, or shoe pressure. Symptoms related by the patient include soreness in the arch when walking, deeper symptoms within the joints of the midfoot complex, localized swelling or soreness in this region of the foot, and pain that radiates distally or proximally.

Soft Tissue Structures

The midfoot/arch is the most common region in the foot for the presence of soft tissue masses, ganglion cysts, and plantar fascia fibromas. The extensor synovial sheaths cross the tarsometatarsal joints here. Underlying arthritic changes in the joints of the midfoot, compression from shoe gear, and direct trauma to the dorsal aspect of the foot can result in injury to the overlying extensor tendons, tendon sheaths, and cutaneous nerves. Moreover, there are several notable tendon insertions functionally important in gait: the tibialis anterior and tibialis posterior at the navicular; the peroneous brevis at the fifth metatarsal base; and the peroneous longus, which inserts plantar to the tarsometarsal

joints medially after wrapping beneath the cuboid.

Plantar Fibromatosis

Plantar fibromatosis lesions are fibrous connective tissue nodules that proliferate along the medial band plantar fascia as single or multiple lesions. They appear with low to intermediate signal intensity on T1- and T2-weighted sequences and usually enhance with contrast. If the lesions are symptomatic adjacent tissue edema may be present, with increased signal intensity indicating inflammation (Fig. 3A, B, C).

Ganglion Cysts

Ganglion cysts can appear in any region of the foot and are most commonly found in regions with synovial tendon sheaths, such as the dorsal foot and the anterior, medial, and lateral ankle. Clinical symptoms associated with these cysts are often due to compression of adjacent nerves, rubbing of the lesion against shoe gear, and concern over the appearance of a possible soft tissue tumor. T2-weighted images demonstrate high intensity within the cyst. T1-weighted fat-suppressed contrast images show no enhancement, indicating a cyst.[8] Enhancement of the thin cyst wall and septations may be seen, if present (Fig. 4A, B).

Tenosynovitis

Tenosynovitis can occur anywhere there are synovial sheaths surrounding tendons within the foot and ankle. This inflammatory condition, which causes fluid to surround the circumference of the tendon, may occur owing to stress on the tendon. Etiologies include stress due to repetitive motion or overuse, inflammatory arthritis, or infection. Stenosing tenosynovitis occurs when there are loculated collections of synovial fluid within the tendon sheath. In the foot this is most commonly seen in the flexor hallucis brevis.

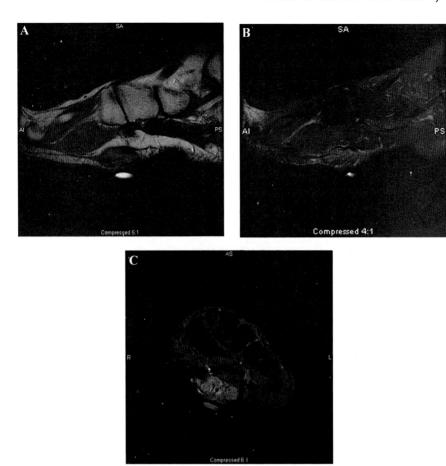

Figure 3. Plantar fibromatosis: Sagittal T1 and T2 fast spin-echo with fat-saturation images show a lobulated soft tissue mass in the plantar soft tissues. The mass is low signal on T1 images with regions of high signal intensity on T2 images. Contrast enhancement, which can be variable in plantar fibromatosis, was seen in this patient

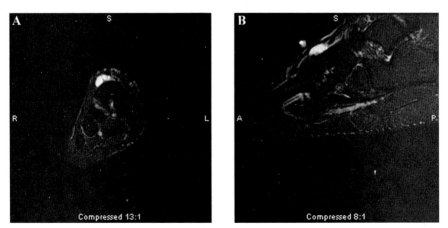

Figure 4. Ganglion cyst: Coronal T2 fast spin-echo with fat-saturation and sagittal STIR images of the foot demonstrate a well-defined, slightly lobulated mass dorsal to the middle cuneiform. On the sagittal image it is seen at the level of the marker placed on the patient's skin denoting the site of the palpable mass. The mass is bright on both sequences, consistent with a fluid-filled ganglion cyst.

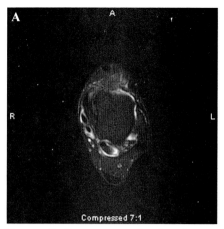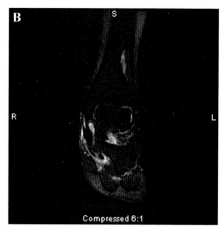

Figure 5. Tenosynovitis: Axial and coronal T2 fast spin-echo with fat-saturation images at the ankle show high T2 signal compatible with fluid surrounding all of the medial tendons at the ankle. The tendons themselves appear normal. The findings represent tenosynovitis.

MRI findings in the presence of tenosynovitis are that there is fluid of low signal intensity on T1-weighted images and high signal intensity on T2-weighted images, that synovial fluid is seen circumferentially around the tendon, and that the tendon may be normal or abnormal in diameter and signal intensity (Fig. 5A, B).[9]

Skeletal Structures

Skeletal origins of midfoot pain include metatarsal stress fractures, navicular fractures, accessory navicular bones, Lis Franc's joint dislocation, avulsion injuries in the tarsometatarsal joints, and arthritic changes in the tarsometatarsal joints.

Metatarsal Stress and Insufficiency Fractures

Stress fractures in the foot most commonly appear in the neck or shaft of metatarsals two, three, and four; however, these fractures can also occur in the metatarsal bases, navicular, and calcaneus. High-energy or abnormal repetitive loading of the normal bone induces stress fractures. Normal levels of activity applied to abnormal bone induce insufficiency fractures. The clinical presentation is typically that of pain in the forefoot or midfoot with weight bearing. There may be accompanying localized edema, erythema, or calor. A diagnosis is usually made by plain film radiographs; however, the cortical break and early callus formation is only evident after approximately 2 weeks. The diagnosis can be made earlier, or in cases with strong clinical suspicion without radiographic findings, with use of a radionucleotide bone scan or an MRI. The latter will reveal an area of low intensity signal on T1 and high intensity on T2 or STIR images. With progression, the fracture line and bone callus become visible. In the elderly or osteoporotic patient, MRI is more sensitive and specific than radionucleotide scans (Fig. 6A, B, C).[10]

Accessory Navicular

An accessory navicular bone can cause symptoms due to degenerative changes or trauma to the fibroligamentous attachment with the primary navicular bone. MRIs that reveal increased marrow edema, evident in coronal and sagittal STIR images, correlate with degenerative changes in this articulation. In the presence of a symptomatic accessory navicular bone, the posterior tibial tendon should be evaluated for tears.[11]

Lis Franc's Injuries

Trauma significant enough to result in joint dislocation or avulsion of the tarsometatarsal

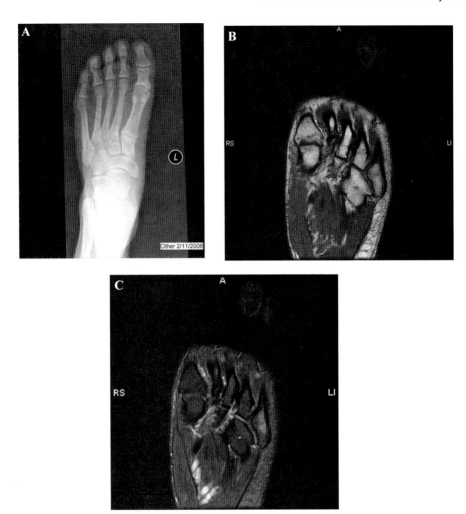

Figure 6. Metatarsal stress fractures: AP view of the foot demonstrates subtle transverse lucent lines through the proximal shafts of the second and fifth metatarsals. The line at the fifth metatarsal is best visualized at the lateral cortex. Axial T1 and axial T2 fast spin-echo with fat-saturation images show a linear low-signal fracture line in the proximal aspect of the fifth metatarsal with surrounding bone marrow edema, which is dark on T1-weighted images and bright on T2-weighted images. A similar appearing stress fracture was seen in the second metatarsal on MRI.

ligaments requires significant force. Plain film radiographs are usually sufficient to diagnosis these injuries. Subtle injuries to Lis Franc's joint can be missed on plain film radiographs. In the case of the neuropathic diabetic patient, Charcot osteoarthropathy may be missed until there is complete joint collapse. Coronal and axial T2 and STIR images may demonstrate disruption of ligaments or displacement at the metatarsal cuneiform joints. In a case of early

Charcot joint (neurotrophic osteoarthropathy), changes are typically of low signal intensity in the bone marrow on T1, T2, and STIR images. In a case of complete joint fragmentation and/or collapse, acute inflammation manifests as high signal intensity with marrow and tissue edema on T2-weighted images.[8] Differentiation from osteomyelitis in this phase may be difficult without an accurate clinical history.

Rearfoot Symptoms

As above, there is considerable overlap of symptoms among regions of the foot. Some patient-described symptoms can be clearly identified as rearfoot, such as plantar or posterior heel pain. However, posterior tibial tendon tears can result in symptoms that localize from the medial malleolus to the navicular, or, in another example, tarsal tunnel syndrome can cause symptoms along the entire plantar aspect of the foot though its origin is at the junction of the foot and ankle. For the purposes of this section, rearfoot pain encompasses symptoms that typically are described by patients as being within the hindfoot.

Plantar Calcaneal Pain: Plantar Fasciitis

Patients typically present with pain in the plantar heel that manifests after periods of rest, especially upon rising after sleep. Initial walking activity usually eases the symptoms temporarily, but then they intensify with prolonged weight bearing. This condition has been attributed to repetitive weight-bearing stress exacerbated by hyperpronation, worn out or poorly made shoes, obesity, intensive sports activities, flatfootedness, or several of these factors combined. Seronegative arthritides such as anklylosing spondylitis, reactive arthritis, psoriatic arthritis, as well as rheumatoid arthritis and gout should all be included in the broad list of differential diagnoses for heel pain. Pain with palpation elicited at the medial calcaneal tubercle plantarly, just distal to the weight-bearing surface, is indicative of insertional fasciitis or fasciosis. Plantar tenderness more proximal than the fascial attachment suggests infracalcaneal bursitis, whereas pain with medial and lateral compression of the heel may indicate a calcaneal stress fracture. In some cases inflammation may be present along the length of the medial band of the plantar fascia, and may have to be differentiated from flexor hallucis longus tendonitis. One should also check for accompanying insertional tenderness of the posterior tibial tendon at the navicular.

MRI of plantar fasciitis is rarely indicated as a primary diagnostic tool, as clinical history and physical examination nearly always lead to a diagnosis of the condition. Should MRIs be sought owing to diagnostic complexities such as lack of clinical response or concomitant diagnoses, the images would reveal thickening (normally 4 mm) of the fascia near its calcaneal insertion, intermediate signal on T1 and high signal on T2.[9] Adjacent tissue edema may be present, with erosions or spur formation at the calcaneus. Rupture of the plantar fascia is rare, but if suspected is best diagnosed with MRI. A fascial rupture is apparent as a separation of the ligament with accompanying edema and hemorrhage, seen as a high signal on T2 images. Calcaneal stress fracture should also be ruled out when evaluating these studies and images should be evaluated for inflamed bursae plantar posteriorly (Fig. 7A, B).

Posterior Calcaneal Pain

Achilles Tendonitis

Tendonitis of the Achilles tendon typically arises from mechanical origins; however, it can also be attributable to multiple arthritides such as rheumatoid arthritis and the spondyloarthropathies. The patient's pain is typically increased after periods of rest and initially decreases with activity. Pain is typically aggravated by dorsiflexing the foot at the ankle, as well as with pressure, with palpation at the calcaneal insertion, or with compression of the tendon between two fingers. The inflammatory changes have been attributed to degenerative changes within the body of the tendon and tendonosis is a more accurate term. The Achilles tendon does not have a synovial sheath. The paratenon is present along the anterior surface of the tendon. Edema visualized on MRIs in this region corresponds to inflammation of this structure, as opposed to tenosynovitis. Advanced degenerative changes or partial tears and ruptures typically occur within a region

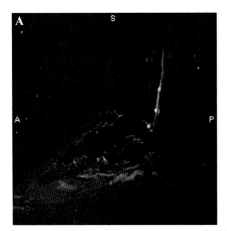 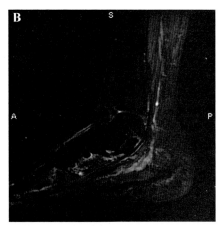

Figure 7. Plantar fasciitis: Two sagittal STIR images show mild thickening of the proximal portion of the plantar fascia near its insertion on the calcaneus. Signal intensity changes are seen in the adjacent subcutaneous soft tissues with increased signal on the STIR images.

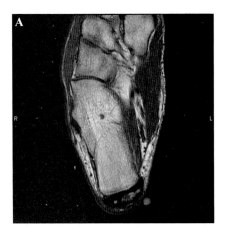 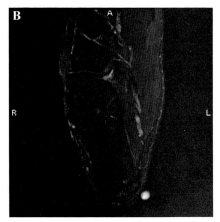

Figure 8. Partial tear of the Achilles tendon: Axial T1 and axial T2 fast spin-echo with fat-saturation images demonstrate thickening of the Achilles tendon with intrasubstance high signal on the T1- and T2-weighted images at the insertion compatible with partial thickness tear.

4 cm proximal to the calcaneal insertion. Retrocalcaneal bursitis and erosive bone changes at the tendon insertion can accompany the condition.

Normal tendon anatomy is revealed on sagittal and axial T1- and T2-weighted images as well as on STIR axial and sagittal images. In axial images the tendon should appear flat or somewhat concave on the anterior surface. A convex appearance indicates abnormal thickening of the tendon. The anterior and posterior surfaces should appear parallel on properly positioned sagittal images.[12] The plantaris tendon is located anteromedially to the Achilles tendon

and can be mistaken for a partially torn Achilles tendon. Tendon changes that may be present include an acute complete tear, an acute partial tear, a chronic partial tear, and tendonosis (Fig. 8A, B).

Retrocalcaneal and Pre-Achilles Bursitis

Inflammation of the retrocalcaneal bursa is revealed with deep palpation of the space anterior to the Achilles tendon just proximal to the calcaneal insertion. Pressing medially and laterally, just proximal to the dorsal calcaneus and anterior to the Achilles tendon, produces pain. MRI findings on sagittal T1-weighted images

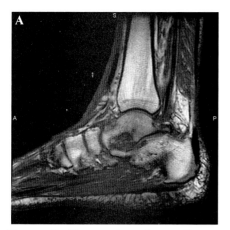 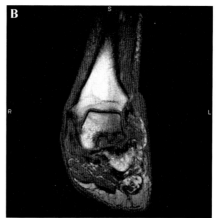

Figure 9. Sinus tarsi syndrome: On sagittal and coronal T1-weighted images there is obliteration of fat in the sinus tarsi. The normally high-signal fat seen on T1 imaging is replaced with fluid or scar tissue that is lower in signal intensity on these images. In advanced cases, associated osteoarthritis at the subtalar joints with subchondral cysts, as was seen in this patient, can occur.

may reveal bone erosion, and T2-weighted images would reveal high-intensity signal corresponding to an enlarged bursa. There may be accompanying Achilles tendon changes such as thickening, inflammation, or calcification in these images.

The pre-Achilles (retro-Achilles) bursa is located subcutaneously, superficial to the Achilles insertion and is tender to light palpation. This bursa is typically aggravated by pressure from the shoe heel counter. Sagittal and axial T2-weighted images reveal signal intensity within the bursae when they are inflamed.

Accompanying the above conditions may be a Haglund's deformity and enlargement of the posteriosuperior calcaneus. This has also been dubbed a "pump-bump" deformity, which often results in inflammation of the pre-Achilles bursae.

Rearfoot Pain

Sinus Tarsi Syndrome

Patients with sinus tarsi syndrome relate lateral foot pain and a feeling of instability in the heel. The condition most commonly occurs as a result of trauma, typically inversion injuries. Inflammatory arthritides, gout, ganglion cysts,

and structural foot deformities are responsible for about 30% of cases. Palpation of the sinus tarsi typically produces pain, and as deep pressure on this space is often perceived as uncomfortable, the clinician should palpate the contralateral sinus tarsi for comparison. The sinus is formed by the space between the talus and the calcaneous laterally. The shape of this canal is wide laterally and tapers medially. Within this space is a fatty plug, a neurovascular bundle that contributes to proprioception in the rearfoot and five ligaments. The most functionally important of these is the talocalcaneal ligament. It has been determined that injury to the ligaments and/or the nerve within the canal is responsible for the symptoms of pain and instability.

Abnormalities within the sinus tarsi are revealed on sagittal and coronal MRIs. T1 images reveal fat obliteration, with intermediate signal instead of high signal with a visible talocalcaneal ligament passing through it, as expected. T2 images reveal inflammatory changes with high signal or chronic fibrosis with low signal (Fig. 9A, B).

Tarsal Tunnel Syndrome

Entrapment or compression of the posterior tibial nerve within the tarsal tunnel can result in plantar symptoms in the heel, forefoot, and the midfoot. In some cases there can be pain in the medial ankle as well. Described symptoms include burning, tingling, electric shooting sensations, and a viselike pressure on the ball of the foot. Anatomically, the tarsal tunnel extends from just proximal to the medial malleolus and then courses distally to the abductor hallucis muscle belly. It is bordered by the flexor retinaculum superficially and the calcaneus on the deep surface. Within this space course the posterior tibial nerve, artery, and vein; the posterior tibial tendon; the flexor digitorum longus tendon; and the flexor hallucis longus tendon. Compression of the posterior tibial nerve as it passes within this space can be due to ganglion cysts, varicosities in the accompanying vein, synovial thickening or tumors in the sheaths of the neighboring tendons, post-traumatic bone or ligament changes; it has also been attributed to hyperpronatory foot types.[13]

The initial diagnosis is made from the patient's history and a physical examination. Percussion of the posterior tibial nerve may result in a Tinel's sign, and sustained dorsiflexion and eversion of the foot may trigger pain symptoms. Nerve conduction velocity testing of the posterior tibial nerve may reveal diminished conduction velocity distal to the tarsal tunnel. MRI is useful when trying to determine etiology, specifically when a space-occupying lesion is suspected. Ganglion cysts and nerve sheath changes are among the most common abnormal MRI findings, both appearing as a homogeneous low signal on T1-weighted images and high signal intensity on T2-weighted images. Use of gadolinium contrast assists in distinguishing between a cyst and changes in the nerve sheath.

Tarsal Coalitions

Coalition of the tarsal bones is present in 2–6% of the population, and is present bilaterally in 50% of cases. Osseous, cartilaginous, or fibrous coalition of the calcaneonavicular joint is the most common, followed by the talocalcaneal joint, with these two accounting for 90% of cases. Symptoms are typically due to disruption of a fibrocartilaginous bridge or fracture of an osseous bridge. Severe pain with motion within the rearfoot may result in spasm of the peroneal musculature and a resultant flatfoot deformity. Initial diagnosis is by characteristic plain film radiographic findings: talar beaking, elongation of the anteriosuperior calcaneus, an osseous bar between bones, and obliteration of calcaneal facets. CT and MRI provide detailed images of the coalition type and anatomic location of the coalition. MRI has the advantage of also revealing accompanying areas of inflammation or impingement. Osseous coalitions produce signal intensity of the bone marrow, low signal on T1 and T2 with fibrous coalitions, and an intermediate signal with cartilaginous coalitions.[8]

Ankle Symptoms

Again, as above, there is considerable overlap of symptoms between the ankle and other regions of the foot. Changes may occur in various structures at the ankle level anatomically and continue into the rearfoot and midfoot or present with symptoms in these more distal regions.

Soft Tissue: Tendonitis

There are four groupings of tendons at the ankle, with 11 tendons crossing the ankle joint: the long flexors and posterior tibial medially, the peroneals laterally, and the tibialis anterior and long extensors anteriorly. The Achilles and plantaris tendons also pass the ankle joint posteriorly, but they have already been discussed. With the exception of the Achilles tendon, all of the ankle tendons are within synovial sheathes. MRI evaluation of these sheathed tendons is similar in all cases, but the posterior tibial, flexor hallucis longus, and peroneal tendons have the greatest clinical significance and receive special attention here. Tendons in the foot and ankle may undergo degenerative changes, tear, or develop synovitis owing to the same host of reasons encountered throughout the body; however, the repetitive stress and microtrauma on key functional tendons in gait are often of clinical significance in both evaluation and treatment of these conditions. Conditions that have been attributed to tendon tears and degeneration include acute trauma, rheumatoid arthritis, diabetes, gout, medications, tumors, xanthomas, and calcific tendonitis.

MRI reveals tendon pathology best in transverse plane images. The exception to this is the Achilles tendon, which is also well imaged in the sagittal plane. Contrast use is not typically indicated. Normal tendon anatomy is revealed as low signal intensity on T1-weighted images owing to water molecules being tightly held by the tendon substrate. Increased signal may be noted at the point of tendon insertion or owing to the fusing of several tendons or the magic angle effect. The synovial sheath is not normally visible and the tendon should appear uniformly round, oval, or flat. When tendon abnormalities are present, changes are seen on T2-weighted images. Specifically these may include high signal within the tendon, suggesting degeneration or partial tear, and high signal around the tendon circumferentially, indicating synovitis. Other findings in symptomatic tendons include complete separation of the tendon, anatomic subluxation, deposits within the tendon (calcium hydroxyapatite, calcium pyrophosphate crystals, gouty tophi, xanthomas), and tumors (giant cell tumor, clear cell sarcoma).[9]

Medial Ankle Tendons

Posterior Tibial Tendon

The posterior tibial tendon is a powerful inverter of the foot that stabilizes the midtarsal joints during gait. When function in this tendon is diminished owing to inflammatory or degenerative changes, unopposed pronatory forces result in progressive dysfunction and arch collapse. Posterior tibial tendon symptomatology shows an increased prevalence in patients with rheumatoid arthritis. However, it is difficult to differentiate between tendon changes that are due to arthritic changes in the rearfoot and those that are caused by inflammatory tendon dysfunction that has resulted in subtalar joint collapse.[14]

The typical clinical presentation and progression of what has been called "posterior tibial tendon dysfunction" syndrome is as follows. Initially pain and localized clinical signs of inflammation present along the course of the posterior tibial tendon at the medial malleolus or navicular insertion. Tears and deformity are not present at this stage, with typical MRI findings being of tenosynovitis. With progression due to continued overuse, increased signal intensity within the tendon may be seen on T1 images with eventual appearance of tendon tears. T2-weighted images demonstrate increased fluid within the tendon sheath.

Clinically, signs of inflammation increase greatly and there may be a lowering of the arch, as tendon integrity is lost. T2 axial views at the ankle best reveal partial tears and surrounding fluid. Progression to a complete tear is not as common as the loss of tendon function and collapse of the foot into a pes-valgo planus attitude. With loss of muscular function, the calcaneus maintains an everted position when bearing weight. When the patient attempts a single-limb heel raise on the affected limb, the heel does not invert as it would normally. Late-stage progression results in degenerative changes in the rearfoot, chronic pain, and a fixed flatfoot deformity. Complete tears of the posterior tibial tendon, whether as a result of trauma or degenerative processes, appear as a gap on axial and sagittal images with surrounding inflammation. With collapse of the arch, the presence of the plantar calcaneonavicular ligament (spring ligament) should be confirmed on short TE spin-echo axial and sagittal images (Fig. 10A, B).[15]

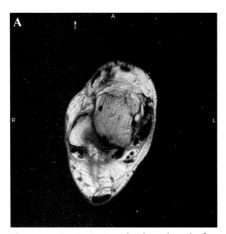
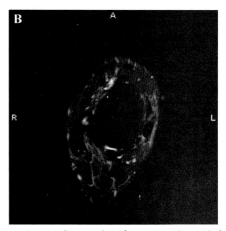

Figure 10. Posterior tibial tendon dysfunction: On axial T1 and T2 fast spin-echo with fat-saturation images the posterior tibialis tendon is enlarged. Linear intrasubstance high signal intensity seen on the T1-weighted image represents a partial tear of the tendon.

Flexor Digitorum Longus

The flexor digitorum longus courses deep to the posterior tibial tendon and superficial to the neurovascular bundle. This tendon is an uncommon source of clinical symptoms. Synovial changes could potentially lead to compression of the posterior tibial nerve.

Flexor Hallucis Longus (FHL)

This medial tendon is rarely injured and seldom a source of clinical symptoms, but it may be stressed by certain activities such as soccer or ballet. Tenosynovitis may be seen at the level of the sesamoids plantar to the first MTP joint or as it passes posterior to the talus. Caution is indicated in diagnosing synovitis of this tendon, as communication of the tendon sheath and the ankle joint posteriorly has a prevalence of 20%. This anatomic characteristic can result in a greater presence of fluid surrounding the FHL in the absence of tendon pathology. Asymmetrical fluid accumulation would indicate stenosing tenosynovitis. This condition can occur when an os trigonum (accessory ossicle at the posterior talus) is present. T2-weighted images in the axial and sagittal planes best reveal fluid surrounding the FHL tendon.

Lateral Ankle Tendons: Peroneal Tendons

MRI of the peroneal tendons is typically performed to evaluate for tenosynovitis and tendon tears or to reveal a subluxed tendon position. The peroneal brevis tendon, coursing behind the head of the fibula, above the peroneal tubercle of the calcaneus, and inserting into the base of the fifth metatarsal, is a powerful everter of the foot. The peroneus longus tendon shares a common tendon sheath as it passes superficially to the peroneus brevis behind and beneath the fibular head. Distal to the superior retinaculum they have their own tendon sheathes. When the limb is in the gait cycle, the peroneus brevis assists in pronation of the foot. The peroneus longus tendon has been described as both a pronator/everter of the foot and as a supinator. The longus tendon inserts on the medial side of the foot, beneath the first metatarsal–medial cuneiform joint, after coursing beneath the cuboid. In closed kinetic chain motion (heel and forefoot on the ground) the longus tendon supinates the foot by plantar-flexing the first ray. In open kinetic chain motion (the heel off of the ground and forefoot weight bearing) the longus tendon may result in eversion while continuing to exert a

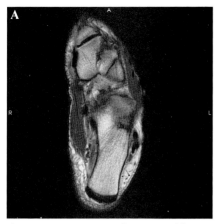
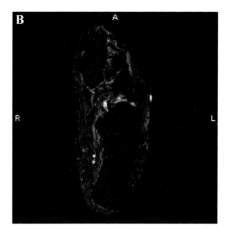

Figure 11. Peroneus brevis and longus tears: Axial T1 and T2 fast spin-echo with fat-saturation images at the level of the hindfoot show splits of the peroneus brevis and longus tendons. The partial tears give the tendons an irregular appearance, which is best appreciated on the T2-weighted image.

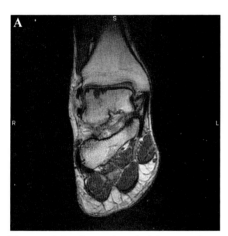
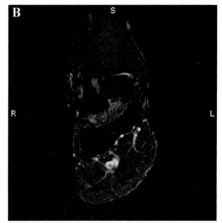

Figure 12. Osteochondral lesion: Coronal T1 and coronal T2 fast spin-echo with fat-saturation images of the ankle demonstrate abnormal bone marrow signal at the lateral talar dome. There are several areas of decreased T1 signal and increased T2 signal in the subchondral bone with preservation of the overlying articular cartilage compatible with a Stage 1 osteochondral injury.

plantar-flexory force on the first ray. When the foot is being thrown into excessive inversion that may result in an ankle sprain, the peroneal muscles, particularly the brevis, activate and strongly contract to regain balance. This action may be responsible for some incidences of synovitis, tendon tears, tendon subluxation, and avulsion fractures at the fifth metatarsal base. T2-weighted axial images may best reveal subluxations or dislocation of the lateral tendons (Fig. 11A, B).

Anterior Ankle Tendons: Tibialis Anterior, Extensor Hallucis, and Digitorum Longus

Tenosynovitis, tears, or ruptures infrequently affect these synovial tendons. As with other tendons, imaging is best accomplished with T2-weighted or STIR in the axial and sagittal planes.

Osteochondral injuries to the cartilage of the talar dome result from inversion or eversion sprains at the ankle. Strong rotational forces that result in ligament sprains or tears can result in contusion or fractures of the subchondral bone of the talus, within the ankle mortise. The Berndt–Hardy classification stages these injuries based on the depth of the lesion and the displacement of the resultant fragment. The clinical presentation is persistent ankle pain and diffuse edema at the joint, usually with a history of prior ankle trauma. MRI detects these lesions well in all stages, whereas plain film radiographs may not reveal changes in the early stages. T2-weighted images show breaks in the cartilage continuity, missing or displaced fragments, and high signal intensity around nondisplaced fragments (Fig. 12A, B).[16]

Conflicts of Interest

The authors declare no conflicts of interest.

References

1. Sanders, T.G., R. Linares & A. Su. 1998. Rheumatoid nodules of the foot. MRI appearances mimicking an indeterminate soft tissue mass. *Skeletal Radiol.* **27:** 457–460.
2. Zanetti, M., T. Ledermann, H. Zollinger & J. Hodler. 1997. Efficacy of MR imaging in patients suspected of having Morton's neuroma. *AJR Am. J. Roentgenol.* **168:** 529–532.
3. Terk, M.R., P.K. Kwong, M. Suthar, *et al*. 1992. Morton's neuroma: Evaluation with MR imaging performed with contrast enhancement and fat suppression. *Radiology* **189:** 239–241.
4. Yu, G.V., M.S. Judge, *et al*. 2002. Predislocation syndrome. *J. Am. Podiatr. Med. Assoc.* **92:** 182–199.
5. Taylor, J.A.M., D.J. Sartoris, G. Huang, *et al*. 1993. Painful conditions of the first metatarsal sesamoid bones. *Radiographics* **13:** 817–830.
6. Zanetti, M., S.C.L. Steiner, B. Seifert, *et al*. 2002. Clinical outcomes of edema-like bone marrow abnormalities of the foot. *Radiology* **222:** 184–188.
7. Yu, J.S. & J.R. Tanner. 2002. Considerations in metatarsalgia and midfoot pain: An MR imaging perspective. *Sem. Musculoskeletal Radiol.* **6:** 91–104.
8. Berquist, T.H. 2006. *MRI of the Musculoskeletal System*, 5th ed.: 499, 515. Lippincott Williams & Wilkins. Philadelphia.
9. Kaplan, P.A. *et al*. 2001. *Musculoskeletal MRI*, 1st ed.: 58–59, 410–413. W.B. Saunders. Philadelphia.
10. Dunfee, W.R., M.K. Dalinka & J.B. Kneeland. 2002. Imaging of athletic injuries to the foot and ankle. *Radiol. Clin. North Am.* **40:** 289–312.
11. Miller, T.T., R.B. Staron, F. Feldman, *et al*. 1995. The symptomatic accessory tarsal navicular bone: Assessment with MR imaging. *Radiology* **195:** 849–853.
12. Miller, T.T., R.B. Staron, F. Feldman, *et al*. 1995. The symptomatic accessory tarsal navicular bone: Assessment with MR imaging. *Radiology* **195:** 849–853.
13. Jenkins, W.J. 2004. Approach to the patient with foot and ankle pain. In *Current Rheumatology Diagnosis and Treatment*. J.B. Imboden *et al*. Eds.: 51–65. McGraw-Hill Professional. New York.
14. Michelson, J., M. Easley, F.M. Wigley & D. Hellman. 1995. Posterior tibial tendon dysfunction in rheumatoid arthritis. *Foot Ankle Int.* **16:** 156–161.
15. Yao, L., A. Gentili & A. Cracchiolo. 1999. MR imaging findings in spring ligament insufficiency. *Skeletal Radiol.* **28:** 245–250.
16. Magee, T.H. & G.W. Hinon. 1998. Usefulness of MR imaging in the detection of talar dome injuries. *AJR Am. J. Roentgenol.* **170:** 1227–1230.

Magnetic Resonance Imaging of the Idiopathic Inflammatory Myopathies

Structural and Clinical Aspects

Rodolfo Victor Curiel,[a] **Robert Jones,**[b] **and Kathleen Brindle**[c]

Departments of [a]*Medicine,* [b]*Pathology, and* [c]*Radiology, The George Washington University, Washington, DC, USA*

Idiopathic inflammatory myopathies are chronic diseases clinically characterized by symmetrical proximal muscle weakness. MRI has assumed a major role in the evaluation and management of these conditions. It is sensitive to the presence of inflammation and edema, especially with incorporation of fat suppression sequences, so it is a useful tool for establishing an early diagnosis, for evaluating the extent and number of lesions, and for determining the right site for biopsy. The noninvasive nature of the procedure makes it ideal for serial studies to evaluate response to treatment. Whole-body MRI can scan a large volume of muscles without prolonged acquisition time and has the potential to identify previously unsuspected sites of involvement. MRI is also an excellent technique for identifying areas of fatty infiltration within the muscles, which usually occurs in the late stages of inflammatory myopathies. In summary, MRI has revolutionized the way muscular diseases are diagnosed and treated.

Key words: MRI; inflammatory myopathies; myopathy

Introduction

Idiopathic inflammatory myopathies (IIM) are chronic systemic connective tissue diseases that are clinically characterized by symmetrical proximal muscle weakness. Although the IIMs share the characteristics of immune-mediated attacks on skeletal muscle with mononuclear cell infiltration, fiber degeneration, and regeneration on pathological examination, they are in fact heterogeneous diseases with distinct histopathological and clinical characteristics. Dermatomyositis is thought to result from humorally mediated vascular injury, with perivascular inflammation and perifascicular atrophy being its most characteristic features. Vessel thrombosis, fiber necrosis, and regeneration can also be seen. In contrast, polymyositis and inclusion body myositis (IBM) are thought to involve cytotoxic T cells in their pathogenesis. In polymyositis, CD8-positive lymphocytes surround and invade the muscle fibers. IBM is likely to be present if the biopsy shows rimmed vacuoles containing basophilic granules and amyloid deposits in addition to inflammation.[1]

The IIMs represent a treatable group of disorders, but their differential diagnosis is wide. Early and accurate diagnosis is essential before commencement of therapy. Although muscle biopsy is the essential and definitive diagnosis modality for IIMs, MRI has assumed a major role in IIM evaluation and management, primarily because this technique is very sensitive to the presence of inflammation and edema, especially with incorporation of fat suppression sequences.[2] MRI is thus very good for early diagnosis of disease, evaluation of

Address for correspondence: Rodolfo Victor Curiel, M.D., The George Washington University–Rheumatology, 2150 Pennsylvania Ave., Washington DC, 20037, USA. Voice: 202 741 2492; fax: 202 741 2490. rcuriel@mfa.gwu.edu

MRI and Ultrasound in Diagnosis and Management: Ann. N.Y. Acad. Sci. 1154: 101–114 (2009).
doi: 10.1111/j.1749-6632.2009.04386.x © 2009 New York Academy of Sciences.

the extent and number of lesions, guidance for locating a biopsy site in an area of active disease, and monitoring therapy responses. Unlike muscle biopsy or electromyograms, MRI is noninvasive, making it possible to perform repeat studies for longitudinal analyses of outcome.[3–5]

Another advantage is that MRIs evaluate much larger areas of muscle tissue than is accessible by surgical or needle biopsies. Long-term studies are facilitated by the fact that the technique can generate the type of quantitative data needed for making accurate comparisons over time.[6,7] Moreover, the procedure itself is less dependent on the operator than ultrasound, making it readily comparable with studies that are obtained at different institutions.[8]

Physics of MRI in Muscle Disorders

The principal sources of the MRI signal are fat and water. Soft tissue contrast of MRI (the ability to differentiate different types of tissue based on their signal intensity) is related to differences in proton resonance within the tissues. The protons within fat resonate differently than those in fluid, and by changing the imaging parameters at the MRI console, differences in these tissue-specific properties can be emphasized. This is known as *weighting the image* (T1-weighted images vs. T2-weighted images). Abnormalities causing a change in fat or water content result in altered T1 and T2 relaxation times.[9]

T1-weighted images are based on differences in T1 relaxation times among different tissues. Healthy muscle has a long T1 relaxation time, whereas fat has a relatively short T1 relaxation time. T1-weighted images are thus very sensitive in detecting fatty deposition in muscle.[9–11] As fatty deposition into muscles reflects chronic disease, T1-weighted images are frequently unhelpful early in the clinical course of IIM (Fig. 1A). Like normal muscle tissue, water has a long T1 relaxation time. As these times are similar, T1-weighted im-

ages are insensitive at detecting increased water in muscle. T2-weighted images distinguish among tissues with different T2 relaxation times.

Healthy muscle has a short relaxation time, whereas both water and fat have long T2 relaxation times. T2-weighted images are, therefore, very sensitive to both fat and water increases within muscle. T2-weighted images may show abnormalities early in the disease course of IIM, likely reflecting increased water content due to inflammation or increased blood flow (Fig. 1B).

Owing to the fact that fat and water content are both bright on T2-weighted images, fat cannot be distinguished from edema solely on the basis of these sequences. Fat suppression sequences are invaluable in this setting. Short tau inversion recovery (STIR) imaging results in the removal of signal originating from fat, allowing visualization of edema and water (Fig. 1C).[12–14]

MRI Changes in Myopathy

There are a limited number of ways in which muscle can respond to injury. The cardinal radiologic abnormalities are altered signal intensity (muscle edema/fatty infiltration) and changes in muscle size or shape (atrophy, hypertrophy, and pseudohypertrophy). Most primary neuromuscular diseases (inflammatory and noninflammatory) that cause MRI abnormalities result in a change in signal intensity. Alterations in muscle signal intensity seen in myopathies usually fall into one of the three recognizable patterns: muscle edema, fatty infiltration, or muscle atrophy.[14]

Muscle Edema

The MRI finding in the edema pattern of abnormal muscle signal intensity is increased signal intensity on T2-weighted images superimposed on an otherwise normal appearance of the involved muscle or muscles. Muscle edema

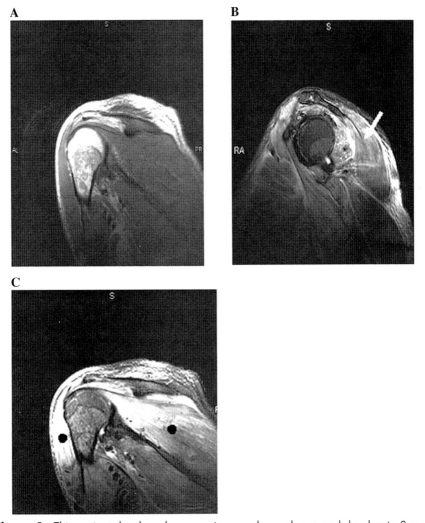

Figure 1. This patient developed progressive muscle weakness and dysphagia 3 months after surgery for testicular cancer. On examination, his proximal strength was diminished, and an erythematous, scaly, and plaquelike rash with a predilection for extensor surfaces was observed. His serum creatine kinase level was 3549 IU/L (normal < 325). MRI of the shoulder revealed multifocal areas of inflammation: (**A**) Coronal T1-weighted image shows a normal appearance. (**B**) A T2-weighted sagittal fat-suppressed image shows patchy areas of increased signal intensity, best seen on this image in the deltoid muscle (white arrow). (**C**) Patchy areas of increased signal on a coronal fat-suppressed STIR image can also be seen (black dots).

may be focal with ill-defined and poorly circumscribed margins or may involve a muscle diffusely. Muscle edema can be quite subtle and detectable only with inversion-recovery or fat-suppressed T2-weighted images. A finding of muscle edema on MRIs is almost always due to increased intracellular or extracellular free water, that is, true muscle edema.

Typical MRI findings early in the course of the inflammatory myopathies are bilateral and symmetric edemas in pelvic and thigh musculature, especially in the vastus lateralis and vastus intermedius muscles. The severity of muscle edema indicated on MRIs has been shown to correlate with the severity of the disease (Fig. 2).

A

B

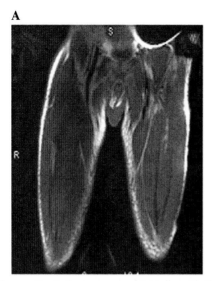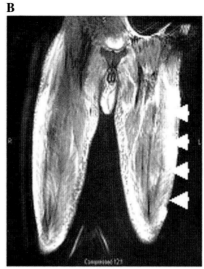

Figure 2. Patient presented initially with 3-month history of progressive muscle weakness affecting the muscles of both thighs and arms. Initially CPK was 14,520 IU/L (<200) and initial aldolase was 38 IU/L (<8): (**A**) Coronal T1-weighted images of both thighs show normal muscle architecture. (**B**) Coronal STIR images show diffuse increased signal intensity affecting muscles and soft tissues (white arrows).

The presence of muscle edema is not exclusive to inflammatory myopathies. It may also be seen in injuries, infectious myositis, muscle infarction, radiation therapy, subacute denervation, compartment syndrome, early myositis ossificans, rhabdomyolysis, and sickle cell crisis, as well as a transient, physiologic finding during and briefly following muscle exercise (Fig. 3).

Fatty Infiltration

Fatty infiltration involves abnormal deposition of fat diffusely within the muscle. It occurs in the late stages of many pathologic conditions involving skeletal muscle and pathologic fatty infiltration is usually seen in association with muscle atrophy. MRIs reveal increased quantities of fat with its characteristic signal intensity within the involved muscle, usually with a decreased volume of muscle tissue. Fatty infiltration may be seen in the chronic stages of muscle denervation, chronic stages of inflammatory myopathies (the hallmark of chronicity being fatty infiltration within the muscle, resulting in increased signal intensity in both T1- and T2-weighted imaging), in chronic disuse, as a late finding after a severe muscle injury or chronic tendon tear, and as a consequence of corticosteroid use (Fig. 4).[13,14]

Muscle Atrophy

Magnetic resonance imaging can quantify muscle atrophy accurately and is likely superior to clinical assessments, which have several limitations. The total muscle bulk in one particular region may remain unchanged owing to compensatory hypertrophy. MRI allows direct visualization of individual muscle bulk, revealing atrophy that may not be apparent otherwise. Comparison to contralateral or normal surrounding muscles may be helpful. When muscle bulk appears hypertrophied, the T1-weighted images should be examined for increased signal intensity indicative of fat deposition, which suggests pseudohypertrophy. The presence of asymmetry or selective muscle atrophy is an important diagnostic clue, as some myopathies have disproportionate involvement of individual muscle groups (e.g., finger flexor musculature in inclusion body myositis).[13,14]

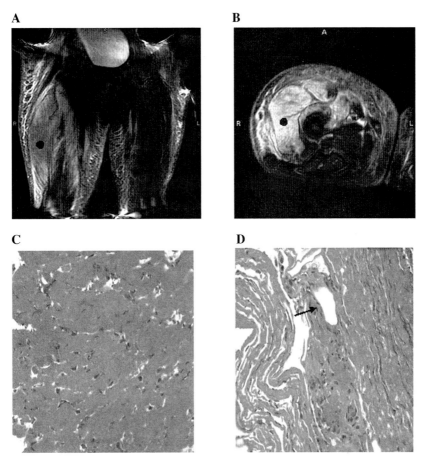

Figure 3. This patient with a medical history significant for diabetes complicated by chronic renal insufficiency, peripheral neuropathy, and retinopathy presented with a 2-week history of progressive pain, swelling, and tenderness involving the right thigh. On examination the thigh was found to be swollen and with exquisite tenderness to palpation. (**A, B**) The right thigh is larger than the left. Increased STIR (black dot) (**A**) and T2 (**B**) signal is seen within the musculature of the right thigh (black dot). This is most prominent at the vastus lateralis muscle, where diffuse increased signal is seen. The muscle is also enlarged. The rectus femoris, the vastus intermedius, and vastus medialis muscles are also involved but to a lesser extent. A significant STIR signal is also noted in the subcutaneous soft tissues of both thighs. (**C**) Glutaraldehyde-fixed, paraffin-embedded tissue, hematoxylin and eosin, 400×. Quadriceps biopsy shows a muscle infarct characterized by pannecrosis: nuclear pyknosis, and loss of sarcoplasmic cross-striations involving all myofibers. (**D**) Glutaraldehyde-fixed, paraffin-embedded tissue, hematoxylin, and eosin, 400×. Small blood vessels in necrotic muscle show mural thickening and hyalinization characteristic of diabetic small vessel damage (black arrow).

Gadolinium

Gadolinium is a paramagnetic compound that demonstrates increased signal intensity on T1-weighted images. Contrast enhancement is best evaluated on T1-weighted fat-saturated images. When administered intravenously, gadolinium results in enhancement proportional to soft tissue vascularity. Originally, it was determined that gadolinium-enhanced sequences did not add to the diagnostic yield of MRI, but these earlier studies were not performed with fat suppression imaging. A more recent study suggests that gadolinium

A   B

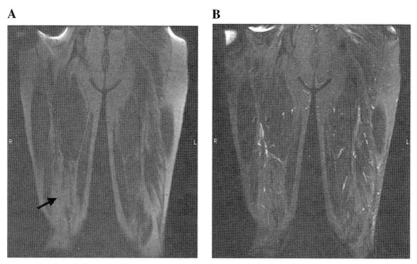

Figure 4. This 24-year-old patient was diagnosed with polymyositis 15 years ago and was treated with methotrexate and prednisone for at least 5 years. His current CPK and aldolase are within normal range. He continues to report proximal muscle weakness: (**A**) Coronal T1-weighted images showed extensive muscle atrophy with fatty replacement (black arrow). (**B**) Coronal STIR image again demonstrates fatty replacement of muscles. No bright signal or acute inflammation is seen.

A   B

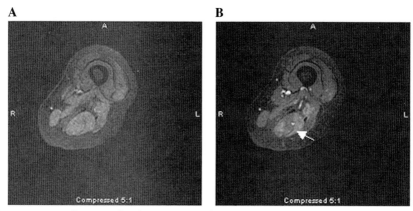

Figure 5. Axial T1-weighted images with fat saturation were performed (**A**) before and (**B**) after gadolinium contrast administration. There is patchy contrast enhancement in the posterior muscles of the thigh (white arrow).

enhancement in combination with fat suppression imaging is superior to routine imaging. The theory behind this is that muscle inflammation results in increased vascularity, so this technique is potentially useful for detecting these scattered areas of inflammation and increased vascularity within different muscles.[15–17] Further experience with gadolinium-enhanced MRI in neuromuscular diseases will help clarify the optional use of this method (Fig. 5).

MRI as Tool for Diagnosis and Management of Idiopathic Inflammatory Myopathies

Although most inflammatory myopathies are diagnosed clinically and confirmed with biopsy, current methods for their diagnosis and evaluation have several limitations. A small percentage of patients will have normal muscle enzyme levels, and up to 10% of patients will have a normal EMG (electromyogram). The so-called myositis-specific autoantibodies (anti-Jo-1, anti-M1–2, and anti-SRP) occur in only about 40% of all inflammatory myopathies.[18–20] The muscle biopsy remains the definitive diagnostic test.

Obtaining a muscle biopsy to make a definitive diagnosis before initiation of therapy is of paramount importance for a number of reasons. First, the treatment involves prolonged immunosuppression and is associated with a significant risk of adverse effects. Second, as there is sometimes a delay between the initiation of therapy and the clinical response, persevering with therapy requires that the clinician have confidence in the diagnosis. Finally, muscle biopsy is required to enable recognition of unusual varieties of inflammatory myopathies, such as inclusion body myositis, and to distinguish them from noninflammatory conditions (muscular dystrophies, metabolic myopathies) that in some instances have similar clinical features. The selection of an appropriate site for a muscle biopsy is important in order to minimize the need for repeat biopsies and thus reduce delays in diagnosis. Severe muscle inflammation does not necessarily imply diffuse inflammation; a patchy distribution on MRI is characteristic and a normal muscle biopsy can be obtained despite severe disease.[20]

In their series of 153 patients with polymyositis and dermatomyositis, Bohan *et al.* reported that blind muscle biopsy was negative in 12.5% of cases [21,22] and a smaller more recent study identified a false negative rate of 45%,[3,23,24] but the use of MRI may overcome some of the problems. MRI can demonstrate areas of active myositis (highlighted by T2-weighted images and STIR imaging) and separate them from areas of fatty infiltration and atrophy (highlighted by T1-weighted images), minimizing the false-negative rate, so the diagnostic yield of the biopsy is increased.

Although the use of MRI to guide biopsy in patients with suspected IIM has been proven to be cost effective and to significantly reduce the number of false-negative biopsy results, it is not widely used in clinical practice, probably owing to cost and limitations in availability. In our institution, MRI is performed on every single patient suspected of having IIM, with the result that our false-negative biopsy rate is close to zero (Fig. 6).

MRI is also an essential tool for differentiating active disease from chronic damage that leads to replacement of muscle with fibrosis or adipose tissue. In patients with long-standing disease, muscle weakness is due to a combination of active inflammation, necrosis, muscle atrophy, and fatty replacement, and sometimes to steroid-induced myopathy. MRI with T1-weighted and STIR sequences can help define the contribution of each of these problems to the patient's weakness, and the results can guide the therapeutic decisions (Fig. 7).

On the other hand, in patients with elevated muscle enzymes whose signs or symptoms do not support the diagnosis of myositis, MRI allows confirmation of the lack of muscle involvement, and the evaluation can be directed elsewhere. MRI is also a useful tool for identifying inflammation in areas that are otherwise difficult to visualize, such as paravertebral muscles, muscles of mastication, and neck flexors (Fig. 8).

Whole-Body MRI

A limitation of conventional MRI has been the inability to scan a large volume of muscles without prolonged acquisition times, but STIR sequencing now allows for rapid whole-body MRI. Whole-body STIR MRI can now be performed in approximately 15 to 30 min total room time and is increasingly available to clinicians. Whole-body MRI has the potential to identify sites of muscle inflammation amenable to biopsy, including those that are not suspected clinically and those not imaged using standard protocols. A recent study using whole-body MRI showed that groups of muscles traditionally deemed not frequently involved in myositis, such as intercostal, obturator

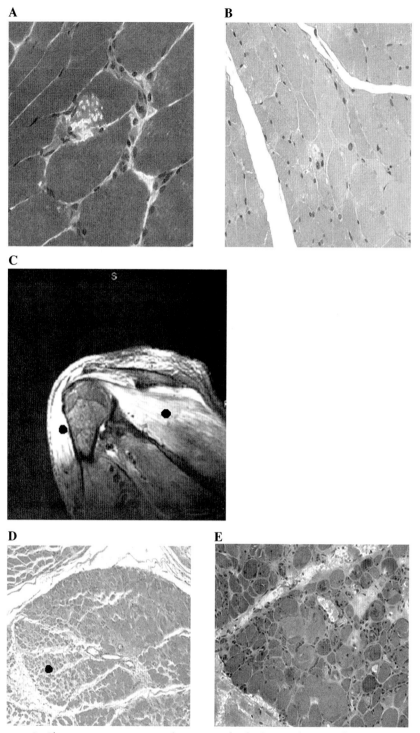

Figure 6. This patient, seen in our department for further evaluation after an inconclusive muscle biopsy, initially presented with generalized muscle weakness affecting predominantly the proximal musculature of the upper and lower extremities. An EMG showed abnormal insertion and spontaneous activity consistent with inflammatory biopsy. A muscle biopsy of the quadriceps was not conclusive: (**A**) Formalin-fixed, paraffin-embedded tissue, hematoxylin and eosin, 400×. Fixed tissue from the left quadriceps shows minimal myopathic changes:

externus, iliacus psoas, and gastrocnemius, depicted increased signal intensity consistent with edema.[25] By identifying the number of muscles involved, this technique can also be utilized to quantify the extent of the disease.

This technique enables analysis of the pattern and the site of involvement in different inflammatory myopathies. A recent, small study showed that the pattern and the extent of the involvement in dermatomyositis differ from that in polymyositis or inclusion body myositis. Dermatomyositis showed inflammation in both muscles and subcutaneous tissues. Subcutaneous edema was diffuse, whereas muscle edema was patchy and diffuse, involving both the proximal and distal extremities. Polymyositis showed muscle inflammation centered in the shoulder and hip girdles, as well as in the neck flexors, erector spinae, and psoas muscle groups. Edema in involved muscles was diffuse in every case, in contrast to the more patchy edema identified in patients with dermatomyositis. No significant subcutaneous edema was seen in polymyositis. Inclusion body myositis showed inflammation in the forearm, thigh (vastus medialis and lateralis), and calf regions in a symmetrical pattern in association with peripheral subcutaneous edema. In this study, ankle dorsiflexors were not involved. Muscle edema was seen to be diffuse in every case.[25–28]

Further studies are needed to determine the sensitivity and specificity of this test, whether it should be part of the routine work-up of myositis, and how the technique performs in relation to standard imaging protocols.

Magnetic Resonance Spectroscopy: Biochemical Assessment

Information on biochemical changes in muscle can be obtained using magnetic resonance spectroscopy (MRS). ^{31}P MRS is most commonly utilized, as it allows the measurement of several metabolites that are important for muscle contraction. Reduced levels of phosphocreatine (PC) and ATP have been demonstrated in myositis patients assessed at rest, and the reductions become even more pronounced after exercise.[29,30] The ratio of inorganic phosphate (Pi) to PC is an excellent indicator of the biochemical status and energy potential of both resting and exercising muscles. An elevated Pi/CP ratio relative to normal values is indicative of myopathy. As biochemical changes usually precede morphologic or functional changes, ^{31}P MRS may have potential as a sensitive indicator of a modified clinical status or as a monitor for early evaluation of therapeutic protocols for inflammatory myopathies. In a few longitudinal studies, positive changes in the levels of

---

variability in myofiber size and shape with rare foci of myofiber segmental necrosis and enlarged internally positioned nuclei containing prominent nucleoli. There is no endomysial, perimysial, or myofiber chronic inflammation; perifascicular atrophy is not present. (**B**) Flash-frozen tissue, hematoxylin and eosin, 400×. In frozen tissue from the left quadriceps rare myofibers show segmental necrosis with scant endomysial mononuclear cells. (**C**) An MRI of the left shoulder was performed. A T2-weighted image with fat suppression shows diffuse increased signal intensity, most prominent in the deltoid muscle (black dot). An MRI-guided muscle biopsy was then performed. (**D**) Formalin-fixed, paraffin-embedded tissue, hematoxylin and eosin, 100×. Fixed tissue from the left deltoid shows prominent perifascicular atrophy involving the left aspect of the illustrated fascicle (black dot). (**E**) Flash-frozen tissue, hematoxylin and eosin, 200×. Frozen deltoid tissue shows active myopathic changes including myofiber segmental necrosis and regeneration and early perifasicular atrophy at the edge of the illustrated fascicle. Perimysial and endomysial chronic inflammatory infiltration is only slight to moderate, most likely reflecting corticosteroid treatment prior to biopsy.

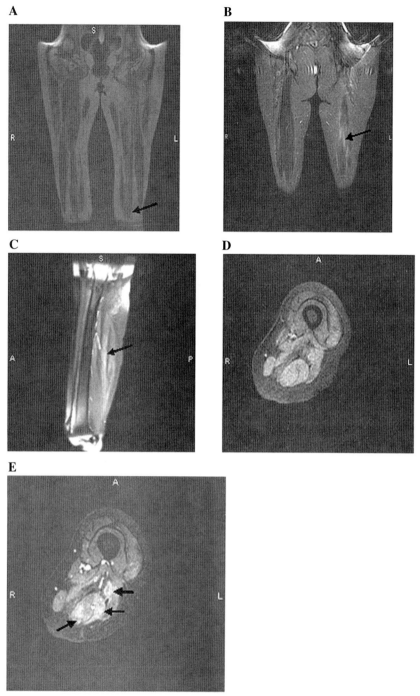

Figure 7. This female patient presented with a 5-year history of biopsy-proven polymyositis. She continued to have persistent weakness of both thighs despite aggressive treatment with corticosteroids, methotrexate, and azathioprine. Coronal T1-weighted image (**A**) demonstrates significant atrophy of the muscles of the thigh with fatty replacement (increased signal). Coronal STIR image of the thighs (**B**) also demonstrates increased signal in the muscles of the thighs compatible with acute inflammation (black arrow). Sagittal T2 fat-saturated image of the left thigh (**C**) also shows acute inflammation in the thigh posteriorly with increased signal seen in the muscles (black arrow). Axial T1-weighted images with fat saturation were performed

energy metabolites were recorded in the muscles of patients with inflammatory myopathies after immunosuppressive treatment, which correlated with clinical improvement.[31,32] In their landmark paper, Park *et al.* demonstrated that the concentrations of ATP and PC in diseased muscles were 30% below normal values. The Pi/PC ratios were significantly increased in the patients' muscles at rest and throughout exercise.[29]

Successful response to therapy has been monitored with ^{31}P MRS in different types of ischemic metabolic disorders, featuring a decreased Pi/PC ratio and faster rates of recovery after exercise. The biochemical changes were accompanied by increased strength and improved muscular performance.[29,31,32]

Magnetic resonance spectroscopy provides quantitative measurements that could be useful for assessing disease progression and response to therapy, as well as for understanding more about the disease mechanisms in longitudinal studies. However, the sensitivity of the technique in relation to identifying change in comparison with other methods still has to be validated, and a drawback for clinical use is its currently limited availability.

The Future: Quantitative Assessment and Response to Treatment

Evaluation of the extent of the disease, reversible versus irreversible, and response to therapy is particularly difficult in IIM owing to the lack of reliable and repeatable measures of disease activity. Although serum CK is the most reliable enzyme for use in routine patient care to predict clinical events, some patients with active biopsy-proven myositis (dermatomyositis > polymyositis and children > adults) have a normal CK and others have circulating inhibitors of CK activity. Recent publications showed a lack of association of disease activity scores with serum CK levels.[4,17] Furthermore, there is

F 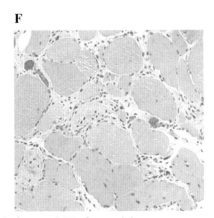   **G**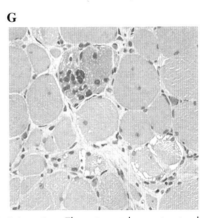

(**D**) before and (**E**) after gadolinium contrast administration. There is patchy contrast enhancement in the posterior muscles of the thigh (black arrow). Given these MRI observed changes (both acute and chronic), an MRI-guided biopsy was performed. (**F**): Formalin-fixed, paraffin-embedded tissue, hematoxylin and eosin, 200×. Fixed quadriceps tissue shows moderate to marked size and shape variation among myofibers consistent with chronic myopathy and atrophy. Scattered myofibers demonstrate segmental necrosis, phagocytosis, and regeneration with slight endomysial chronic inflammatory cell infiltration. (**G**) Formalin-fixed, paraffin-embedded tissue, hematoxylin and eosin, 400×. Myofiber segmental necrosis, phagocytosis, and regeneration with minimal endomysial chronic inflammation are seen at another site from the fixed quadriceps tissue.

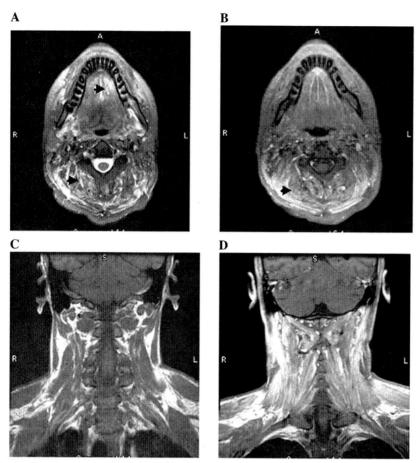

Figure 8. This patient developed dysphagia while being evaluated for presumptive myositis. MRI showed increased signal on axial T2-weighted images with fat saturation in the tongue, masticator, pharyngeal, and paravertebral muscles (black arrows) (**A**). Contrast enhancement was also seen on axial T1-weighted images after gadolinium administration (black arrow) (**B**). Coronal T1 (**C**) and T2 fat-saturated (**D**) images of the neck were also performed. Increased signal intensity is best appreciated on the T2-weighted images, consistent with muscle edema and inflammation.

considerable racial variation in CK concentrations and one cannot apply reference values from white populations to persons of Afro-Caribbean descent, in whom the upper limit of normal CK is increased. On the other hand, muscle weakness in chronic patients may just reflect muscular atrophy and fibrosis related to continuous or chronic-recurrent inflammatory disease or glucocorticosteroid usage, rather than ongoing active inflammation.[33]

MRI appears to be suitable for quantifying the extent of disease and differentiating active (edema, increased signal on T2-weighted images) from chronic, nonreversible (fat replacement on T1-weighted images) muscle damage. Although conclusive research is lacking, MRI also appears to be an objective method for quantifying the degree of inflammation. In several small clinical trials, the extent (number of muscles involved) and the intensity (brightness of the image, pixel values) of the "MRI affection" were shown to correlate with disease activity. Bartlett *et al.* demonstrated that quantitative histogram analysis of MRIs correlated with clinical assessment of disease activity; and Tomasova *et al.* (and other researchers) showed that signal intensity on MRI scanning was the best predictor of disease activity.[16,34,35]

In summary, MRI seems to be the best technique for evaluating the total inflammatory burden in inflammatory myopathies.

Conclusions

MRI has revolutionized the practice of rheumatology. It is difficult to imagine managing a patient with an inflammatory myopathy without an MRI. It has been shown to raise the diagnostic yield and to lower the rate of false-negative biopsies, resulting in more rapid diagnoses with decreased cost and fewer potentially painful invasive procedures. The noninvasive nature of this method makes it ideal for repeat studies to evaluate response to treatment and the extent of the disease. New and emerging MRI techniques show significant potential for expanding clinical applications in muscle diseases.

Conflicts of Interest

The authors declare no conflicts of interest.

References

1. Coyle, K.M. *et al.* 2008. Why isn't my myositis patient getting better? *The Rheumatologist* **2:** 18–22.
2. Lovitt, S. *et al.* 2006. The use of MRI in the evaluation of myopathy. *Clin. Neurophysiol.* **117:** 486–495.
3. Schweitzer, M.E. *et al.* 1995. Cost-effectiveness of MR imaging in evaluating polymyositis. *AJR Am. J. Roentgenol.* **165:** 1469–1471.
4. Lundberg, I.E. *et al.* 2007. Technology insight: Tools for research, diagnosis and clinical assessment of treatment in idiopathic inflammatory myopathies. *Nat. Clin. Pract. Rheumatol.* **3:** 282–290.
5. Hernandez, R.J. *et al.* 1993. MR imaging in children with dermatomyositis: Musculoskeletal findings and correlation with clinical laboratory findings. *AJR Am. J. Roentgenol.* **161:** 359–366.
6. Olsen, N.J. *et al.* 2005. Imaging and skeletal muscle disease. *Curr. Rheumatol. Rep.* **7:** 106–114.
7. Lovell, D.J. *et al.* 1999. Development of validated disease activity and damage indices for the juvenile idiopathic inflammatory myopathies. *Arthritis Rheum.* **42:** 2213–2219.
8. Kuo, G.P. *et al.* 2007. Skeletal muscle imaging and inflammatory myopathies. *Curr. Opin. Rheumatol.* **19:** 530–535.
9. Lang, P. 2008. Magnetic resonance imaging. In *Rheumatology*, 4th ed. M.C. Hochberg *et al.*, Eds.: pp. 339–348. Elsevier. Philadelphia.
10. Adams, E.M. *et al.* 1995. The idiopathic inflammatory myopathies: Spectrum of MR imaging findings. *Radiographics* **15:** 563–574.
11. Olsen, N.J. *et al.* 2005. Imaging and skeletal muscle disease. *Curr. Rheumatol. Rep.* **7:** 106–114.
12. Chang, W.P. *et al.* 2002. MR imaging of primary skeletal muscle diseases in children. *AJR Am. J. Roentgenol.* **179:** 989–997.
13. Farber, J.M. *et al.* 2002. MR imaging in nonneoplastic muscle disorders of the lower extremity. *Radiol. Clin. North Am.* **40:** 1013–1031.
14. May, D.A. 2000. Abnormal signal intensity in skeletal muscle at MR imaging: Patterns, pearls and pitfalls. *Radiographics* **20:** S295–S315.
15. Chahin, N. *et al.* 2008. Correlation of muscle biopsy, clinical course, and outcome in PM and sporadic IBM. *Neurology* **70:** 418–424.
16. Tomasova, S.J. *et al.* 2007. The role of MRI in the assessment of polymyositis and dermatomyositis. *Rheumatology* **46:** 1174–1179.
17. Pachman, L.M. *et al.* 2006. Duration of illness is an important variable for untreated children with juvenile dermatomyositis. *J. Pediatr.* **148:** 247–253.
18. Connor, A. *et al.* 2007. STIR MRI to direct muscle biopsy in suspected idiopathic inflammatory myopathy. *J. Clin. Rheumatol.* **13:** 341–345.
19. Nascif, A.K. *et al.* 2006. Inflammatory myopathies in childhood: Correlation between nailfold capillaroscopy findings and clinical and laboratory data. *J. Pediatr. (Rio J)* **82:** 4045.
20. Wong, E.H. *et al.* 2005. MRI in biopsy-negative dermatomyositis. *Neurology* **64:** 750.
21. Bohan, A.P. *et al.* 1975. Polymyositis and dermatomyositis (Pt. 1). *N. Engl. J. Med.* **292:** 344–347.
22. Bohan, A.P. *et al.* 1975. Polymyositis and dermatomyositis (Pt. 2). *N. Engl. J. Med.* **292:** 403–407.
23. Gerami, P. *et al.* 2007. A systematic review of juvenile-onset clinically amyopathic dermatomyositis. *Br. J. Dermatol.* **157:** 637–644.
24. Esteves, M.O. *et al.* 2000. Juvenile idiopathic myopathies: The value of magnetic resonance imaging in the detection of muscle involvement. *Sao Paulo Med. J.* **118:** 35–40.
25. O'Connell, T.P. *et al.* 2001. Whole-body MR imaging in the diagnosis of polymyositis. *AJR Am. J. Roentgenol.* **179:** 967–971.
26. Cantwell, C. *et al.* 2005. A comparison of inflammatory myopathies at whole-body turbo STIR MRI. *Clin. Radiol.* **60:** 261–267.

27. El-Noueam, K.I. *et al*. 1997. The utility of contrast-enhanced MRI in diagnosis of muscle injuries occult to conventional MRI. *J. Comput. Assist. Tomogr.* **21:** 965–968.

28. Yosipovitch, G. *et al*. 1999. STIR magnetic resonance imaging: A noninvasive method for detection and follow-up of dermatomyositis. *Arch. Dermatol.* **135:** 721–723.

29. Park, J.H. *et al*. 1990. Dermatomyositis: Correlative MR imaging and P-31 MR spectroscopy for quantitative characterization of inflammatory disease. *Radiology* **177:** 473–479.

30. Gordon, B.A. *et al*. 1995. Pyomyositis: Characteristics at CT and MR imaging. *Radiology* **197:** 279–286.

31. King, L.E. *et al*. 1995. Phosphorus 31 magnetic resonance spectroscopy for quantitative evaluation of therapeutic regimens in dermatomyositis. *Arch. Dermatol.* **131:** 522–529.

32. Constantinides, C.D. *et al*. 2000. Human skeletal muscle: Sodium MR imaging and quantification—Potential applications in exercise and disease. *Radiology* **216:** 558–568.

33. Hochberg, M.C. *et al*. Eds. 2008. *Inflammatory Muscle Disease*, 4th ed.: 1433–1448. Elsevier. Philadelphia.

34. Bartlett, M.L. *et al*. 1999. Quantitative assessment of myositis in thigh muscles using magnetic resonance imaging. *Magn. Reson. Imaging* **17:** 183–191.

35. Maillard, S.M. *et al*. 2004. Quantitative assessment of MRI T_2 relaxation time of thigh muscles in juvenile dermatomyositis. *Rheumatology* **43:** 603–608.

MRI in Degenerative Arthritides

Structural and Clinical Aspects

Jian Zhao and Thomas M. Link

*Department of Radiology, University of California, San Francisco,
San Francisco, California, USA*

Owing to the potential to image not only bone but also cartilage, bone marrow, and the surrounding internal soft tissue structures, MRI is particularly useful for the assessment of degenerative arthritides. Cartilage-sensitive MRI techniques have been shown to have a significant correlation with arthroscopic grading scores. MRI is also helpful in differentiating osteoarthritis from avascular necrosis, labral pathology, and pigmented villonodular synovitis. This chapter describes advanced imaging techniques, including driven equilibrium Fourier transform (DEFT) and steady-state free precision (SSFP) imaging, direct MRI arthrography, and 3D-T1rho-relaxation mapping.

Key words: magnetic resonance imaging; osteoarthritis; degenerative disease

Introduction

Osteoarthritis (OA) is an increasingly common disease, encompassing degenerative changes that are mostly age related and affect all joint tissues, in particular the weight-bearing knee and hip joints. It frequently occurs in mechanically overloaded joints and very often in subjects with a genetic predisposition.[1] The knee joint is the most significant site, with considerable pain and loss of clinical function as well as disability. Osteoarthritis affects 10% of adults over the age of 50, and approximately 17 million people in the United States are affected.[2,3] Osteoarthritis-related complaints are among the most common reasons for individuals to seek medical care, causing serious logistical problems for health systems throughout the world.[4,5] Proper diagnosis and management of OA are major clinical and economic issues in health care for an aging population demanding an active lifestyle without joint pain.

Osteoarthritis is a condition that can be defined in different ways. The currently more widely used definitions of OA include pathogenetic features (mechanical and biological events) and morphological features (changes in articular cartilage and subchondral bone), as well as clinical features (joint pain, stiffness, tenderness, limitation of movement, crepitus and occasionally inflammation, effusion).[6]

This chapter discusses structural and clinical aspects of degenerative arthritis focusing on MRI. Given MRI's potential to image not only bone but also cartilage, bone marrow, and the surrounding internal soft tissue structures, it has evolved as the most powerful imaging technique for noninvasively assessing early degenerative disease as well as monitoring disease progression and therapy-related changes. It not only assesses morphological changes in joint tissues but also provides an understanding of their function on a molecular level using advanced imaging techniques. This chapter presents required imaging techniques, joint related findings, semiquantitative techniques for assessing OA, and new advanced imaging modalities for characterizing joint tissues on a molecular level.

Address for correspondence: Jian Zhao, University of California, San Francisco (UCSF), Radiology, 185 Berry St. Lobby 7, San Francisco, CA 94107, USA. jianzhao@radiology.ucsf.edu

MRI and Ultrasound in Diagnosis and Management: Ann. N.Y. Acad. Sci. 1154: 115–135 (2009).
doi: 10.1111/j.1749-6632.2009.04387.x © 2009 New York Academy of Sciences.

Imaging Techniques for Osteoarthritis

Conventional radiography is widely used in the evaluation of OA and its long-term progression. Typically, for the knee, weight-bearing extended, anteroposterior, and lateral views are used. For semiquantitative grading, clinicians generally use the Kellgren–Lawrence (KL) scale to rate the extent of degenerative joint disease at the knee and hip (Fig. 1).[7]

In epidemiological studies and clinical trials, the traditional radiographic method for assessing OA progression estimates cartilage loss indirectly by measuring the narrowed joint space width. However, there are a number of other findings frequently associated with OA that can only be visualized with MRI, such as bone marrow edema pattern, cartilage loss, and meniscal pathology, as well as lesions of ligaments and synovial tissue. These changes were frequently demonstrated on MRIs in patients with advanced OA but clinical findings were inconsistently correlated with these results, except, to some extent, for cartilage lesions[8,9] and bone marrow edema pattern.[10,11]

Although computed tomography (CT) and bone scintigraphy may be useful in the differential diagnosis of joint disorders, they do not play a significant role in the assessment of OA.

MRI Technique for Osteoarthritis

MRI is a noninvasive modality that allows all components of the joint and the subcortical bone marrow to be visualized directly. Osteoarthritis should be considered a disease of organ failure, not one of just cartilage loss or osteophyte formation and MRI can examine the joint as a whole organ.[10] Promising results in therapeutic research in OA have created a new demand for better and earlier imaging of degenerative joint disease. At the same time, more sophisticated cartilage repair techniques and pharmacological therapies to prevent and treat OA are developing rapidly. Optimized MRI for diagnosis, for planning therapy, and

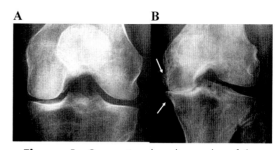

Figure 1. Conventional radiographs of knees (anteroposterior position): (**A**) Knee with a KL score of 2 with small osteophytes and normal joint space. (**B**) Knee with a KL score of 4 with substantially impaired medial joint space and severe osteophytes (arrows).

for monitoring of these interventions is of growing importance,[8,12] and MRI-based techniques to visualize cartilage are prerequisites for guiding and monitoring these therapies.

Field Strength

At present, standard imaging is performed at 1.5 T, as 3.0-T systems are not yet widely available. Initial studies have suggested that higher field strength may improve diagnostic outcome, in particular for the visualization of cartilage.[13] Low-field systems should not be used for cartilage imaging, as studies have shown that low-field MRI machines operating at field strengths of 0.18–0.20 T have substantial limitations compared to high-field systems (1.5 T).[14,15] The 3.0-T systems have shown promise in optimizing cartilage imaging (Fig. 2). The great appeal of 3.0-T MRI for musculoskeletal scanning is the improvement in image quality and spatial resolution. As the signal-to-noise ratio (SNR) correlates in an approximately linear fashion with field strength, it is roughly twice as great at 3.0 T as at 1.5 T. The time necessary to acquire satisfactory images can be substantially reduced, minimizing motion artifacts and possibly speeding patient turnover. Alternatively, the same acquisition time can be used to obtain images at higher spatial resolution. Finally, higher field strength provides greater contrast.

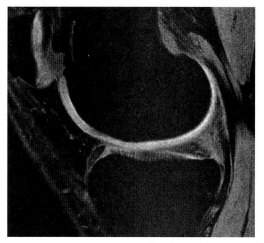

Figure 2. MRI scan obtained at 3 T in a 25-year-old normal volunteer using a 3D-fast spin-SPGR sequence. This high-resolution technique enables visualization of the radial zone with parallel organized collagen fibers at the tibia.

All of the above features are particularly attractive for cartilage imaging, in particular for smaller joints. However, acquisition of imaging studies with a higher-field machine clearly mandates considerable adjustment in MRI practice, including revision of many imaging protocols. Higher SNR and more contrast come at a price. First, tissues differ in their magnetic susceptibility, and this effect is exacerbated at higher field strengths. Second, there are safety concerns: the energy deposited in the patient's tissues is fourfold higher at 3 T than at 1.5 T. Third, 3-T images are more subject to flow artifacts, which may be a particular problem when scanning the knee joint. Furthermore, there is doubling of the chemical shift when the field strength is doubled. Hence, imaging parameters have to be adjusted to the higher field strength, which includes increasing repetition time (TR) and bandwidth as well as decreasing echo time (TE) and flip angles.[16–18]

Coils

Dedicated phased array coils for knee imaging are currently state of the art. These provide a high SNR with excellent image quality and allow the use of parallel imaging to speed up examination time or to improve spatial resolution. In order to optimize imaging, dedicated coils should also be used for other joints, including the shoulder, ankle, and wrist. New multichannel coils are also available for imaging of the hip.

MRI Sequences

Standard MRI sequences for the joints and the spine include T1-weighted spin echo [TR/TE (400–500)/20 ms], proton density-weighted fast spin-echo [TR/TE (2000–3000)/(20–40) ms], and T2-weighted fast spin-echo (FSE) [TR/TE (3000–4000)/(50–90)] sequences. These are usually obtained in coronal, sagittal, and axial orientations. In addition, fast low-angle shot (FLASH) and three-dimensional spoiled gradient echo (3D-SPGR) sequences (TR/TE/flip angle, 30/16 ms/30°) have been used to image cartilage with high spatial resolution. Usually T2-weighted sequences are obtained with fat saturation to improve visualization of bone marrow lesions as well as tendon and ligament pathology. Alternatively, short tau inversion recovery (STIR) sequences are very sensitive to fluid within the bone marrow but use a different mechanism of fat saturation. Figure 3 shows MRI sequences used for scanning cartilage.

Cartilage Imaging

Cartilage-sensitive MRI techniques have been shown to have a significant correlation with arthroscopic grading scores and can be used for an effective, noninvasive evaluation of knee joint cartilage.[19,20] While 3D-SPGR and FLASH sequences are well suited to quantify cartilage volume, PD-w (proton density-weighted) and T2-w FSE sequences show cartilage surface lesions and internal pathology because of the more intermediate signal of the cartilage and hence higher intrinsic cartilage contrast compared to surrounding joint fluid.[8] Many institutions tend to use

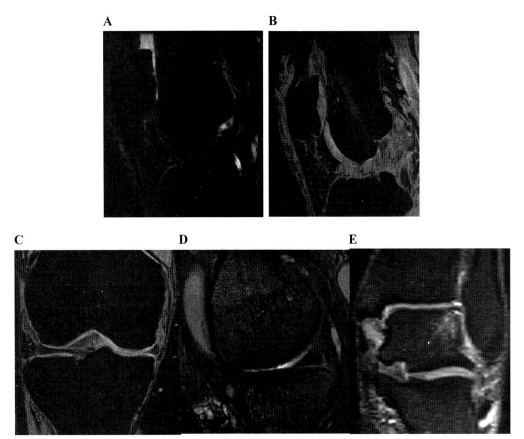

Figure 3. Dedicated cartilage sequences used to image OA: (**A**) Sagittal fat-saturated intermediate-weighted FSE (4300/51 ms; TR/TE) of the knee. (**B**) Spectral selective fat-saturated SPGR sequence of the knee (21/12.5 ms, flip angle 15°). (**C**) Coronal water excitation SPGR sequence of the knee (20/7.5 ms, 12°). (**D**) Sagittal Fiesta (fast imaging employing steady-state acquisition, 9/4.1 ms, 15°) of the knee. (**E**) Coronal DESS (25.7/9 ms) sequence of the ankle.

intermediate-weight FSE sequences with a mixed PD/T2 contrast, which are thought to provide higher intrinsic contrast and be less prone to so-called magic-angle effects as compared with "true" PD-w pulse sequences obtained at shorter echo times.

In addition to these sequences, the three-dimensional double-echo steady-state sequence (3D-DESS) has also shown good results in assessing cartilage. This mixed T1/T2*-w sequence provides high spatial resolution with the cartilage appearing more intermediate in signal. Steady-state free precision (SSFP) imaging is an efficient, high-signal method for obtaining three-dimensional images and may be useful for depicting cartilage, as cartilage signal contrast was found to be higher than in con-

ventional sequences. Preliminary studies found that SSFP-based techniques show a greater increase in SNR and CNR (contrast-to-noise) efficiency compared with SPGR sequences.[21] However, there have not yet been any large clinical studies using this sequence. The DESS is also a steady-state sequence and thus has cartilage signal features similar to the SSFP sequences; yet the parameters are to some extent different.[18,22]

Imaging of Bone Marrow

Bone marrow edema pattern also defined as bone marrow lesions can be clearly shown on fat-suppressed T2-w images or PD-w FSE sequences. Non-fat-saturated T2 and PD-w

FSE sequences do not show bone marrow edema pattern well enough. STIR sequences have also been used to assess bone marrow pathology, as they are very sensitive to fluid, are less susceptible to metal artifacts, and usually provide more homogeneous fat suppression (due to a different fat-suppression mechanism). However, anatomical detail in these sequences is usually inferior to that found in the FSE sequences. T1-w sequences can also visualize this pathology with low signal intensity.

Imaging of Tendon, Ligaments, and Muscle

T1-w and PD or T2-w FSE sequences are used to image tendons, ligaments, and muscles. Owing to the magic-angle effects[23] on short-TE images (which can mimic inflammation and tears), ligaments and tendons are best examined with long-TE MRI techniques. Indeed, the magic-angle phenomenon must be considered in all collagen-containing structures, including articular cartilage and the menisci. In the knee, the anterior cruciate ligament and posterior cruciate ligament are typically assessed in the sagittal plane, whereas the medial and lateral collateral ligament are assessed in the coronal plane.[24]

MRI Findings Associated with Osteoarthritis in Specific Joint Areas

There is a significant relationship between the radiographic stages of OA and the extent of associated MRI findings, including cartilage defects, bone marrow changes, and meniscal and ligamentous lesions (Fig. 4). MRI, however, gives substantial information by visualizing cartilage and bone marrow directly. In addition, a number of other pathologies, such as those of the menisci, synovium, and ligaments typically associated with OA have been described.

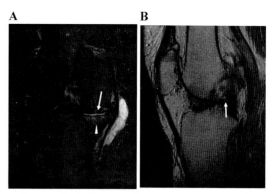

Figure 4. MRI scans of a patient with severe knee OA: (**A**) A coronal fat-saturated T2-w (4300/46.5 ms; TR/TE) sequence shows cartilage defects (arrow), bone marrow edema pattern (arrowhead), and meniscal extrusion. A periarticular cyst can be seen adjacent to the medial collateral ligament. (**B**) A sagittal T1-w (550/10.5 ms; TR/TE) sequence demonstrates a degenerative tear of the ACL.

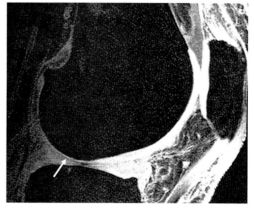

Figure 5. Sagittal SPGR (21/12.5 ms, flip angle 15°) image of the knee shows more than 50% diffuse cartilage thinning (arrow) and full thickness cartilage loss at the tibia.

Knee

Cartilage

One of the most prominent signs of OA on MRIs is a change in the hyaline cartilage, which is one of the most important biomarkers in degenerative and traumatic joint disease (Fig. 5). As there is a loss of cartilage even in the early stages of OA, MRI has been established as the standard cartilage imaging modality (Fig. 6). Cartilage loss can be diffuse or focal, and while diffuse loss is more typically due to degenerative

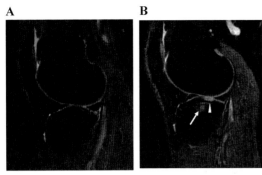

Figure 6. Focal cartilage degeneration demonstrated in a patient with mild OA in a 9-month follow-up examination. Both images were obtained using an intermediate-weight FSE sequence (3600/34.1 ms). In (**A**) a mild amount of cartilage inhomogeneity is shown at the tibia, whereas in (**B**) substantial cartilage signal abnormality with defect (arrowhead) and focal bone marrow edema pattern (arrow) are found.

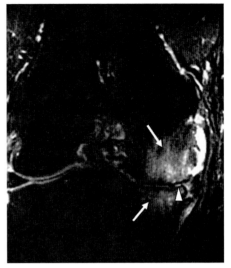

Figure 8. Coronal fat-suppressed T2-w FSE sequence (3000/70 ms) showing bone marrow edema pattern (arrows) in both femur and tibia. Meniscal pathology (arrowhead) with extrusion and destruction of the meniscus is shown. A tear of the MCL was also found.

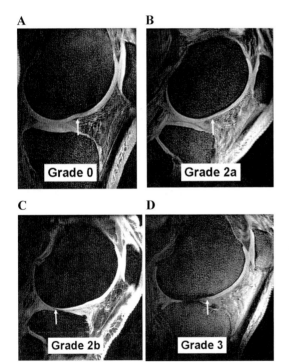

Figure 7. Different grades of cartilage lesions of knee OA obtained with a fat-suppressed SPGR sequence (30/8 ms, 30°): (**A**) Grade 0, normal. (**B**) Grade 2a, cartilage defects that involve less than half of the articular cartilage thickness (arrow in **B**). (**C**) Grade 2b, cartilage defects involving more than half of the cartilage but less than full thickness (arrow in **C**). (**D**) Grade 3, cartilage defects exposing the bone (arrow in **D**).

changes, focal loss may indicate a traumatic component.

According to Recht *et al.* three different grades of cartilage lesions are defined (Fig. 7)[25]: grade I lesions demonstrate areas of inhomogeneous signal intensity; grade IIa lesions are cartilage defects that involve less than half of the articular cartilage thickness; grade IIb lesions involve more than half but less than full thickness of the cartilage; and grade III lesions expose the bone. A previous study found that the grade of cartilage lesions increased with increasing KL scores.[8] Whereas 81% of knees with a KL score of 4 showed full-thickness cartilage lesions, less than 10% of knees with a KL score of 1 or 2 showed cartilage lesions.

Bone Marrow Edema Pattern/Bone Marrow Lesions

In addition to cartilage lesions, another important finding in OA is bone marrow edema pattern (Fig. 8), which is defined as diffuse subchondral low signal intensity on T1-w images and high signal intensity on T2-w images. A previous study correlating MRI

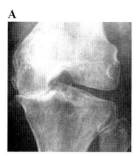 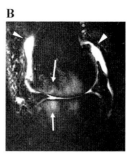

Figure 9. Radiographs and MRIs of a patient with severe OA and a KL score of 4: (**A**) Antero-posterior radiograph shows advanced signs of OA with medial joint space narrowing, osteophytes, and subchondral sclerosis. (**B**) Sagittal fat-suppressed T2-w FSE (3000/70 ms) image shows bone marrow edema pattern (arrows in **B**) at the femur and the tibia and a large joint effusion (arrowheads in **B**).

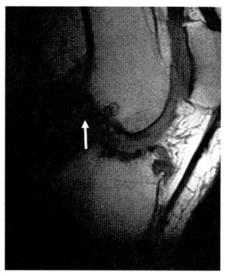

Figure 10. ACL tear in a patient with advanced OA. The sagittal T1-w FSE (500/9 ms) sequence shows an absent ALC (arrow) consistent with a tear as a sign of severe degenerative changes.

findings and histology found that bone marrow edema pattern in OA knees represents a number of noncharacteristic histological abnormalities, which include bone marrow necrosis, bone marrow fibrosis, and trabecular abnormalities, but, in fact, only a small amount of bone marrow edema.[26] Thus "edema" is not a major constituent of MRI signal intensity abnormalities in OA knees. Rather than the term "bone marrow edema," it has been suggested that the terms "bone marrow lesions" or "bone marrow edema pattern" be used instead.

A number of grading systems have been described, including the WORMS score, which is discussed below. Other investigators have used grading based on the diameter of the edema pattern: a diameter of less than 1 cm in the long axis on fat-suppressed T2-w images is graded as mild; a diameter is 1–2 cm is considered moderate; and a diameter larger than 2 cm in the long axis is graded severe.[8]

In one study a correlation between KL score and bone marrow edema pattern was found in fat-suppressed T2-w images (Fig. 9)[8]; only 33% of the knees with a KL score of 1 or 2 showed bone marrow edema pattern, whereas there was such a pattern in 81% of the knees with a KL score of 4.

Ligaments

A connection has been demonstrated between ligamentous pathology and the degree of OA.[8] Mostly, changes are seen in the anterior cruciate ligament (ACL) (Fig. 10) and to a lesser extent in the collateral ligaments. ACL tears were absent in knees with early and mild OA, but ACL lesions were found in 38% of patients with moderate OA and in 56% of the patients with severe OA.[8] ACL tears in this study were diagnosed when either the ligament was interrupted by abnormal signal intensity on T2-w images or the ligament had abnormal alignment (or was completely absent).

Collateral ligament sprains were found in 10% of the patients with early OA and in 25% of the patients with severe OA.[8] Collateral ligament sprains included tears and edematous changes, which were located at the most severely damaged joint compartment (mostly medially) and may be explained by stress due to altered biomechanical loading of the knee.

Menisci

In addition to cartilage lesions, bone marrow edema, and ligament tears, meniscal lesions

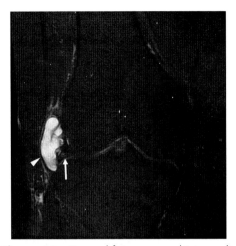

Figure 11. Coronal fat-suppressed intermediate-weighted FSE (3500/50 ms) image of the right knee showing a tear of the lateral meniscal body (arrow) with a parameniscal cyst at the lateral femorotibial joint compartment adjacent to the iliotibial band.

are also associated with OA. Meniscal lesions include meniscal tears and intrasubstance degeneration and extrusion; sometimes parameniscal cysts are found (Figs. 8 and 11). Meniscal tears range from minor disruptions that do not change the shape of the menisci to severe tears in which the meniscus is substantially deformed or can no longer be depicted. Intrasubstance degeneration is defined as signal intensity changes of the meniscus without tears or linear signal abnormalities that extend to the meniscal surface. In a previous study,[8] meniscal tears were found in 50% of patients with early OA, in 92% of patients with moderate OA, and in all patients with severe OA.

A previous study found that meniscal extrusion contributes significantly to radiographic narrowing in patients with OA, particularly early in the disease.[27] Seventeen patients with OA were studied and mild joint space narrowing was found to be associated with meniscal extrusion in all cases, whereas thinning of articular cartilage was not observed in any of these patients. Meniscal extrusion appears to precede other pathologies in patients developing OA. Early joint space narrowing on conventional radiographs appears to reflect meniscal

derangement, often in the absence of disease of the cartilage.

Osteophytes

Osteophytes are usually well visualized with standard radiographs. However, MRI may better visualize central osteophytes. One study has shown that patients with central osteophytes have significantly higher Western Ontario and McMasters University Osteoarthritis Index (WOMAC) stiffness scores than did those without central osteophytes,[8] but WOMAC pain and function scores showed no significant differences between patients with and without central osteophytes.

Grading Systems for Osteoarthritis in the Knee

WORMS Score. Semiquantitative whole-organ MRI scoring (WORMS) is a method for performing multifeature assessment of OA in the knee using MRI. It can be used to capture different patterns of regional cartilage loss and more information about the extent of surface involvement.[24] The WORMS method takes into account a variety of features that are currently believed to be relevant to the functional integrity of the knee and potentially involved in the pathophysiology of OA. These features are (i) articular cartilage integrity, (ii) subarticular bone marrow abnormality, (iii) subarticular cysts, (iv) subarticular bone attrition, (v) marginal osteophytes, (vi) medial and lateral meniscal integrity, (vii) anterior and posterior cruciate ligament integrity, (viii) medial and lateral collateral ligament integrity, (ix) synovitis, (x) intra-articular loose bodies, and (xi) periarticular cysts/bursitis. Intraclass correlation coefficients (ICC) were determined for each feature as a measure of interobserver agreement and an early study found good performance.[24]

Boston–Leeds Osteoarthritis Knee Score (BLOKS). The Boston–Leeds osteoarthritis knee score (BLOKS) is a novel expert-based semiquantitative scoring system specific for knee OA.[28] It is a descriptive score for each morphological feature including (i) cartilage integrity, (ii) attrition, (iii) bone marrow lesions and cysts, (iv) osteophytes, (v) ligaments, (vi) meniscus, and (vii) synovitis. Hunter *et al.*[28] explored the validity of assessment of different pathologies using the BLOKS instrument and found that it demonstrated reasonable reliability and validity.

Hip

Osteoarthritis is the most common disease of the hip joint seen in adults.[29] The diagnosis of OA is based on a combination of radiographic findings of joint degeneration and characteristic subjective symptoms. The earliest changes in articular cartilage may be asymptomatic in the hip joint. However, as the disease progresses with changes in subchondral bone and the development of osteophytes, there are often accompanying symptoms,[30] which include generalized hip pain, pain in the lateral and anterior thigh or groin, and pain with prolonged ambulation.[31,32]

Radiography is the most useful imaging technique for epidemiologic studies of knee and hip OA. Plain radiographs have been used as the primary diagnostic method for hip OA for many decades and radiographs of a hip with established idiopathic OA are so characteristic that other forms of imaging are seldom necessary. The radiological findings of OA include osteophyte formation, joint space narrowing, subchondral sclerosis, and subchondral cyst formation. If plain radiographs are inconclusive, MRI and/or multidetector row CT (MDCT), especially if combined with arthrography, may offer a direct demonstration of the state of the cartilage and illustrate erosions as well as bone marrow edema pattern and labral tears.[29] Kellgren–Lawrence scoring is the most widely used classification of disease severity.[33,34] However, this classification is not specific and sensitive enough to evaluate the changes in short-term clinical or long-term prospective studies because measurements of knee and hip joint space width in millimeters are more sensitive for detecting OA than the KL scale.[33–35]

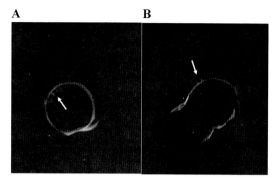

Figure 12. Sagittal (**A**) and coronal (**B**) images of an MRI arthrogram of the right hip joint (FSE sequences with fat saturation): (**A**) shows subchondral cysts anteriorly in the femoral head (arrow in **A**) with overlying cartilage loss. (**B**) The coronal image demonstrates a superolateral labral tear (arrow in **B**) with a bump at the head–neck junction indicating femoroacetabular impingement.

Typical MRI findings associated with OA include loss of cartilage with concomitant joint space narrowing, bone marrow edema pattern, and subchondral cysts. Typically associated with hip OA are labral degeneration and tears, which may be best visualized with MR arthrography. Femoroacetabular impingement syndrome (FAI) is one of the important predisposing factors for degenerative arthritis of the hip.[36] FAI is an abutment conflict occurring between the proximal femur and the acetabular rim arising from morphologic abnormalities affecting the acetabulum or/and the proximal femur. Typical MRI findings include articular cartilage damage, acetabular labral tearing, and a bump at the head–neck junction (Fig. 12).[37]

Pincer and Cam Femoroacetabular Impingement

There are two types of FAI, pincer and cam. In pincer-type FAI the femoral head–neck junction contacts the acetabular rim, typically as a result of an underlying acetabular abnormality, such as an acetabular fossa that is too deep. In cam-type FAI there is abnormal morphology at the anterior femoral head–neck junction, such as a bump, that directly injures the labrum. In a study by Kassarjian *et al.*[37] abnormal head–neck morphology, anterosuperior cartilage abnormality, and anterosuperior labral tear were found in MR arthrographic scans of patients with cam impingement of the hip. The abnormal morphology of the anterior femoral head–neck junction can be best evaluated with MRI arthrography in the oblique sagittal plane, running parallel to the femoral neck. The labrum and cartilage are delineated as distinct entities by internal contrast in MRI arthrography, whereas the cartilage and labral abnormalities associated with head–neck morphology would be more difficult to see in nonarthrographic MRI.

In general, however, MRI is rarely used to assess advanced OA, as findings are well visualized on radiographs. Mostly MRI is used to assess additional and differential pathologies, including avascular necrosis, labral pathology, a tear in the ligamentum capitis femoris, and pigmented villonodular synovitis.

Osteoarthritis of the Hand

Osteoarthritis of the hand is most often seen in postmenopausal women. The estimated prevalence of this disorder in patients more than 65 years of age ranges from 70 to 99% in women and 64 to 78% in men.[38,39] In descending order, the distal interphalangeal (DIP) joints, the base of the thumb, the proximal interphalangeal (PIP) joints, and the metacarpophalangeal (MCP) joints are the joints most commonly involved, and there is a relative symmetry of distribution in both hands.[39]

MRI is rarely used in the diagnosis of hand OA. However, it has a role in assessing the differential diagnostic considerations including rheumatoid arthritis (RA), and ligamentous and tendon pathologies. MRI of the hand is challenging and requires dedicated surface coils with high SNR. High-resolution MRI has recently been used to a limited extent to assess OA in the hand, and it was found to be better for defining the microanatomic basis for early hand-joint involvement.[40,41] In the case of early hand OA, gadolinium contrast agent en-

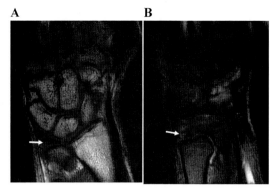

Figure 13. Coronal T1-w (500/9 ms) (**A**) and fat-saturated PD-w (3500/50 ms) (**B**) MRI scans of the left hand showing degenerative changes and a tear of the triangular fibrocartilage (arrow).

hancement was found to reflect inflammatory and destructive changes. Interestingly joint ligament abnormalities are especially common in normal joints adjacent to OA joints.[40] Kirkhus *et al.* found that dynamic contrast-enhanced MRI may play a role in differentiating synovitis in RA from synovitis in OA and also in measuring synovial activity in OA and RA.[42] Among the pathologies causing accelerated OA that can be visualized with MRI are lesions of the triangular fibrocartilage (Fig. 13) as well as tears of the scapholunate and lunotriquetral joint space.

Osteoarthritis of Other Joints

Compared with weight-bearing joints, primary OA of the shoulder is uncommon and usually occurs in the elderly. On the other hand, secondary OA is more common. Chondromalacia, osteophyte formation, subchondral cysts, and synovitis characterize degenerative arthritis of the shoulder. MRI is a useful tool for accessing the cartilage, labral pathology, subchondral bone marrow edema, synovitis, subarticular cysts, and ligamentous/tendon pathologies associated with OA (Fig. 14). In T1-w images sclerosis and edema show decreased signal. Subchondral cysts with low signal and sometimes marrow fat signal extending into osteophytes can also be found. Subchondral cysts, bone marrow edema pattern, and synovitis

A   B

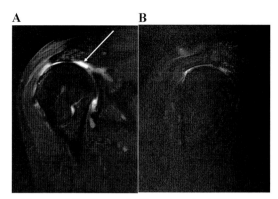

Figure 14. Coronal (**A**) and sagittal (**B**) fast spin T2-w FSE images of the right shoulder showing a complete rotator cuff tear with a high-riding humeral head. Cartilage thinning at the humeral head (arrow) and a moderate joint effusion are also demonstrated.

show high signal on T2-w images, especially in fat-suppressed sequences.

Shoulder OA can be divided into two groups: nontraumatic and posttraumatic. Nontraumatic OA may occur as a result of such conditions as RA, calcium pyrophosphate dihydrate arthropathy, chronic rotator cuff tear, avascular necrosis, or congenital malformations. The posttraumatic group encompasses traumatic dislocation and fractures of the humeral head or glenoid.[43,44] The most frequent abnormality in glenohumeral OA is osteophyte formation along the articular margin of the humeral head and the line of attachment of the labrum to the glenoid fossa. Degenerative changes in the rotator cuff can also lead to instability of the glenohumeral joint and arthritis. The acromioclavicular (AC) joint is commonly involved in degenerative changes and is routinely assessed with conventional radiography, as well as MRI. De Abreu *et al.*[45] found that AC joint disease is more frequently diagnosed with MRI than with radiography. MRI also enables the assessment of adjacent soft tissue structures and their effect on the underlying rotator cuff.[45] Typical MRI findings in OA of the AC joint are hypertrophy of the joint and surrounding soft tissues, with substantial amounts of edema.

Osteoarthritis of the ankle is usually secondary to previous fractures or ligamentous injury, chronic repetitive stresses, or occupational or sports activities.[46] Asymmetric cartilage space loss, subchondral sclerosis, and cystic changes and osteophytosis can be found on radiographs. The weight-bearing position contributes to demonstrating cartilage space loss.[47] MRI is helpful for determining potential causes of ankle OA and is useful for assessing additional and differential pathologies, including trauma, ligamentous and tendon abnormalities, osteochondritis dissecans, avascular necrosis, and anterolateral and anteromedial impingement. MRI arthrography is reported to be an accurate technique for assessing subtle cartilage abnormalities and soft tissue changes in patients with impingement syndrome.[48] Secondary OA is usually caused by underlying cartilage damage from trauma, arthritis, infection, metabolic conditions, or other causes. Most of these underlying conditions may be better characterized with MRI imaging.

Degenerative Spine Disease

As far as techniques are concerned, conventional radiographs play an important role as an initial imaging test in the diagnosis of degenerative spine disease.[49] MRI is widely used for the clinical diagnosis of disc disorders, as well as pathologies of the spinal canal and the neuroforamen. MRI is, in principle, capable of providing information both on the morphology of the disc and on its molecular composition. Contrast administration is very rarely needed in degenerative spine disease. Sodium images have been used to assess the GAG content of the intervertebral disc.[50] T1rho MRI has also been used not only to determine degenerative changes in human discs *in vivo*, but also to quantify proteoglycan content in cadaveric discs.[51,52]

Disc herniation is one of the most frequent causes of spinal degenerative disorders.[53] The first step in disc degeneration is dehydration of the nucleus pulposus and consequent rigidity. Degeneration can be detected early as signal decrease on T2-w MRIs and is especially

A　　　　　　B

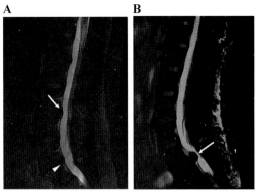

Figure 15. Degenerative changes of the intervertebral discs: (**A**) Sagittal T2-w fat-saturated FSE sequence shows decreased signal of the L3/4 and L5/S1 intervertebral discs as well as a protrusion at L3/4 (arrow) and an extrusion at L5/S1(arrowhead). (**B**) Sagittal T2-w fat-suppressed FSE shows decreased signal of the L3/4, L4/5, and L5/S1 intervertebral discs, as well as a large disc extrusion at the level of L5/S1, which causes severe central canal narrowing (arrow).

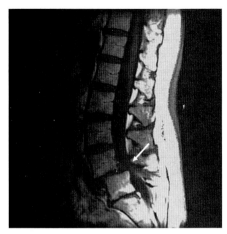

Figure 16. Degenerative spondylolisthesis at the L4/5 level of the lumbar spine. Sagittal T1-w image (700/8.8 ms) shows a grade 1–2 anterolisthesis of L4 on L5 with severe spinal canal stenosis (arrow).

obvious on fat-suppressed sequences. Later, fissures within the disc appear. Almost all individuals older than 40 have transverse intranuclear clefts. The rupture of collagen bridges among the peripheral fibers produces annular weakness and a disc bulge, and the rupture of the fibers and a radial tear of the annular fibers produces disc herniation. The presence of a radial tear is detectable by MRI and consists of a focal bright signal on T2-w sequences. These findings comprise the so-called high intensity zone.[54]

Herniation is defined as a localized displacement of disc material beyond the limits of the intervertebral disc space. Herniated discs may take the form of protrusion or extrusion, based on the shape of the displaced material. Protrusion is a focal or asymmetric extension of the disc beyond the interspace, whereas extrusion is a more extreme extension of the disc beyond the interspace (Fig. 15).[55] Destruction and collapse of the disc can be caused by the loss of water content and annular fissures in the intervertebral disc. In some degenerative diseases gas and calcifications can also be found within the disc.[53]

Vertebral body bone marrow changes, spondylosis, degenerative facet joint disease, degenerative spondylolisthesis, and stenosis are also found in degenerative spine diseases. Modic *et al.*[56] classified signal intensity changes noted in the bone marrow adjacent to the degenerated disc and identified three types: Modic type 1 changes show decreased signal intensity on T1-w spin-echo images and increased signal intensity on T2-w spin-echo images consistent with bone marrow edema pattern. Type 2 represents increased signal intensity on T1-w spin-echo images with slightly increased signal intensity on T2-w images consistent with fatty changes. Type 3 changes show decreased signal intensity on both T1- and T2-w images consistent with bony sclerosis.

Imaging findings in degenerative disease of the facet joints includes joint space narrowing, bony sclerosis, and osteophytosis. Juxta-articular cysts sometimes form next to degenerated facet joints. Degenerative spondylolisthesis is a dislocation of the vertebral body anteriorly owing to the degeneration of the supporting structures of the intervertebral disc, intervening muscles and ligaments, capsules, and facet joints (Fig. 16). Chaput *et al.*[57] found an association between facet joint effusion seen on

MRI and the presence of spondylolisthesis indicated on standing lateral flexion-extension radiographs. The prevalence of spondylolysis increases with age and occurs most frequently at the L5 segment. Degenerative spinal stenosis can be congenital, acquired (degenerative), or mixed. Acquired spinal stenosis is typically caused by spondylosis, disc bulges or herniations, ligamentous degeneration, spondylolisthesis, or a combination of these disorders. Calcification and ossification of spinal ligaments may also cause spinal stenosis.

Clinical findings must be carefully evaluated in conjunction with the results of MRI studies. The preferred term for description of imaging manifestations alone or imaging manifestations of uncertain relationship to symptoms is degenerated disc rather than degenerative disc disease.[55] It has been suggested that bulges and protrusions on MRI scans in patients with low back pain may be coincidental, as previous studies have found that many people without back pain have disc bulges or protrusions (but not extrusions).[58]

Erosive (Inflammatory) Osteoarthritis

Erosive OA is a disorder that most often involves the hands of postmenopausal women and is manifested by acute inflammation with swelling, painful joints, warmth, and limitation of function. DIP joints are the most frequently involved, followed by PIP joints. The radiological changes of erosive OA are characterized by a combination of bony proliferation and erosions. Osteophytosis may occur in the absence of erosive changes, predominating at the margins of the DIP and PIP joints. Joint space narrowing and associated subchondral sclerosis also are common.

Generally, erosions occur at the central portion of the articulation in the form of defects with sharp margins. Marginal erosions are less common and may occur between the edge of the articular cartilage and the joint capsule.

The central erosions are most commonly seen in the interphalangeal joints. However, clinical symptoms and osteophytosis may occur even before the appearance of erosions.[59-61] High-resolution MRI has recently been used to assess erosions of hand OA in both central and marginal locations.[40,41] Grainger and co-workers compared conventional radiography (CR) and MRI when investigating erosion numbers and morphology of hand OA. Using MRI, they found that 80% of the joints examined showed one or more erosions, compared with 40% using CR, which indicates that MRI may show evidence of erosive OA even when radiographs indicate a nonerosive form of the disease.[62] These investigators found that erosions in OA, and particularly marginal erosions similar to those seen in inflammatory arthritis, are a more common feature of small-joint OA than had been previously indicated by conventional radiographs. The distribution of joint involvement is nearly identical to non-inflammatory OA of the hand.[63,64] Large-joint involvement is rarely reported in the shoulder, hips, knees, or spine.[60,65,66]

Differential Diagnosis of Osteoarthritis

Radiographic and MRI findings of OA should be differentiated from other articular diseases, such as rheumatoid arthritis, seronegative spondyloarthritis, Reiter's syndrome, gouty arthritis, calcium pyrophosphate dihydrate crystal deposition disease, osteonecrosis, and neuropathic osteoarthropathy.

MRI is a useful technology for differentiating OA from other diseases, such as avascular necrosis, labral pathology, and pigmented villonodular synovitis. But it is difficult to differentiate the abnormal MRI appearance of ligaments in OA from milder cases of traumatic injury. Bergin *et al.*[67] described medial collateral ligament (MCL) edema in association with OA of the medial compartment in patients without trauma to the knee, and they found a correlation with the grade of osteophytes, as well as with the presence of meniscal extrusion. They postulated that the MCL edema might be a result of local friction caused by the osteophytes rubbing against the capsular ligament and tibial collateral ligament during knee movement. Wen *et al.*[68] described a group of patients who had no prior knee trauma, but whose MRI scans demonstrated MCL edema, and compared their MRIs with a group of patients with varying grades of traumatically injured MCLs. They concluded that differentiating between atraumatic MCL edema and trauma-related MCL injury can be difficult when only minor MCL signal abnormality is present. Another typical finding in knee OA is signal and morphological abnormality of the ACL, which also may be difficult to differentiate from traumatic injury.

Radiographs remain important for differential diagnoses since they may better visualize juxta-articular osteoporosis or small bone abnormalities such as traumatic avulsions. MRIs always have to be analyzed in concert with radiographs to better assess potential differential pathologies.

New Advanced Imaging Techniques

A number of studies have been developed to improve visualization of cartilage and quantification of its biochemical composition. New morphological sequences that have been developed and are currently being investigated include driven equilibrium Fourier transform (DEFT) and steady-state free precision (SSFP) imaging. DEFT imaging makes use of a much higher cartilage-to-fluid contrast; the signal of synovial fluid is higher than in SPGR sequences and the signal of cartilage is higher than in T2-w FSE. Some investigators found that the 3D-DEFT sequences provided excellent synovial fluid-to-cartilage contrast while preserving signal from cartilage, giving this method a high cartilage SNR. Furthermore,

3D-DEFT showed the full cartilage thickness better than T2-FSE, but T2-FSE had superior fat saturation and fewer artifacts.[18,69,70] As an efficient, high-signal method for obtaining three-dimensional images, SSFP imaging may be useful for depicting cartilage, as cartilage signal was found to be higher than in conventional sequences. It should be noted that the previously described DESS sequence is also a steady-state sequence and thus has cartilage signal features similar to those of SSFP, but the parameters are, to some extent, different.

Direct MRI arthrography with the use of T1-w pulse sequences following the intra-articular injection of diluted gadolinium chelates has been shown to be a reliable imaging technique for the detection of surface lesions of articular cartilage with sensitivities and specificities ranging from 85 to 100%.[71] The injected fluid produces high contrast within the joint space and, at the same time distends the joint, thus improving the separation of corresponding joint surfaces, such as the chondral surfaces of the femur and the tibia. A simple method of producing artificial arthrographic contrast in a T1-like FSE sequence using a driven equilibrium pulse (DRIVE) has recently been described. In contrast to the 3D-DEFT sequence mentioned above, this two-dimensional technique provides bright signal intensity of joint fluid with otherwise unchanged signal intensities compared with a normal T1-w FSE sequence at high spatial resolution and short scan times.[72] Driven equilibrium pulses can also be used to increase the contrast and/or spatial resolution of intermediate-weighted FSE images. However, this new technique and its value for cartilage imaging are still being evaluated clinically.

MRI at 3.0 T

High-field MRI at 3.0 T improves visualization of cartilage and the related pathology relative to lower field strengths. In one *in vitro* study,[73] assessment of the diagnostic value of MRI sequences at 1.5 and 3.0 T in detecting cartilage lesions was carried out using receiver operator characteristics (ROC) analysis. Eighty-four cartilage lesions were created in porcine knees and imaged with three cartilage-specific sequences: SPGR sequence and two fat-saturated PD-w FSE sequences (low and high spatial resolution). All the images were analyzed by three radiologists independently. In this study, it was shown that 3.0-T MRI with optimized high-resolution sequences significantly improved the diagnostic performance of all three radiologists in assessing focal cartilage lesions compared to 1.5-T MRI. Moreover, imaging times can be reduced with optimized sequences, as has been shown in this study with the SPGR sequence. Additional *in vitro* ankle studies showed similar results.[13]

Cartilage Volume

Volumetric quantitative cartilage MRI was developed as a tool to assess the evolution of OA and its structural changes in human joints and to evaluate new pharmacological cartilage protective therapies. Quantitative MRI of cartilage volume was improved by applying three-dimensional postprocessing techniques.[74–76] Assessment of cartilage volume at the knee joint is done primarily for scientific studies and has no role in routine knee MRI. For the introduction of cartilage volume calculation into the daily clinical routine, fast and accurate determination modalities are required. Maataoui *et al.*[12] investigated the accuracy and time saving using a so-called Argus application in the assessment of cartilage volume in OA knees and noted that the calculation was a simple, fast, and reliable alternative to other volumetric tools. Piplani *et al.*[75] found that articular cartilage volume in cadaveric specimens can be reliably determined by means of semiautomated three-dimensional processing of MRI scans. Accurate serial measurements of articular cartilage volumes could play a role as an objective indicator of disease progression in patients with degenerative arthropathy. Eckstein *et al.*[74] found that with three-dimensional image processing, MRI can provide accurate data on cartilage volume and thickness on the human knee joint surfaces.

Molecular Imaging Techniques

Molecular and biochemical changes in the joints, including loss of proteoglycans (PG) from the extracellular matrix of articular cartilage, are distinctive characteristics of OA. To detect these changes *in vivo* is a prerequisite for the early diagnosis of OA and monitoring of treatment efficacy. Several techniques have been developed and are described in more detail below. In particular, sodium MRI has been suggested for quantification of early OA. Wheaton *et al.*[77] found that sodium MRI can serve as a quantitative method for measuring *in vivo* changes in PG content in an animal model of OA.

T1rho Mapping

Three-dimensional-T1rho-relaxation mapping is a new technique that is sensitive and specific to slow macromolecular interactions and has been proposed for measuring cartilage composition. It describes spin-lattice relaxation in the rotating frame. Changes in the extracellular matrix of cartilage, such as the loss of GAG, are reflected in measurements of T1rho owing to the less-restricted activity of water protons.

Initial results were published by Regatte *et al.*,[78,79] who studied T1rho-weighted MRI of symptomatic OA patients and found that 3D-T1rho spatial mapping performed with a 1.5-T clinical MRI instrument can achieve a good SNR, with a reasonable acquisition time and without exceeding FDA guidelines for a specific radiofrequency energy absorption rate. T1rho-w MRI provided a noninvasive marker for quantitation of early degenerative changes of cartilage *in vivo*. The study demonstrated *in vivo* feasibility of quantifying early biochemical changes in symptomatic OA subjects employing a 1.5-T clinical scanner.

A significant difference in the average T1rho within patellar and femoral cartilage between healthy volunteers and early OA patients was found by Li *et al.* using 3-T MRI.[80] They also discerned a significant correlation between T1rho and T2 relaxation measurements, but the difference in T2 measurements was not significant between controls and OA patients. According to these preliminary results, using T1rho relaxation times to detect early cartilage degeneration prior to morphologic changes may allow us to critically monitor the course of OA and injury progression and to evaluate the efficacy of treatment in the early stages of OA. Further studies are clearly mandated to correlate T1rho measurements with early OA (determined by arthroscopy as a standard of reference) in larger symptomatic populations.[18]

T2 Mapping

Another approach that has been used to measure cartilage composition is T2 mapping. It has been shown that increasing T2 relaxation time is proportional to the distribution of cartilage water and is sensitive to small water content changes.[81] In an early study, Dardzinski *et al.*[82] examined the spatial variation of *in vivo* cartilage T2 in young asymptomatic adults and found a reproducible pattern of increasing T2 that was proportional to the known spatial variation in cartilage water and inversely proportional to the distribution of proteoglycans. They postulated that the regional T2 differences were secondary to the restricted mobility of cartilage water within an anisotropic solid matrix. Thus, measurement of the spatial distribution of the T2 (reflecting areas of increased and decreased water content) may be used to quantify cartilage degeneration before morphologic changes are appreciated.

Mosher *et al.*[83] found that aging is associated with an asymptomatic increase in T2 of the transitional zone of articular cartilage. The results of their study indicated that this diffuse increase in T2 in senescent cartilage is different in appearance than the focally increased T2 observed in damaged articular cartilage. In an additional study,[84] they obtained T2 maps

at 3.0 T of the weight-bearing femoral and tibial articular cartilage in seven young healthy men before and immediately after 30 min of running. They found no statistically significant change in T2 profiles of tibial cartilage, but a statistically significant decrease in T2 of the superficial 40% of weight-bearing femoral cartilage after exercise. These data support the hypothesis that cartilage compression results in greater anisotropy of superficial collagen fibers.

Dunn *et al.*[85] analyzed 55 subjects who were categorized with radiography as healthy or as having mild or severe OA. They found that all cartilage compartments except the lateral tibia showed significant increases in T2 relaxation time between healthy and diseased knees. The correlation of T2 values with clinical symptoms and cartilage morphology was found predominantly in the medial compartment. Quantitative cartilage imaging may enhance our ability to detect subtle, early matrix changes associated with cartilage degeneration when used in conjunction with standardized cartilage-sensitive imaging.

Delayed Gadolinium-Enhanced MRI of Cartilage and Menisci

Delayed gadolinium-enhanced MRI of cartilage (dGEMRIC) was successfully employed to quantify degenerative changes in cartilage, including PG depletion (Fig. 17). The ability to measure the loss of glycosaminoglycans *in vitro* with dGEMRIC has been validated,[86–88] and the technique has been used in a number of clinical studies.[89–92] Variations of this measurement have been shown in patients with OA, trials of autologous chondrocyte implants, and subjects with sedentary lifestyles versus those engaged in regular exercise. Williams *et al.*[92] examined 31 patients with knee OA using MRI with a dGEMRIC protocol at 1.5 T as well as semiflexed-knee and full-limb radiographs to assess alignment. They found that compartments of the knee joint without joint space narrowing had a higher dGEMRIC index than

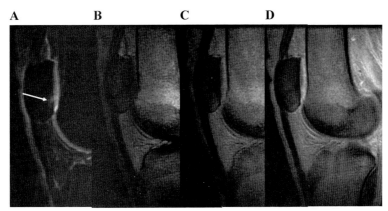

Figure 17. Sagittal T2-w fat-saturated FSE sequence (**A**) and dGEMRIC images obtained 90 min postinjection (**B–D**) of the knee showing an area of cartilage pathology at the inferior aspect of the patella with bone marrow edema pattern (arrow in **A**). dGEMRIC images show increased enhancement in the area of the cartilage pathology consistent with loss of proteoglycans in this area.

those with any level of narrowing. These quantitative findings may have a particularly important role in evaluating early OA.

Diffusion Tensor Imaging

Diffusion tensor imaging (DTI) has been used to analyze the microstructural properties of articular cartilage in addition to T2 and T1rho mapping. Not only the degree, but also the main direction of the free mobility of water protons can be assessed. In one study, human patellar cartilage-on-bone samples were imaged at 9.4 T using a diffusion-weighted spin-echo sequence.[93] They found that the DTI-derived parameter fractional anisotropy (FA) and eigenvector maps might reflect the macromolecular environment and the predominant alignment of the collagenous fiber network, respectively. However, further studies are required to establish DTI at clinical high-field strength systems for use in human subjects.

Future Needs Concerning MRI in Degenerative Arthritis

A number of cartilage-dedicated sequences are available to depict cartilage lesions, but these only show damage at stages when car-

tilage is irreversibly lost. The future goal of MRI is to diagnose cartilage matrix changes at stages when the damage is still reversible and may be better treated. This is an ambitious goal, yet promising tools, such as dGEMRIC, T1rho, and T2 relaxation time mapping are already available, and future research will show how clinically feasible these new biomarkers are as measures of early cartilage degeneration. Together with new pharmacological therapies, they may revolutionize management of early OA and could have a tremendous impact on population health.[18]

Conflicts of Interest

The authors declare no conflicts of interest.

References

1. Dieppe, P. & J. Kirwan. 1994. The localization of osteoarthritis. *Br. J. Rheumatol.* **33:** 201–203.
2. Centers for Disease Control and Prevention. 1995. Prevalence and impact of arthritis among women–United States, 1989–1991. *JAMA* **273:** 1820–1822.
3. Felson, D.T. 1988. Epidemiology of hip and knee osteoarthritis. *Epidemiol. Rev.* **10:** 1–28.
4. Lawrence, R.C., C.G. Helmick, F.C. Arnett, *et al.* 1998. Estimates of the prevalence of arthritis and

selected musculoskeletal disorders in the United States. *Arthritis Rheum.* **41:** 778–799.

5. Guccione, A.A., D.T. Felson, J.J. Anderson, *et al.* 1994. The effects of specific medical conditions on the functional limitations of elders in the Framingham Study. *Am. J. Public Health* **84:** 351–358.

6. Hinton, R., R.L. Moody, A.W. Davis & S.F. Thomas. 2002. Osteoarthritis: Diagnosis and therapeutic considerations. *Am. Fam. Physician* **65:** 841–848.

7. Kellgren, J.H. & J.S. Lawrence. 1957. Radiological assessment of osteo-arthrosis. *Ann. Rheum. Dis.* **16:** 494–502.

8. Link, T.M., L.S. Steinbach, S. Ghosh, *et al.* 2003. Osteoarthritis: MR imaging findings in different stages of disease and correlation with clinical findings. *Radiology* **226:** 373–381.

9. Zhai, G., F. Cicuttini, C. Ding, *et al.* 2007. Correlates of knee pain in younger subjects. *Clin. Rheumatol.* **26:** 75–80.

10. Felson, D.T., C.E. Chaisson, C.L. Hill, *et al.* 2001. The association of bone marrow lesions with pain in knee osteoarthritis. *Ann. Intern. Med.* **134:** 541–549.

11. Felson, D.T., J. Niu, A. Guermazi, *et al.* 2007. Correlation of the development of knee pain with enlarging bone marrow lesions on magnetic resonance imaging. *Arthritis Rheum.* **56:** 2986–2992.

12. Maataoui, A., H. Graichen, N.D. Abolmaali, *et al.* 2005. Quantitative cartilage volume measurement using MRI: Comparison of different evaluation techniques. *Eur. Radiol.* **15:** 1550–1554.

13. Barr, C., J.S. Bauer, D. Malfair, *et al.* 2007. MR imaging of the ankle at 3 Tesla and 1.5 Tesla: Protocol optimization and application to cartilage, ligament and tendon pathology in cadaver specimens. *Eur. Radiol.* **17:** 1518–1528.

14. Woertler, K., M. Strothmann, B. Tombach & P. Reimer. 2000. Detection of articular cartilage lesions: Experimental evaluation of low- and high-field-strength MR imaging at 0.18 and 1.0 T. *J. Magn. Reson. Imaging* **11:** 678–685.

15. Vahlensieck, M. & O. Schnieber. 2003. Performance of an open low-field MR unit in routine examination of knee lesions and comparison with high field systems. *Orthopade* **32:** 175–178.

16. Gold, G.E., E. Han, J. Stainsby, *et al.* 2004. Musculoskeletal MRI at 3.0 T: Relaxation times and image contrast. *AJR Am. J. Roentgenol.* **183:** 343–351.

17. Gold, G.E., B. Suh, A. Sawyer-Glover & C. Beaulieu. 2004. Musculoskeletal MRI at 3.0 T: Initial clinical experience. *AJR Am. J. Roentgenol.* **183:** 1479–1486.

18. Link, T.M., R. Stahl & K. Woertler. 2007. Cartilage imaging: Motivation, techniques, current and future significance. *Eur. Radiol.* **17:** 1135–1146.

19. Roemer, F.W., A. Guermazi, J.A. Lynch, *et al.* 2005. Short tau inversion recovery and proton density-

weighted fat suppressed sequences for the evaluation of osteoarthritis of the knee with a 1.0 T dedicated extremity MRI: Development of a time-efficient sequence protocol. *Eur. Radiol.* **15:** 978–987.

20. Libicher, M., M. Ivancic, M. Hoffmann & W. Wenz. 2005. Early changes in experimental osteoarthritis using the Pond-Nuki dog model: Technical procedure and initial results of in vivo MR imaging. *Eur. Radiol.* **15:** 390–394.

21. Kornaat, P.R., S.B. Reeder, S. Koo, *et al.* 2005. MR imaging of articular cartilage at 1.5T and 3.0T: Comparison of SPGR and SSFP sequences. *Osteoarthr. Cartilage* **13:** 338–344.

22. Hargreaves, B.A., G.E. Gold, C.F. Beaulieu, *et al.* 2003. Comparison of new sequences for high-resolution cartilage imaging. *Magn. Reson. Med.* **49:** 700–709.

23. Erickson, S.J., R.W. Prost & M.E. Timins. 1993. The "magic angle" effect: Background physics and clinical relevance. *Radiology* **188:** 23–25.

24. Peterfy, C.G., A. Guermazi, S. Zaim, *et al.* 2004. Whole-Organ Magnetic Resonance Imaging Score (WORMS) of the knee in osteoarthritis. *Osteoarthr. Cartilage* **12:** 177–190.

25. Recht, M.P., D.W. Piraino, G.A. Paletta, *et al.* 1996. Accuracy of fat-suppressed three-dimensional spoiled gradient-echo FLASH MR imaging in the detection of patellofemoral articular cartilage abnormalities. *Radiology* **198:** 209–212.

26. Zanetti, M., E. Bruder, J. Romero & J. Hodler. 2000. Bone marrow edema pattern in osteoarthritic knees: Correlation between MR imaging and histologic findings. *Radiology* **215:** 835–840.

27. Adams, J.G., T. McAlindon, M. Dimasi, *et al.* 1999. Contribution of meniscal extrusion and cartilage loss to joint space narrowing in osteoarthritis. *Clin. Radiol.* **54:** 502–506.

28. Hunter, D.J., G.H. Lo, D. Gale, *et al.* 2008. The development and reliability of a new scoring system for knee osteoarthritis MRI: BLOKS (Boston Leeds Osteoarthritis Knee Score). *Ann. Rheum. Dis.* **67:** 206–211.

29. Karachalios, T., A.H. Karantanas & K. Malizos. 2007. Hip osteoarthritis: What the radiologist wants to know. *Eur. J. Radiol.* **63:** 36–48.

30. Altman, R.D. & D. Dean. 1989. Pain in osteoarthritis: Introduction and overview. *Semin. Arthritis Rheum.* **18:** 1–3.

31. Altman, R., G. Alarcon D. Appelrouth, *et al.* 1991. The American College of Rheumatology criteria for the classification and reporting of osteoarthritis of the hip. *Arthritis Rheum.* **34:** 505–514.

32. Gupta, K.B., J. Duryea & B.N. Weissman. 2004. Radiographic evaluation of osteoarthritis. *Radiol. Clin. North Am.* **42:** 11–41.

33. Ravaud, P., B. Giraudeau, G.R. Auleley, *et al*. 1996. Radiographic assessment of knee osteoarthritis: Reproducibility and sensitivity to change. *J. Rheumatol*. **23:** 1756–1764.

34. Croft, P., C. Cooper, C. Wickham & D. Coggon. 1990. Defining osteoarthritis of the hip for epidemiologic studies. *Am. J. Epidemiol*. **132:** 514–522.

35. Dieppe, P.A. 1995. Recommended methodology for assessing the progression of osteoarthritis of the hip and knee joints. *Osteoarthr. Cartilage* **3:** 73–77.

36. Beall, D.P., C.F. Sweet, H.D. Martin, *et al*. 2005. Imaging findings of femoroacetabular impingement syndrome. *Skeletal Radiol*. **34:** 691–701.

37. Kassarjian, A., L.S. Yoon, E. Belzile, *et al*. 2005. Triad of MR arthrographic findings in patients with cam-type femoroacetabular impingement. *Radiology* **236:** 588–592.

38. Hart, D.J. & T.D. Spector. 2000. Definition and epidemiology of osteoarthritis of the hand: A review. *Osteoarthr. Cartilage* **8**(Suppl. A): S2–S7.

39. Chaisson, C.E., Y. Zhang, T.E. McAlindon, *et al*. 1997. Radiographic hand osteoarthritis: Incidence, patterns, and influence of pre-existing disease in a population based sample. *J. Rheumatol*. **24:** 1337–1343.

40. Tan, A.L., A.J. Grainger, S.F. Tanner, *et al*. 2005. High-resolution magnetic resonance imaging for the assessment of hand osteoarthritis. *Arthritis Rheum*. **52:** 2355–2365.

41. Tan, A.L., A.J. Grainger, S.F. Tanner, *et al*. 2006. A high-resolution magnetic resonance imaging study of distal interphalangeal joint arthropathy in psoriatic arthritis and osteoarthritis: Are they the same? *Arthritis Rheum*. **54:** 1328–1333.

42. Kirkhus, E., A. Bjornerud, J. Thoen, *et al*. 2006. Contrast-enhanced dynamic magnetic resonance imaging of finger joints in osteoarthritis and rheumatoid arthritis: An analysis based on pharmacokinetic modeling. *Acta Radiol*. **47:** 845–851.

43. Ogawa, K., A. Yoshida & H. Ikegami. 2006. Osteoarthritis in shoulders with traumatic anterior instability: Preoperative survey using radiography and computed tomography. *J. Shoulder Elbow Surg*. **15:** 23–29.

44. Phillips, W.C. Jr. & S.V. Kattapuram. 1991. Osteoarthritis: With emphasis on primary osteoarthritis of the shoulder. *Del. Med. J*. **63:** 609–613.

45. de Abreu, M.R., C.B. Chung, M. Wessely, *et al*. 2005. Acromioclavicular joint osteoarthritis: Comparison of findings derived from MR imaging and conventional radiography. *Clin. Imaging* **29:** 273–277.

46. Harrington, K.D. 1979. Degenerative arthritis of the ankle secondary to long-standing lateral ligament instability. *J. Bone Joint Surg. Am*. **61:** 354–361.

47. Keats, T.E. & R.B. Harrison. 1979. Hypertrophy of the talar beak. *Skeletal Radiol*. **4:** 37–39.

48. Robinson, P., L.M. White, D.C. Salonen, *et al*. 2001. Anterolateral ankle impingement: MR arthrographic assessment of the anterolateral recess. *Radiology* **221:** 186–190.

49. Almen, A., A. Tingberg, J. Besjakov & S. Mattsson. 2004. The use of reference image criteria in X-ray diagnostics: An application for the optimisation of lumbar spine radiographs. *Eur. Radiol*. **14:** 1561–1567.

50. Insko, E.K., D.B. Clayton & M.A. Elliott. 2002. In vivo sodium MR imaging of the intervertebral disk at 4 T. *Acad. Radiol*. **9:** 800–804.

51. Auerbach, J.D., W. Johannessen, A. Borthakur, *et al*. 2006. In vivo quantification of human lumbar disc degeneration using T(1rho)-weighted magnetic resonance imaging. *Eur. Spine J*. **15**(Suppl. 3): S338–S344.

52. Johannessen, W., J.D. Auerbach, A.J. Wheaton, *et al*. 2006. Assessment of human disc degeneration and proteoglycan content using T1rho-weighted magnetic resonance imaging. *Spine* **31:** 1253–1257.

53. Gallucci, M., E. Puglielli, A. Splendiani, *et al*. 2005. Degenerative disorders of the spine. *Eur. Radiol*. **15:** 591–598.

54. Saifuddin, A., E. McSweeney & J. Lehovsky. 2003. Development of lumbar high intensity zone on axial loaded magnetic resonance imaging. *Spine* **28:** E449–E451; discussion E451–E452.

55. Fardon, D.F. & P.C. Milette. 2001. Nomenclature and classification of lumbar disc pathology. Recommendations of the Combined Task Forces of the North American Spine Society, American Society of Spine Radiology, and American Society of Neuroradiology. *Spine* **26:** E93–E113.

56. Modic, M.T., P.M. Steinberg, J.S. Ross, *et al*. 1988. Degenerative disk disease: Assessment of changes in vertebral body marrow with MR imaging. *Radiology* **166:** 193–199.

57. Chaput, C., D. Padon, J. Rush, *et al*. 2007. The significance of increased fluid signal on magnetic resonance imaging in lumbar facets in relationship to degenerative spondylolisthesis. *Spine* **32:** 1883–1887.

58. Jensen, M.C., M.N. Brant-Zawadzki, N. Obuchowski, *et al*. 1994. Magnetic resonance imaging of the lumbar spine in people without back pain. *N. Engl. J. Med*. **331:** 69–73.

59. Belhorn, L.R. & E.V. Hess. 1993. Erosive osteoarthritis. *Semin. Arthritis Rheum*. **22:** 298–306.

60. Utsinger, P.D., D. Resnick, R.F. Shapiro & K.B. Wiesner. 1978. Roentgenologic, immunologic, and therapeutic study of erosive (inflammatory) osteoarthritis. *Arch. Intern. Med*. **138:** 693–697.

61. Ehrlich, G.E. 2001. Erosive osteoarthritis: Presentation, clinical pearls, and therapy. *Curr. Rheumatol. Rep*. **3:** 484–488.

62. Grainger, A.J., J.M. Farrant, P.J. O'Connor, *et al.* 2007. MR imaging of erosions in interphalangeal joint osteoarthritis: Is all osteoarthritis erosive? *Skeletal Radiol.* **36:** 737–745.

63. Cobby, M., J. Cushnaghan, P. Creamer, *et al.* 1990. Erosive osteoarthritis: Is it a separate disease entity? *Clin. Radiol.* **42:** 258–263.

64. Smith, D., E.M. Braunstein, K.D. Brandt & B.P. Katz. 1992. A radiographic comparison of erosive osteoarthritis and idiopathic nodal osteoarthritis. *J. Rheumatol.* **19:** 896–904.

65. Kidd, K.L. & J.B. Peter. 1966. Erosive osteoarthritis. *Radiology* **86:** 640–647.

66. Ehrlich, G.E. 1972. Inflammatory osteoarthritis: I. The clinical syndrome. *J. Chronic Dis.* **25:** 317–328.

67. Bergin, D., C. Keogh, M. O'Connell, *et al.* 2002. Atraumatic medial collateral ligament oedema in medial compartment knee osteoarthritis. *Skeletal Radiol.* **31:** 14–18.

68. Wen, D.Y., T. Propeck, S.M. Kane, *et al.* 2007. MRI description of knee medial collateral ligament abnormalities in the absence of trauma: Edema related to osteoarthritis and medial meniscal tears. *Magn. Reson. Imaging* **25:** 209–214.

69. Yoshioka, H., K. Stevens, B.A. Hargreaves, *et al.* 2004. Magnetic resonance imaging of articular cartilage of the knee: Comparison between fat-suppressed three-dimensional SPGR imaging, fat-suppressed FSE imaging, and fat-suppressed three-dimensional DEFT imaging, and correlation with arthroscopy. *J. Magn. Reson. Imaging* **20:** 857–864.

70. Gold, G.E., S.E. Fuller, B.A. Hargreaves, *et al.* 2005. Driven equilibrium magnetic resonance imaging of articular cartilage: Initial clinical experience. *J. Magn. Reson. Imaging* **21:** 476–481.

71. Gagliardi, J.A., E.M. Chung, V.P. Chandnani, *et al.* 1994. Detection and staging of chondromalacia patellae: Relative efficacies of conventional MR imaging, MR arthrography, and CT arthrography. *AJR Am. J. Roentgenol.* **163:** 629–636.

72. Woertler, K., E.J. Rummeny & M. Settles. 2005. A fast high-resolution multislice T1-weighted turbo spin-echo (TSE) sequence with a DRIVen equilibrium (DRIVE) pulse for native arthrographic contrast. *AJR Am. J. Roentgenol.* **185:** 1468–1470.

73. Link, T.M., C.A. Sell, J.N. Masi, *et al.* 2006. 3.0 vs 1.5 T MRI in the detection of focal cartilage pathology–ROC analysis in an experimental model. *Osteoarthr. Cartilage* **14:** 63–70.

74. Eckstein, F., J. Westhoff, H. Sittek, *et al.* 1998. In vivo reproducibility of three-dimensional cartilage volume and thickness measurements with MR imaging. *AJR Am. J. Roentgenol.* **170:** 593–597.

75. Piplani, M.A., D.G. Disler, T.R. McCauley, *et al.* 1996. Articular cartilage volume in the knee: Semi-automated determination from three-dimensional reformations of MR images. *Radiology* **198:** 855–859.

76. Eckstein, F., M. Reiser, K.H. Englmeier & R. Putz. 2001. In vivo morphometry and functional analysis of human articular cartilage with quantitative magnetic resonance imaging–from image to data, from data to theory. *Anat. Embryol. (Berl)* **203:** 147–173.

77. Wheaton, A.J., A. Borthakur, G.R. Dodge, *et al.* 2004. Sodium magnetic resonance imaging of proteoglycan depletion in an in vivo model of osteoarthritis. *Acad. Radiol.* **11:** 21–28.

78. Regatte, R.R., S.V. Akella, A.J. Wheaton, *et al.* 2004. 3D-T1rho-relaxation mapping of articular cartilage: In vivo assessment of early degenerative changes in symptomatic osteoarthritic subjects. *Acad. Radiol.* **11:** 741–749.

79. Regatte, R.R., S.V. Akella, A. Borthakur, *et al.* 2003. In vivo proton MR three-dimensional T1rho mapping of human articular cartilage: Initial experience. *Radiology* **229:** 269–274.

80. Li, X., E.T. Han, C.B. Ma, *et al.* 2005. In vivo 3T spiral imaging based multi-slice T(1rho) mapping of knee cartilage in osteoarthritis. *Magn. Reson. Med.* **54:** 929–936.

81. Liess, C., S. Lusse, N. Karger, *et al.* 2002. Detection of changes in cartilage water content using MRI T2-mapping in vivo. *Osteoarthr. Cartilage* **10:** 907–913.

82. Dardzinski, B.J., T.J. Mosher, S. Li, *et al.* 1997. Spatial variation of T2 in human articular cartilage. *Radiology* **205:** 546–550.

83. Mosher, T.J., B.J. Dardzinski & M.B. Smith. 2000. Human articular cartilage: Influence of aging and early symptomatic degeneration on the spatial variation of T2—preliminary findings at 3 T. *Radiology* **214:** 259–266.

84. Mosher, T.J., H.E. Smith, C. Collins, *et al.* 2005. Change in knee cartilage T2 at MR imaging after running: A feasibility study. *Radiology* **234:** 245–249.

85. Dunn, T.C., Y. Lu, H. Jin, *et al.* 2004. T2 relaxation time of cartilage at MR imaging: Comparison with severity of knee osteoarthritis. *Radiology* **232:** 592–598.

86. Bashir, A., M.L. Gray, R.D. Boutin & D. Burstein D. 1997. Glycosaminoglycan in articular cartilage: In vivo assessment with delayed Gd(DTPA) (2-)-enhanced MR imaging. *Radiology* **205:** 551–558.

87. Trattnig, S., V. Mlynarik, M. Breitenseher, *et al.* 1999. MRI visualization of proteoglycan depletion in articular cartilage via intravenous administration of Gd-DTPA. *Magn. Reson. Imaging* **17:** 577–583.

88. Burstein, D., J. Velyvis, K.T. Scott, *et al.* 2001. Protocol issues for delayed Gd(DTPA)(2-)-enhanced MRI

(dGEMRIC) for clinical evaluation of articular cartilage. *Magn. Reson. Med.* **45:** 36–41.

89. Burstein, D. & M. Gray. 2003. New MRI techniques for imaging cartilage. *J. Bone Joint Surg. Am.* **85-A**(Suppl. 2): 70–77.

90. Gillis, A., A. Bashir, B. McKeon, *et al.* 2001. Magnetic resonance imaging of relative glycosaminoglycan distribution in patients with autologous chondrocyte transplants. *Invest. Radiol.* **36:** 743–748.

91. Williams, A., A. Gillis, C. McKenzie, *et al.* 2004. Glycosaminoglycan distribution in cartilage as determined by delayed gadolinium-enhanced MRI of cartilage (dGEMRIC): Potential clinical applications. *AJR Am. J. Roentgenol.* **182:** 167–172.

92. Williams, A., L. Sharma, C.A. McKenzie, *et al.* 2005. Delayed gadolinium-enhanced magnetic resonance imaging of cartilage in knee osteoarthritis: Findings at different radiographic stages of disease and relationship to malalignment. *Arthritis Rheum.* **52:** 3528–3535.

93. Filidoro, L., O. Dietrich, J. Weber, *et al.* 2005. High-resolution diffusion tensor imaging of human patellar cartilage: Feasibility and preliminary findings. *Magn. Reson. Med.* **53:** 993–998.

Section III. Ultrasound

Ultrasound and Structural Changes in Inflammatory Arthritis

Synovitis and Tenosynovitis

Marina Backhaus

Department of Rheumatology and Clinical Immunology University Hospital Charité, Berlin, Germany

Accurate assessment of disease activity and joint damage in rheumatological diseases is important for monitoring treatment efficacy and predicting the disease outcome, and such assessment requires sensitive imaging tools. Conventional radiography is insensitive to soft tissue lesions and to early erosive bone lesions. Musculoskeletal ultrasonography has become an important diagnostic technique in rheumatological diseases, as it can detect both early inflammatory soft tissue lesions (e.g., synovitis, tenosynovitis, and bursitis) and early erosive bone lesions in arthritic joint diseases. Studies show good correlation in this regard between ultrasound and magnetic resonance imaging. Owing to good soft tissue contrast, ultrasound enables differentiation between exudative and proliferative synovial changes and may also direct further diagnostic and therapeutic procedures and color and power Doppler ultrasonography help to differentiate active from inactive joint processes. Specifically, the use of contrast agents increases the sensitivity for the detection of a thickened, hypervascular, and inflamed joint capsule and enables better quantification of inflammatory disease by estimating ultrasound signal intensity changes. At present, contrast-enhanced ultrasonography is of particular interest for clinical studies in monitoring the new anti-inflammatory drugs used to treat rheumatological diseases.

Key words: ultrasound; synovitis; tenosynovitis

Introduction

Sensitive imaging tools are needed for the detection and the accurate assessment of disease activity and joint damage in rheumatological diseases needed to monitor treatment efficiency and predict disease outcome. Conventional radiography (CR) is the most well established imaging technique for identifying progressive joint damage (e.g., in rheumatoid arthritis), but it is not sensitive to soft tissue lesions or early erosive bone lesions. Musculoskeletal ultrasonography has become an important diagnostic technique in rheumatological diseases, as it can detect both early inflammatory soft tissue lesions (e.g., synovitis, tenosynovitis, and bursitis) and early erosive bone lesions in arthritic joint diseases.[1-6] Studies have shown good correlations between ultrasound (US) and MRI. Synovitis plays an important role in joint damage. No bone destruction occurs without the presence of synovitis.

Owing to good soft tissue contrast, US can differentiate between exudative and proliferative synovial changes, and early detection of synovial proliferation is important for timely diagnosis of arthritis. Moreover, it can guide further diagnostic and therapeutic procedures.[7] Color and power Doppler ultrasonography are helpful in differentiating active from inactive joint processes, and recent studies using US

Address for correspondence: Marina Backhaus, Department of Rheumatology and Clinical Immunology, University Hospital Charité, Charité Platz 1, D-10117 Berlin, Germany. Voice: +49 30 450 513 137; fax: +49 30 450 513 939. marina.backhaus@charite.de

MRI and Ultrasound in Diagnosis and Management: Ann. N.Y. Acad. Sci. 1154: 139–151 (2009).
doi: 10.1111/j.1749-6632.2009.04388.x © 2009 New York Academy of Sciences.

contrast media have demonstrated its benefits in the differentiation of inflammatory disorders. Contrast agents increase the sensitivity for detection of a thickened, hypervascular, and inflamed joint capsule and enable better quantification of inflammatory disease by way of US signal intensity changes. At present, contrast-enhanced ultrasonography (CE-US) is of particular interest for clinical studies in monitoring the new anti-inflammatory drugs now being used to treat rheumatological diseases.

Technical Requirements

Modern US devices utilize multifrequency transducers. The frequency of the sound wave determines how deeply it will penetrate the tissue. The frequency also impacts the resolution. For the best resolution, the highest possible US frequency should be used. Musculoskeletal US is generally performed with linear transducers, with the choice of transducer depending on the joint region to be examined. For the wrist, hand, and toe joints, frequencies of 10–18 MHz are recommended. Middle-size joints are examined at 10–12 MHz, and deep-lying joints such as those of the hip are scanned with linear transducers at 5–7.5 MHz or, for deeper penetration, with curved array transducers at 3.5 MHz.

Several joint regions are examined in a standard fashion according to the guidelines of the German Society for Ultrasound in Medicine (DEGUM) and the European League Against Rheumatism (EULAR).[8,9] Joint US is performed in multiplanar scans, where the transducer navigates dynamically from proximal to distal in transverse scans and from medial to lateral in longitudinal scans, a procedure that scans the joint completely. Dynamic imaging is necessary for the detection of small fluid collections. In this case, the transducer should be held in a fixed position on top of the joint region of interest while the joint is moved by the examiner or by isometric contraction of muscles in relation to the joint region.

Although technical developments such as "tissue harmonic imaging" or "sono-CT/cross-beam sonography" can improve image quality, the scan results depend on the techniques utilized and the competence and experience of the examiner. Special knowledge is needed for musculoskeletal US and relevant courses at different levels of expertise are offered under the auspices of EULAR. Interobserver reliabilities, sensitivities, and specificities of musculoskeletal US in comparison with MRI are moderate to good.[10–12]

Ultrasound images can be recorded, stored digitally, and copied onto CD or DVD. Prints can be made using a connected black-and-white thermal printer.

Differentiation of Soft Tissue Lesions by Musculoskeletal Ultrasonography

The inflammatory soft tissue lesions include synovitis with effusion, synovial proliferation, tenosynovitis with effusion and/or synovial proliferation of the tendon sheath, tendinitis, as well as bursitis with effusion and/or synovial proliferation. Synovial proliferation of the joint capsule often occurs in combination with inflammatory effusion and the combination is termed synovitis.

During the Seventh OMERACT Conference (Outcome Measurement Rheumatoid Arthritis Clinical Trial) in Monterrey, California, May 2004, the international US study group described the sonographical definitions as follows[13]:

- *Effusion:* Effusion is a hypoechoic or anechoic intra-articular material, which is displaceable and compressible and without signs of a Doppler signal. Echo texture is relative to the subdermal fat pad (Fig. 1C).
- *Synovial Hypertrophy/Synovial Proliferation:* An abnormal hypoechoic intra-articular tissue, which is not displaceable and hardly

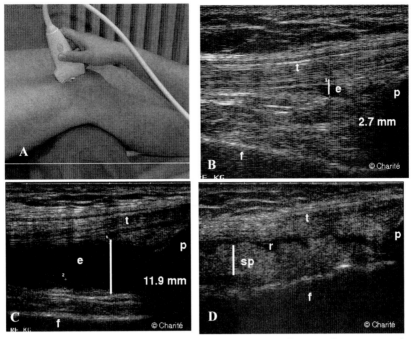

Figure 1. Effusion and synovial hypertrophy of suprapatellar pouch: (**A**) US probe position; (**B**) longitudinal scan at suprapatellar pouch of normal knee, (**C**) knee with effusion; and (**D**) knee with synovial hypertrophy (f = femur, p = patellar, t = tendon, e = effusion, sp = synovial hypertrophy).

compressible, with signs of Doppler signal. Echo texture is impacted by the subdermal fat pad and can at times also be echoic or hyperechoic (Fig. 1D).

- *Tenosynovitis:* An abnormal hypoechoic or anechoic material, with or without fluid inside the tendon sheath and with possible signs of Doppler signals in two perpendicular planes (Fig. 2).
- *Enthesopathy:* Abnormal hypoechoic (loss of normal fibrillar architecture) and/ or thickened tendon or ligament at its bony attachment seen in two perpendicular planes, which may exhibit Doppler signal and/or changes including enthesophytes, erosions or irregularity (Fig. 3).

Clinical studies have shown that musculoskeletal US is more sensitive in the detection of inflammatory signs than a clinical examination.[1-4] Signs of synovitis can be detected more frequently in the palmar proximal area

of the finger joints (PIP and MCP) than from the dorsal aspect (Figs. 4 and 5).[14] Synovitis scores have been developed for the finger joints in arthritic processes.[14,15] The synovitis score according to Szkudlarek grades the inflammatory soft tissue lesions separately for effusion and synovial proliferation,[15] and the one according to Scheel and Backhaus combines both effusion and synovial proliferation in one scoring system.[14,16] The latter authors showed that the best results for joint combinations were achieved using the "sum of four fingers" (second through fifth MCP and PIP joints) and "sum of three fingers" (second through fourth MCP and PIP joints) methods. Comparison of MRI results and semiquantitative US scores (grade 0 = normal; grade 1 = minimal effusion/ synovial hypertrophy; grade 2 = moderate effusion/synovial hypertrophy; grade 3 = severe effusion/synovial hypertrophy) revealed good agreement with the quantitative synovitis scores (measurements of joint capsule distance

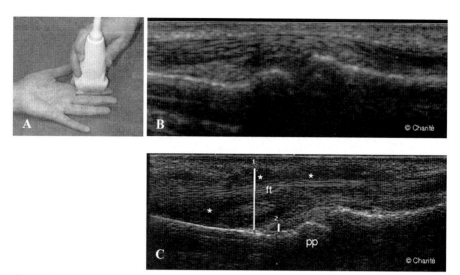

Figure 2. Tenosynovitis of flexor digitorum tendon: (**A**) US probe position; (**B**) longitudinal scan at palmar aspect of normal PIP joint; (**C**) tenosynovitis of flexor tendon (u = ulna, c = carpal bone, t = tendon, s = synovitis, * = tenosynovitis).

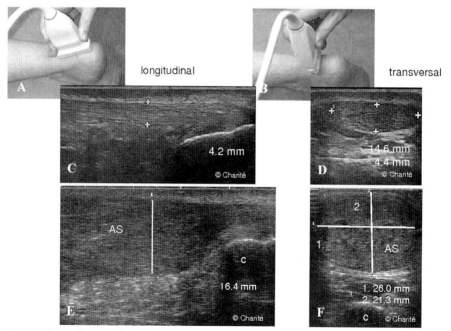

Figure 3. Enthesiopathy of the Achilles tendon: US probe position in longitudinal (**A**) and transverse (**B**) orientation; longitudinal and transverse scan at the normal Achilles tendon (**C, D**), and with tenonitis of the Achilles tendon in longitudinal scan (**E**) and transverse scan (**F**). Thickening of the Achilles tendon is seen (AS = Achilles tendon, c = calcaneus).

to bone margin in millimeters) (Fig. 6). Ultrasonography can also detect synovitis in the toes (especially in MTP joints),[4] as well as in many other joints.[17–24]

The tendon sheath of the long biceps tendon has a connection with the glenohumeral joint and when there is inflammation in the shoulder joint a small amount of fluid is seen

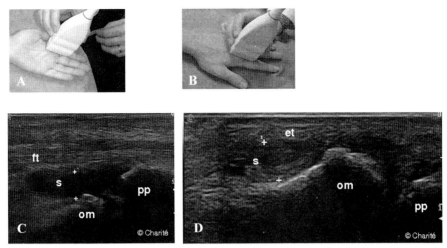

Figure 4. Synovitis of MCP joint: US probe position in longitudinal orientation at palmar (**A**) and dorsal aspect (**B**) longitudinal scan at palmar (**C**) and dorsal aspect (**D**) of MCP joint, with synovitis at palmar and dorsal aspect (ft = flexor tendon, s = synovitis, om = os metacarpale, pp = phalanx proximalis, et = extensor tendon).

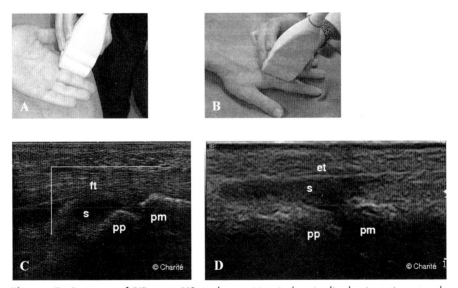

Figure 5. Synovitis of PIP joint: US probe position in longitudinal orientation at palmar (**A**) and dorsal aspect (**B**) longitudinal scan at palmar (**C**) and dorsal aspect (**D**) of PIP joint, with synovitis at palmar and dorsal aspect (ft = flexor tendon, s = synovitis, pp = phalanx proximalis, pm = phalanx medialis, et = extensor tendon).

that sheath (Fig. 7). A tenosynovitis of the extensor carpi ulnaris tendon is an early inflammatory sign in rheumatoid arthritis that can be easily detected by US (Fig. 8).[17] In the case of tendinitis, a hypo- to anechoic rim is seen along the hyperechoic tendon (Fig. 9). Ultrasonography is better than clinical examination in the detection of entheseal abnormality of lower limbs in spondyloarthropathies.[25-27]

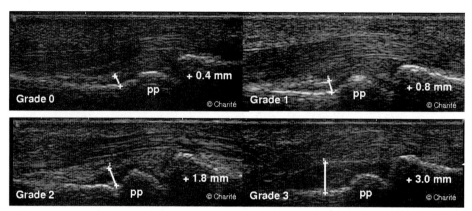

Figure 6. Semiquantitative scoring in B-mode of PIP joints at palmar aspect in rheumatoid arthritis (grades 0–3) (pp = phalanx proximalis).

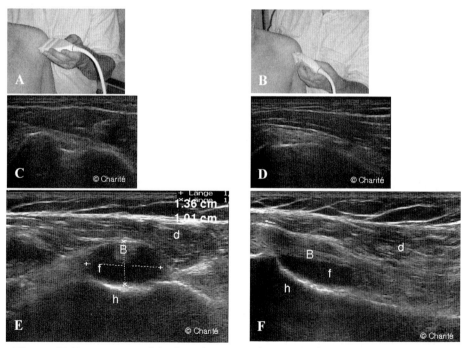

Figure 7. Tenosynovitis of the long biceps tendon: US probe position in transverse (**A**) and longitudinal (**B**) orientation; transverse and longitudinal scan at the normal long biceps tendon sheath (**C, D**), with tenosynovitis of long biceps tendon in transverse scan (**E**) and longitudinal scan (**F**) (h = humerus, b = biceps tendon, f = fluid, d = delta muscle).

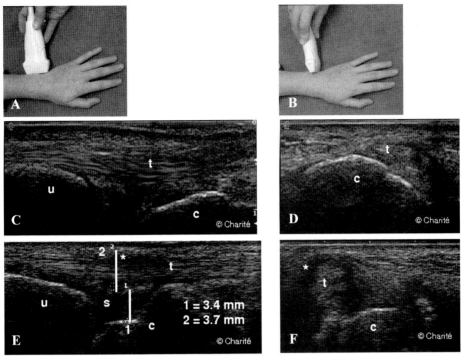

Figure 8. Tenosynovitis of extensor carpi ulnaris tendon: US probe position in longitudinal (**A**) and transverse (**B**) orientation; longitudinal and transverse scan at ulnar aspect of normal wrist (**C, D**), and of wrist with tenosynovitis of extensor carpi ulnaris tendon in longitudinal scan (**E**) and transverse scan (**F**) (u = ulna bone, c = carpal bone, t = tendon extensor carpi ulnaris, s = synovitis, * = tenosynovitis).

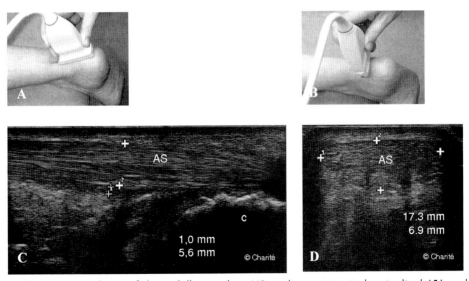

Figure 9. Tendinitis of the Achilles tendon: US probe position in longitudinal (**A**) and transverse (**B**) orientation; longitudinal and transverse scan at the Achilles tendon (**C, D**) showing tendinitis. An anechoic rim is seen along the tendon (AS = Achilles tendon, c = calcaneus).

Color and Power Doppler Sonography in the Diagnosis of Early Arthritis

The echo texture in gray-scale US (B-mode) allows a preliminary assessment of the activity of inflammation. The echo texture of synovial tissue of an active joint process is more hypoechoic and in the case of an inactive joint process more echoic to hyperechoic. The use of color and power Doppler US facilitates a differentiation between active and inactive synovitis.[28] Power Doppler sonography demonstrates the hypervascularization of inflammatory synovial tissue. The vessels of inflammatory tissue are expanded and new vessels are constituted, all of which is detectable with the Doppler technique. With regard to the vessel density of an inflammatory joint, it is possible to illustrate color pixels in different accumulations.

The demonstration of physiological vascularization of healthy joints without signs of inflammation is only possible with very sensitive US devices and high-resolution scanning techniques, and even then only in a very few cases. The principles of diagnostic US are based on different reflections of high-frequency US waves at the interfaces of tissues within the body. In the case where US waves reflect off a moving border, the frequency of the reflected waves is either high or low, depending, respectively, on whether they are moving toward or away from their source. The change in wave frequency on moving tissue—the Doppler effect—is a known physical phenomenon commonly used to demonstrate blood flow.

The reflection of US waves on the surface of corpuscular parts of blood leads to a shift of frequency (Doppler frequency or shift), which is measurable and detectable. The Doppler frequencies are shown in different colors. Normally, red means a movement of waves in the direction of the transducer and blue a movement away from the transducer. A description of blood flow in the location and direction toward the anatomical structures is also possible.

Modern devices use a pulse wave (PW) Doppler, which, unlike the continuous wave (CW) Doppler, sends rhythmical waves with a defined frequency (pulse repetition frequency/PRF) in the form of several "US wave packages." Doppler frequency analysis allows the measurement of the respective fluid speed of blood flow. A correction for the angle of the determinate Doppler fluid curve should be made. A combination of B-mode and Doppler sonography is called duplex sonography. Normally power Doppler sonography has no direction code for blood flow, which consequently allows for a higher sensitivity in the detection of blood flow at lower speed, especially in small blood vessels (such as in the case of inflamed joints). Newer high-quality US devices use a bidirectional power Doppler mode, which is also able to show a direction code of blood flow as with color Doppler US, but at higher resolution. Adding bidirectional mode to power Doppler sonography is therefore able to represent the vascularization of pannus tissue.

Finally, a semiquantitative grading system of color pixels can be used to describe the activity of the joint process (Fig. 10)[29]:

- Grade 0 = No Doppler signal (color pixel)/no flow.
- Grade 1 = Single Doppler signal/little flow (three single spots or two single spots plus one confluent spot).
- Grade 2 = Several Doppler signals/ coherent Doppler signal/clear flow ($\leq$50% color pixels of the intra-articular area).
- Grade 3 = Nearly complete joint area with coherent Doppler signal/strong flow ($\geq$50% color pixels of the intra-articular area).

The intra-articular and intrasynovial color pixels are important in describing joint inflammation. Periarticular color pixels are seen owing to hyperemia in arthritic processes. Several studies employing color and power Doppler sonography in rheumatoid arthritis in hand,

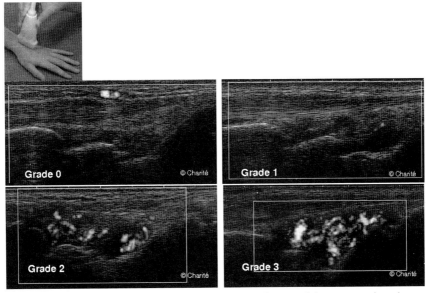

Figure 10. Semiquantitative scoring in power Doppler US of the wrist at dorsal aspect in rheumatoid arthritis (grades 0–3) (r = radius, c = carpal bone, t = tendon, s = synovitis).

wrist, and knee joints have demonstrated good correlation with clinical examination, contrast-enhanced MRI, and histopathology.[29-31] Power Doppler sonography is also useful for monitoring therapy with new antirheumatic drugs (biologicals).[32,33]

Use of Echo Contrast Agent in Diagnosis of Early Arthritis

Differentiation between effusion and synovial proliferation using only gray-scale US may be difficult because both can be similar in their echo texture (ranging from hypoechoic to echoic). Color and power Doppler sonography are limited in their ability to detect slow blood flow or blood flow in very small vessels. The use of echo-contrast-enhanced US enables functional imaging of synovial vascularization and thus an assessment of disease activity (Fig. 11). Low-volume blood flow in very small vessels can be detected owing to improved signal ratio.[34,35]

A multicenter study might show an improvement in the measurement of synovial thickness and activity of synovial processes in patients with rheumatoid arthritis by using echo-contrast-enhanced US.[36] The contrast agents, which are administered intravenously, are stable gas microbubbles with good reflex behavior that binds to red blood cells. Different sizes of bubbles are employed and they may be nonrespirable or respirable. Depending on their oscillation behavior, there are echo contrast agents of either first or second generation. Second-generation echo contrast agents (e.g., SonoVue®, Bracco, Italy) are especially useful in arthritis diagnosis studies. Contrast microbubbles are smaller than erythrocytes (3 μm), do not leave the intravascular space, and are exhaled through the lungs approximately 6 min after intravenous application. Therefore, severe diseases of heart and/or lung (e.g., lung fibrosis, coronary heart diseases NYHA stage III and IV) are contraindications for the use of contrast-enhanced sonography. A semiquantitative grading system[36] or a quantitative analysis with so-called time intensity curves, can be applied for assessment of activity detected by contrast-enhanced sonography.

The comparison of contrast agent behavior of intra- and extra-articular structures also

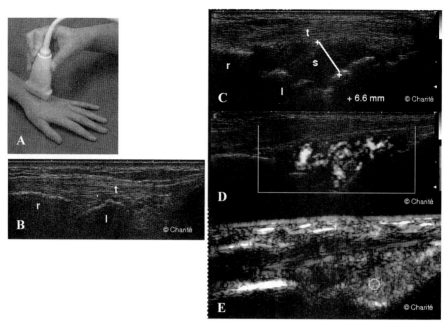

Figure 11. Echo contrast-enhanced US of the wrist in comparison to B-mode and power Doppler US: US probe position in longitudinal (**A**); orientation longitudinal scan at dorsal aspect of a normal wrist in B-mode (**B**), with severe synovitis of the wrist in B-mode (grade 3) (**C**), in power Doppler US (grade 3) (**D**), and in contrast-enhanced US (grade 3) (**E**) (r = radius, c = carpal bone, t = tendon, s = synovitis).

enables a qualitative analysis of inflammatory joint activity. However, for therapeutic response studies, an objective quantification of contrast-enhanced sonography is preferred.

Contrast-enhanced sonography allows better differentiation between effusion and synovial proliferation and leads to a better assessment of disease activity of synovial processes.[37,38] This differentiation is helpful in studies of new treatment procedures involving disease processes acting on the microvascular level. For instance, fibrosis in inactive pannus tissue shows no vascularization and no accumulation of contrast agent. Current studies use contrast-enhanced sonography to evaluate the inflamed synovium of rheumatoid arthritis. A study with Levovist®, a first-generation contrast agent, on knee and MCP joints in rheumatoid arthritis showed good correlation with clinical findings, laboratory tests, and contrast-enhanced MRI.[39-42] No correlation was found between Levovist® in shoulder joints as com-

pared to MRI (as studied in a population of patients with rheumatoid arthritis).[43]

A study with SonoVue®, a second-generation contrast agent, showed good correlation with contrast-enhanced MRI in the detection of synovitis of the suprapatellar recess in knee osteoarthritis.[44,45] Contrast-enhanced sonography is inexpensive compared to contrast-enhanced MRI and has the same high resolution. The time needed for US investigation is about 20 min, including preparation time. Another advantage of US as compared to contrast-enhanced MRI is the fact that echo contrast agents do not leave the vascular space and do not get into the synovial fluid, so they are able to reflect changes within the intravascular compartment precisely.

Echo-contrast-enhanced ultrasonography is helpful in the differentiation and evaluation of inflammatory joint processes. It is especially of interest in testing the efficacy of new antirheumatic drugs. Further studies are necessary to evaluate this new technique in the assessment of joint diseases.

Conclusion

In summary, for the screening of arthritic joint processes, the following procedures are recommended:

1. Longitudinal and transverse scan of the wrist (dorsal, ulnar, palmar aspect) for signs of synovitis, tenosynovitis, and erosions.
2. Longitudinal and transverse scan of the MCP joints and the PIP joints II–IV (dorsal, palmar aspect) for signs of synovitis, tenosynovitis/tendinitis, and erosions.
3. Longitudinal and transverse scan of the MCP joint II (radial) and MCP joint V (ulnar) for signs of erosions.
4. Longitudinal and transverse scan of MTP joints II and V joints (dorsal, plantar aspect) for signs of synovitis and erosions.
5. Longitudinal and transverse scan of MTP joint V (lateral) for signs of erosions.
6. Scans of other symptomatic joints as needed.

Musculoskeletal ultrasonography is helpful in the diagnosis of early arthritis, especially in cases showing normal conventional radiographs but suspicious clinical findings. It enables early detection of inflamed synovial processes such as effusion and/or synovial hypertrophy, tenosynovitis, bursitis, and erosions and is a suitable imaging technique for followup and therapy monitoring. It is also of value in diagnostic and therapeutic joint injection procedures. The use of color and power Doppler US as well as contrast-enhanced sonography reveals additional information about the activity of inflamed joint processes. Ultrasonography is a patient-friendly technique that is now an established method for diagnosis and monitoring of arthritic diseases such as rheumatoid arthritis.

Conflicts of Interest

The authors declare no conflicts of interest.

References

1. Backhaus, M., T. Kamradt, D. Sandrock, *et al.* 1999. Arthritis of the finger joints: A comprehensive approach comparing conventional radiography, scintigraphy, ultrasound, and contrast-enhanced magnetic resonance imaging. *Arthritis Rheum.* **42:** 1232–1245.
2. Backhaus, M., G.-R. Burmester, D. Sandrock, *et al.* 2002. Prospective two-year follow-up study comparing novel and conventional imaging procedures in patients with arthritic finger joints. *Ann. Rheum. Dis.* **61:** 895–904.
3. Scheel, A.K., K.G. Hermann, S. Ohrndorf, *et al.* 2006. Prospective long term follow-up imaging study comparing radiography, ultrasonography and magnetic resonance imaging in rheumatoid arthritis finger joints. *Ann. Rheum. Dis.* **65:** 595–600.
4. Szkudlarek, M., E. Narvestad, M. Klarlund, *et al.* 2004. Ultrasonography of the metatarsophalangeal joints in rheumatoid arthritis: Comparison with magnetic resonance imaging, conventional radiography, and clinical examination. *Arthritis Rheum.* **50:** 2103–2112.
5. Szkudlarek, M., E. Narvestad, M. Court-Payen, *et al.* 2004. Ultrasonography of the RA finger joints is more sensitive than conventional radiography for detection of erosions without loss of specificity, with MRI as a reference method. *Ann. Rheum. Dis.* **63:** 82–83.
6. Wakefield, R.J., W.W. Gibbon, P.G. Conaghan, *et al.* 2000. The value of sonography in the detection of bone erosions in patients with rheumatoid arthritis. *Arthritis Rheum.* **43:** 2762–2770.
7. Karim, Z., R.J. Wakefield, P.G. Conaghan, *et al.* 2001. The impact of ultrasonography on diagnosis and management of patients with musculoskeletal conditions. *Arthritis Rheum.* **44:** 2932–2933.
8. Konermann, W. & G. Gruber. 2000. *Musculoskeletal Sonography. Guidelines of the German Society for Ultrasound in Medicine (DEGUM).* Thieme. Stuttgart.
9. Backhaus, M., G.-R. Burmester, T. Gerber, *et al.* 2001. Guidelines for musculoskeletal ultrasound in rheumatology. *Ann. Rheum. Dis.* **60:** 641–649.
10. Scheel, A.K., W.A. Schmidt, K.G. Hermann, *et al.* 2005. Interobserver reliability of rheumatologists performing musculoskeletal ultrasonography: Results from a EULAR "Train the Trainers" course. *Ann. Rheum. Dis.* **64:** 1043–1049.
11. Naredo, E., I. Moller, C. Moragues, *et al.* 2006. EULAR Working Group for Musculoskeletal Ultrasound. Interobserver reliability in musculoskeletal

ultrasonography: Results from a "Teach the Teachers" rheumatologist course. *Ann. Rheum. Dis.* **65:** 14–19.

12. Szkudlarek, M., M. Court-Payen, S. Jacobsen, *et al.* 2003. Interobserver agreement in ultrasonography of the finger and toe joints in rheumatoid arthritis. *Arthritis Rheum.* **48:** 955–962.

13. Wakefield, R.J., P. Balint, M. Szkudlarek, *et al.* 2005. OMERACT 7 Special Interest Group: Musculoskeletal ultrasound including definitions for ultrasonographic pathology. *J. Rheumatol.* **32:** 2485–2487.

14. Scheel, A.K., K.G. Hermann, E. Kahler, *et al.* 2005. A novel ultrasonographic synovitis scoring system suitable for analyzing finger joint inflammation in rheumatoid arthritis. *Arthritis Rheum.* **52:** 681–686.

15. Szkudlarek, M., M. Court-Payen, C. Strandberg, *et al.* 2001. Power Doppler ultrasonography for assessment of synovitis in the metacarpophalangeal joints of patients with rheumatoid arthritis: A comparison with dynamic magnetic resonance imaging. *Arthritis Rheum.* **44:** 2018–2023.

16. Scheel, A.K. & M. Backhaus. 2004. Ultrasonographic assessment of the finger and toe joint inflammation in rheumatoid arthritis: Comment on the article by Szkudlarek et al. [letter]. *Arthritis Rheum.* **50:** 1008.

17. Backhaus, M., W.A. Schmidt, H. Mellerowicz, *et al.* 2002. Technique and diagnostic value of musculoskeletal ultrasonography in rheumatology: Pt. 6. Ultrasonography of the wrist/hand. *Z. Rheumatol.* **61:** 674–687.

18. Backhaus, M., W.A. Schmidt, H. Mellerowicz, *et al.* 2002. Technical aspects and value of arthrosonography in rheumatologic diagnosis: Pt. 4. Ultrasound of the elbow. *Z. Rheumatol.* **61:** 415–425.

19. Joshua, F., M. Lassere, G.A. Bruyn, *et al.* 2007. Summary findings of a systematic review of the ultrasound assessment of synovitis. *J. Rheumatol.* **34:** 839–847.

20. Hauer, R.W., W.A. Schmidt, M. Bohl-Bühler, *et al.* 2001. Technique and value of arthrosonography in rheumatologic diagnosis: Pt 1. Ultrasound diagnosis of the knee joint. *Z. Rheumatol.* **60:** 139–147.

21. Mellerowicz, H., W.A. Schmidt, R.W. Hauer, *et al.* 2002. Technique and diagnostic value of musculoskeletal ultrasonography in rheumatology: Pt. 5. Ultrasonography of the shoulder. *Z. Rheumatol.* **61:** 577–589.

22. Schmidt, W.A., R.W. Hauer, D. Banzer, *et al.* 2002. Technique and value of arthrosonography in rheumatologic diagnosis: Pt. 2. Ultrasound diagnosis of the hip area. *Z. Rheumatol.* **61:** 180–188.

23. Schmidt, W.A., R.W. Hauer, D. Banzer, *et al.* 2002. Technique and value of arthrosonography in rheumatologic diagnosis: Pt. 3. Ultrasound diagnosis

24. Sattler, H. 2006. Sonography in rheumatology: Standard scans and dynamic examination of musculoskeletal system. *Akt. Rheumatol.* **31:** 123–127.

25. D'Agostino, M.A., R. Said-Nahal, C. Hacquard-Bouder, *et al.* 2003. Assessment of peripheral enthesitis in the spondylarthropathies by ultrasonography combined with power Doppler: A cross-sectional study. *Arthritis Rheum.* **48:** 523–533.

26. Balint, P.V., D. Kane, H. Wilson, *et al.* 2002. Ultrasonography of entheseal insertions in the lower limb in spondyloarthropathy. *Ann. Rheum. Dis.* **61:** 905–910.

27. Kiris, A., A. Kaya, S. Ozgocmen, *et al.* 2006. Assessment of enthesitis in ankylosing spondylitis by power Doppler ultrasonography. *Skeletal Radiol.* **35:** 522–528.

28. Strunk, J. 2006. Color Doppler: Musculoskeletal sonography. *Akt. Rheumatol.* **31:** 148–156.

29. Szkudlarek, M., M. Court-Payen, C. Strandberg, *et al.* 2001. Power Doppler ultrasonography for assessment of synovitis in the metacarpophalangeal joints of patients with rheumatoid arthritis: A comparison with dynamic magnetic resonance imaging. *Arthritis Rheum.* **44:** 2018–2023.

30. Terslev, L., S. Torp-Pedersen, A. Savnik, *et al.* 2003. Doppler ultrasound and magnetic resonance imaging of synovial inflammation of the hand in rheumatoid arthritis: A comparative study. *Arthritis Rheum.* **48:** 2434–2441.

31. Walther, M., H. Harms, V. Krenn, *et al.* 2001. Correlation of power Doppler sonography with vascularity of the synovial tissue of the knee joint in patients with osteoarthritis and rheumatoid arthritis. *Arthritis Rheum.* **44:** 331–829.

32. Filippucci, E., A. Iagnocco, F. Salaffi, *et al.* 2006. Power Doppler sonography monitoring of synovial perfusion at wrist joint in rheumatoid patients treated with adalimumab. *Ann. Rheum. Dis.* **65:** 1433–1437.

33. Ribbens, C., B. Andre, S. Marcelis, *et al.* 2003. Rheumatoid hand joint synovitis: Gray-scale and power Doppler US quantifications following antitumor necrosis factor-alpha treatment—pilot study. *Radiology.* **229:** 562–569.

34. Goldberg, B.B., J.B. Liu & F. Forsberg. 1994. Ultrasound contrast agents: A review. *Ultrasound Med. Biol.* **20:** 319–333. Review.

35. Blomley, M.J., J.C. Cooke, E.C. Unger, *et al.* 2001. Microbubble contrast agents: A new era in ultrasound. *BMJ.* **322:** 1222–1225. Review.

36. Klauser, A., J. Demharter, A. De Marchi, *et al.* 2005. Contrast-enhanced gray-scale sonography in assessment of joint vascularity in rheumatoid arthritis:

Results from the IACUS Study Group. *Eur. Radiol.* **15:** 2404–2410.

37. Kleffel, T., J. Demharter, W. Wohlgemuth, *et al*. 2005. Comparison of contrast-enhanced low mechanical index (low MI) sonography and unenhanced B-mode sonography for the differentiation between synovitis and joint effusion in patients with rheumatoid arthritis. *RöFo* **177:** 835–841.

38. Magarelli, N., G. Guglielmi, L. Di Matteo, *et al*. 2001. Diagnostic utility of an echo-contrast agent in patients with synovitis using power Doppler ultrasound: A preliminary study with comparison to contrast-enhanced MRI. *Eur. Radiol.* **11:** 1039–1046.

39. Klauser, A., F. Frauscher, M. Schirmer, *et al*. 2002. The value of contrast-enhanced color Doppler ultrasound in the detection of vascularization of finger joints in patients with rheumatoid arthritis. *Arthritis Rheum.* **46:** 647–653.

40. Szkudlarek, M., M. Court-Payen, C. Strandberg, *et al*. 2003. Contrast-enhanced power Doppler ultrasonography of the metacarpophalangeal joints in rheumatoid arthritis. *Eur. Radiol.* **13:** 163–168.

41. Carotti, M., F. Salaffi, P. Manganelli, *et al*. 2002. Power Doppler sonography in the assessment of synovial tissue of the knee joint in rheumatoid arthritis: A preliminary experience. *Ann. Rheum. Dis.* **61:** 877–882.

42. Zunterer, H., M. Schirmer & A. Klauser. 2006. Contrast enhance sonography in rheumatic joint diseases. *Akt. Rheumatol.* **31:** 157–161.

43. Wamser, G., K. Bohndorf, K. Vollert, *et al*. 2003. Power Doppler sonography with and without echo-enhancing contrast agent and contrast-enhanced MRI for the evaluation of rheumatoid arthritis of the shoulder joint: Differentiation between synovitis and joint effusion. *Skeletal Radiol.* **32:** 351–359.

44. Song, I.H., C.E. Althoff, K.G. Hermann, *et al*. 2007. Knee OA efficacy of a new method of contrast-enhanced musculoskeletal ultrasonography in detection of synovitis in patients with knee osteoarthritis in comparison with magnetic resonance imaging. *Ann. Rheum. Dis.* [Epub ahead of print]

45. Song, I., C.E. Althoff, K. Hermann, *et al*. 2008. Contrast-enhanced ultrasound in monitoring the efficacy of a bradykinin receptor-2 antagonist in painful knee osteoarthritis compared to magnetic resonance imaging. *Ann. Rheum. Dis.* [Epub ahead of print]

Arthrocentesis and Synovial Fluid Analysis in Clinical Practice

Value of Sonography in Difficult Cases

Leonardo Punzi and Francesca Oliviero

Rheumatology Unit, Department of Clinical and Experimental Medicine, University of Padova, Italy

Joint aspiration, or arthrocentesis, is one of the most useful and commonly performed procedures for the diagnosis and treatment of joint diseases. The synovial fluid aspirated may be examined to evaluate the degree of inflammation and, mainly, to detect the presence of some relevant pathogenic agents, such as crystals or microorganisms. In these cases, synovial fluid analysis still represents the best diagnostic procedure. Arthrocentesis is thus particularly required for the diagnosis and management of the acute "hot red joint," which may be considered a true medical emergency because of the morbidity and mortality related to septic arthritis. The most recent recommendations on arthrocentesis confirm the need for the procedure in the presence of synovial effusion of unknown origin, especially if septic or crystal arthritis is suspected. Owing to the importance of this analysis, it is clearly recommended that ultrasonography should be used to facilitate arthrocentesis in difficult cases. Furthermore, ultrasonography may be useful in revealing the presence of synovial fluid before the joint aspiration and, subsequently, distinguishing some aspects characteristic of crystal-induced arthropathies.

Key words: arthrocentesis; synovial fluid; sonography

Introduction

Joint aspiration, or arthrocentesis, is one of the most useful and commonly performed procedures for the diagnosis and treatment of joint diseases.[1,2] The simple joint aspiration may help in the diagnosis by revealing an excessive pathologic amount of synovial fluid (SF) and may be therapeutic by reducing the intra-articular pressure.[1] Moreover, the aspirated SF may be examined to evaluate the degree of inflammation and, mainly, to detect the presence of some relevant pathogenic agents, such as crystals or microorganisms.[1–3] It is important to underscore the fact that in recent years, despite progress in research in the field of articular diseases, no convincing alternatives to SF analysis are yet available for a definitive diagnosis of crystal arthropathy or septic arthritis.[1] Arthrocentesis is particularly required for the diagnosis and management of the acute "hot red joint," which may be considered a true medical emergency because of the morbidity and mortality related to septic arthritis.[3–6]

Although arthrocentesis is a safe and simple procedure, in some cases it may be problematic because of the limited experience of the physician or the technical difficulties in approaching the joint correctly, as in the case of the hip.[1,2] Furthermore, some general practitioners or specialists interested in joint diseases are circumspect about performing arthrocentesis and intra-articular injections owing to potential legal consequences. In fact, despite its relevance in clinical practice, very few guidelines or recommendations concerning arthrocentesis

Address for correspondence: Dr. Leonardo Punzi, Professor of Rheumatology, Chief, Rheumatology Unit, Department of Clinical and Experimental Medicine, University of Padova, Via Giustiniani 2, 35128 Padova, Italy. Voice: +39 049 8212190; fax: +39 049 8212191. punzireu@unipd.it

MRI and Ultrasound in Diagnosis and Management: Ann. N.Y. Acad. Sci. 1154: 152–158 (2009).
doi: 10.1111/j.1749-6632.2009.04389.x © 2009 New York Academy of Sciences.

TABLE 1. Recommendations of Italian Society of Rheumatology (Modified)

1. Arthrocentesis—fluid aspiration from joint, bursae, or tophi—is an important skill for specialists interested in the field of musculoskeletal diseases and is indicated for diagnostic or therapeutic purposes.
2. Arthrocentesis is always indicated in the presence of synovial effusion of unknown origin, especially if septic or crystal arthritis is suspected, and owing to its importance, ultrasonography should be used to facilitate arthrocentesis in difficult joints.
3. The fluid evacuation often has a therapeutic effect by reducing intra-articular pressure; it may facilitate the success of the subsequent intra-articular injection.
4. Before the arthrocentesis, the patient should be clearly informed of the benefits and risks of the procedure in order to give an informed consent.
5. Careful skin disinfection and the use of sterile, disposable material are mandatory for avoiding septic complications.
6. During arthrocentesis, disposable, nonsterile gloves should always be used by the operator.
7. Topical anesthetics may be useful for children and anxious subjects; it is better to avoid injection of anesthetics.
8. Contraindications to the arthrocentesis are the presence of skin lesions or infections in the area of the puncture.
9. The patient's anticoagulant treatment is not a contraindication, providing the therapeutic range is not exceeded.
10. Joint rest after arthrocentesis is not indicated.

have been published to date. The most recent are those proposed by the Italian Society of Rheumatology (SIR) (Table 1).[7] These confirm the need to perform arthrocentesis in the presence of synovial effusion of unknown origin, especially if septic or crystal arthritis is suspected. Owing to the importance of this analysis, it is clearly recommended that ultrasonography should be used to facilitate arthrocentesis in difficult joints, even when therapeutically anticoagulated. It is relevant that several of these recommendations were based on expert opinion rather than on published evidence. In general, the guidelines reinforce the conclusion that the potential for complications of arthrocentesis is very low and, in particular, infectious complication rates are less than 1/10.000 if normal antiseptic procedure is observed.[7]

Synovial Fluid Analysis

As noted above, a major indication for arthrocentesis is the possibility of analyzing the SF.[8] In some cases, this opportunity is so central to the diagnostic process that arthrocentesis should be considered mandatory. In most cases even few drops of SF may be sufficient to improve the diagnostic process.[8–10] Unfortunately, the SF obtained by arthrocentesis is not always saved, whereby an important opportunity is wasted. This is due in part to the fact that in many countries SF analysis is not performed as a routine procedure, which is, of course, an issue of physician education. It is widely recommended that for the initial evaluation of patients with arthritis and joint effusions, arthrocentesis and subsequent SF analysis should be pursued.[3,6,9,11]

Routine SF analysis should include macroscopic assessment to evaluate viscosity, color, and clarity, as well as microscopic assessment for cell count and crystal detection.[8–10] The SF should be subdivided into aliquots: one sterile tube (with anticoagulant) for bacteriologic studies (cultures and Gram stain); one tube (with EDTA) for routine cytology, including WBC total and differential count; and another in a tube without anticoagulant for crystal analysis; the remaining fluid may be centrifuged and the supernatant utilized for special studies, including protein and/or biomarker determinations, if indicated.

The immediate observation of macroscopic aspects of SF freshly aspirated may early offer some relevant information. In this context, the color is probably the most useful. Normal SF is clear and pale yellow, whereas inflammatory

TABLE 2. Main Causes of Hemarthrosis

Trauma
Bleeding diatheses
Tumors
Pigmented villonodular synovitis
Hemangiomas
Scurvy
Iatrogenic (postprocedure)
Arteriovenous fistula
Calcium pyrophosphate dihydrate (CPPD) arthropathy
Milwaukee shoulder/knee syndrome
Charcot's joint

fluids range from yellow to greenish yellow; in gout or pseudogout it may be white and in septic arthritis greenish or gray-green or frankly purulent. Bloody fluid has to be carefully considered owing to a number of possible causes of hemarthrosis (Table 2).[1,8–10] Additional information may be derived from changes in viscosity and turbidity, usually both in proportion to the degree of local inflammation. The volume of SF effusions is usually considered of little relevance for the diagnosis, although high volumes (>50 ml) are essentially found in inflammatory conditions, and those that are very high (>100 ml) are frequently associated with psoriatic arthritis.[12]

Cytological Analysis

The cytological analysis includes the total and the differential cell count. The total cell count can be easily estimated utilizing a counting chamber with normal optic microscopy. Synovial fluid from healthy subjects contains fewer than 200 WBC/mm^3, mostly mononuclear cells. In the presence of articular damage (especially when inflammatory in nature), the total number of WBCs rises along with the polymorphonuclear (PMN) cell percentage. Although the value of SF cytological examination has never been validated, the total and differential WBC count is helpful in distinguishing between disease categories (inflammatory vs. noninflammatory) (Table 3).[10–13]

Almost all SF from diseased joints fits one of four distinct patterns, but within each group it is usually impossible to distinguish among specific diseases. The WBC cutoff of 2000 cells/mm^3 is widely accepted to distinguish inflammatory from noninflammatory conditions and the cutoff of 50,000 cells/mm^3 is generally used to rule out septic arthritis. However, a recent retrospective study showed that the evaluation of SF using a 50,000 WBC/mm^3 cutoff for septic arthritis is not accurate and suggested that a sensitivity of 61% (95% CI, 48–75%) is far too low as a basis for reliable clinical decisions.[14] A larger study that considered the sensitivities and the specificity values of the laboratory tests for septic arthritis in 156 patients showed a sensitivity for a 50,000 WBC/mm^3 cutoff of 50% (95% CI, 21–79%) and a specificity of 88% (95% CI, 80–93%). However, the diagnostic cutoff that maximized the combination of sensitivity and specificity was a WBC count of 17,500 cells/mm^3, with a sensitivity of 83% and a specificity of 67%.[15] The researchers concluded that as an adjunctive measure in the diagnosis of septic arthritis, the SF WBC count is the best diagnostic test.[15]

The identification of various types of WBCs can be easily obtained by means of supravital stain. The most prevalent populations are PMN and monocytes. It has been observed that the presence of mast cells and cytophagocytic mononuclear cells (CPMs) might be useful for differentiating spondyloarthropathies among the inflammatory group of synovial effusions.[16] Indeed, fluids containing more than 10% of CPMs may derive from patients with ankylosing spondylitis, reactive arthritis, enteropathic arthritis, and psoriatic arthritis. Synovial fluid sediment analysis with Congo red may represent a simple, yet sensitive, test for the diagnosis of amyloid arthropathy. Under polarized microscopy, the amyloid appears as an amorphous material with strong Congo red uptake and typical apple-green birefringence. The high sensitivity (88%) of SF examination as compared to synovial biopsy, along with the good reproducibility of the method, shows that the finding

TABLE 3. Traditional Classification of SF Degree of Inflammation in Acute Monoarthritis[a]

	Normal	Noninflammatory	Inflammatory	Septic
Total WBC count/mm^3	<100	<2000	2000–50,000	>50,000
PMN (%)	<25	<25	>50	>75

[a]WBC = white blood cells; PMN = polymorphonuclear.

of amyloid in SF is sufficient for a diagnosis of synovial amyloidosis.[17]

Crystal Detection

There are few doubts that SF analysis is the best tool for a definitive diagnosis of crystal-induced arthritis.[1,3,4] The recently published EULAR (evidence-based) recommendations for the diagnosis of gout points out that although the rapid development of severe pain, swelling, and tenderness that reaches its maximum within just 6–12 h is highly diagnostic of crystal inflammation, it is not specific for gout.[18] For typical presentations of gout, such as recurrent podagra with hyperuricemia, a clinical diagnosis alone is reasonably accurate, but still not definitive without crystal confirmation. Only a demonstration of monosodium urate (MSU) crystals in SF or tophus aspirates permits a definitive diagnosis of gout.[18] This recommendation is supported by evidence showing that SF analysis is associated with a sensitivity (95% CI) of 0.84 (0.77–0.92), a specificity of 1.00 (0.99–1.00), and a likelihood ratio (LR)(95%CI) of 566.60 (35.46 to 9053.50).[18] No other diagnostic markers reach this absolute specificity.

Other EULAR recommendations suggest that a routine search for MSU crystals be undertaken in all SF samples obtained from undiagnosed inflamed joints and that the identification of MSU crystals from asymptomatic joints may allow definite diagnosis in intercritical periods.[18] This latter recommendation is very important for improving diagnostic procedures in patients with gout and its value has been confirmed in other studies.[19–23] Arthrocentesis in the first metatarsophalangeal joint,

even during the intercritical nonsymptomatic phase, may satisfy this aim.[22] In a study of 37 gout patients who had not received urate-lowering therapy, MSU crystals were identified in 36/37 (97%) asymptomatic but previously inflamed knees. The authors further found crystals in 7/37 (26%) knees that had never suffered acute gout in that joint.[23] A study carried out by Swiss rheumatologists showed that fine-needle aspiration of digit joints can diagnose crystal deposition arthropathy in about 30% of cases.[24] A more recent study conducted in a hospital-based rheumatology service in Singapore demonstrated that SF analysis led to a definite diagnosis in 44% of patients, with septic arthritis occurring in 9.3%, gout in 32%, and pseudogout in 2.3%.[25]

Another relevant value of SF analysis is in the diagnosis of calcium pyrophosphate dihydrate (CPPD) crystal arthritis, one of the most frequent causes of arthritis in the elderly.[1,3,4,26] As with MSU, SF CPPD crystals may be detected in noninflamed states, such as asymptomatic knees affected by chondrocalcinosis plus the structural changes of osteoarthritis. These crystals are frequently intracellular and may be associated with modest elevation of SF cell counts.[4]

Crystals are demonstrated in SF by placing a drop of the fluid on a slide and covering it with a thin glass coverslip. Under polarizing microscopy, birefringent materials demonstrate two refractive indices when a plane of polarized light passes through them. The birefringence is termed positive when the crystals (which then appear blue) are aligned parallel to the slow rays of the retardation plate (first-order red plate compensator) and negative when the crystals appear yellow in parallel alignment (and blue when perpendicular). In polarization microscopy, the MSU crystals demonstrate strong negative birefringence and are usually long and needlelike in appearance. They may occur extracellularly or within PMN or mononuclear cells. The CPPD crystals, which are often broader than MSU crystals, may show a faint "line" down their center, appear as parallelepipeds, and exhibit a weak positive birefringence in the polarizing microscope.

Other crystals identified in SF include hydroxyapatite or basic calcium phosphate crystals, which are minute and identified only with special techniques, mainly electron microscopy. Platelike cholesterol crystals seen in some rheumatoid effusions and the rare corticosteroid crystals found after intra-articular steroid treatment are both capable of inducing a synovitis.

Microbiologic Studies

An important disease for which the SF analysis is frequently decisive is septic arthritis. Although potentially severe, it is less frequently seen than crystal-induced arthritis.[27,28] Prompt microscopic analysis and culture of SF are fundamental diagnostic tools in the evaluation of possible joint sepsis. Some centers stain SF by Gram's and acid-fast methods in order to obtain early information on possible infection. However, culture is more sensitive than microscopy alone, as SF Gram staining is positive in only 50% of cases.[29]

Thus, the best rapid and reliable confirmation of the diagnosis of suspected septic arthritis is microbiological examination of the SF. In recent years, culture methods have increasingly improved their performance in terms of sensitivity and specificity. Therefore, when there is of a suspicion of septic arthritis, arthrocentesis is mandatory, and freshly aspirated SF fluid should be sent to the laboratory for immediate analysis. In clinical practice, it is important to keep in mind that the organism that is the most common cause of septic arthritis is a staphylococcus species that

accounts for from 60 to more than 80% of all such cases.[14,26,27] Other common causative organisms are coagulase-negative staphylococcus, streptococcus, and gonococcus. Coagulase negative staphylococcus is common in patients who have undergone recent joint replacement surgery.[14,26] The joint most commonly involved in septic arthritis is the knee (36–65%), followed by the shoulder (14%) and the hip (12%).[14]

Patients generally present with the complaint of a painful, swollen joint, frequently associated with systemic symptoms such as fever and chills. Multiple studies have shown that SF WBC, erythrocyte sedimentation rate (ESR), and Gram's stain have poor sensitivity or specificity for identifying septic arthritis.

Value of Sonography

Ultrasonography (US) is an increasingly important tool for the diagnosis of joint diseases because it easily demonstrates most articular lesions and allows a better approach to arthrocentesis, especially in difficult cases.[7] Thus over the past few years, there has been a growing interest in US use in rheumatology. There are other relevant advantages as well, including the absence of radiation, low cost, repeatability, patient friendliness, multiplanar imaging capability, high resolution, dynamic assessment, and efficacy as a guide for invasive procedures.[30]

Some of the most relevant aims of US are to reveal or confirm the presence of intra-articular effusion and subsequently to facilitate the ability to place a needle within the joint to perform arthrocentesis or joint injection.[31,32] It has been demonstrated that the clinical palpation traditionally used by rheumatologists to guide needle placement has a poor accuracy even with large joints such as the knee.[33] Balint *et al.* used US to guide needle placement in a range of joints and soft tissue structures, obtaining successful aspiration in 31 of 32 attempts, whereas with palpation guidance, successful aspiration was achieved in only 10 of 32 cases.[34] In another study, using high-frequency US to guide needle placement, the needle tip was placed intra-articularly in 96% of cases on initial needle passage.[35]

Ultrasonography may also reveal some characteristic of SF useful for diagnosis.[36] In this context, the most promising observations seem to be those related to crystal-induced arthritis.[37] Ultrasonography is also a useful tool for detecting crystalline and calcific material in soft tissues because it visualizes tissues as acoustic reflections. Crystalline material found in gouty joints reflects US waves more strongly than surrounding tissues such as unmineralized hyaline cartilage or synovial fluid and can thus be readily distinguished.[30] Ultrasonography interrogation may reveal the double-contour sign due to deposition of MSU crystals on cartilaginous surfaces that is found almost exclusively in gout. It may also reveal tophi, both formed and unformed, even in difficult joints such as metatarsophalangeals. Tophi are frequently associated with bony erosions.

It is important to differentiate US findings in gout patients from those in patients with chondrocalcinosis (or pseudogout) caused by CPPD crystals. In these conditions, US may show characteristic features including deposits not identified by standard radiographs. Ultrasonography can provide useful information on the structure of the deposit based on the presence of posterior acoustic shadowing or the grade of echogenicity and may permit an exact localization of the deposit, helping to indicate its probable nature.[37,38] Although it is still unclear if US has a role in the diagnosis of early CPPD crystal deposition disease, in some cases SF may reveal characteristic aggregates of variable shape.

Conflicts of Interest

The authors declare no conflicts of interest.

References

1. Courtney, P. & M. Doherty. 2005. Joint aspiration and injection. *Best Pract. Res. Clin. Rheumatol.* **19:** 345–369.

2. Samuelson, C.O. Jr., G.W. Cannon & J.R. Ward. 1985. Arthrocentesis. *J. Fam. Practice* **20:** 179–184.

3. Johnson, M.W. 2000. Acute knee effusions: A systematic approach to diagnosis. *Am. Fam. Physician* **61:** 2391–2400.

4. Baker, D.G. & H.R. Schumacher Jr. 1993. Acute monoarthritis. *N. Engl. J. Med.* **329:** 1013–1020.

5. American College of Rheumatology ad hoc Committee on Clinical Guidelines. 1996. Guidelines for the initial evaluation of the adult patient with acute musculoskeletal symptoms. *Arthritis Rheum.* **39:** 1–8.

6. Coakley, G., C. Mathews, M. Field, *et al.* 2006. On behalf of the British Society for Rheumatology Standards, Guidelines and Audit Working Group. BSR & BHPR, BOA, RCGP and BSAC guidelines for management of the hot swollen joint in adults. *Rheumatology* **45:** 1039–1041.

7. Punzi, L., M.A. Cimmino, L. Frizziero, *et al.* 2007. Italian Society of Rheumatology (SIR) recommendations for performing arthrocenthesis. *Reumatismo* **59:** 227–234.

8. Eisenberg, J.M., H.R. Schumacher, P.K. Davidson & L. Kaufmann. 1984. Usefulness of synovial fluid analysis in the evaluation of joint effusions. Use of threshold analysis and likelihood ratios to assess a diagnostic test. *Arch. Intern. Med.* **144:** 715–719.

9. Gatter, R.A., R.P. Andrews, *et al.* 1995. American College of Rheumatology guidelines for performing office synovial fluid examinations. *J. Clin. Rheumatol.* **1:** 194–196.

10. Swan, A., H. Amer & P. Dieppe. 2002. The value of synovial fluid assays in the diagnosis of joint disease: A literature survey. *Ann. Rheum. Dis.* **61:** 493–498.

11. British Society for Rheumatology. 1992. Guidelines and a proposed audit protocol for the initial management of an acute hot joint. Report of a joint working group of the British Society for Rheumatology and the Research Unit of the Royal College of Physicians. *R. Coll. Physicians (London)* **26:** 83–85.

12. Punzi, L., N. Bertazzolo, M. Pianon, *et al.* 1995. The volume of synovial fluid effusion in psoriatic arthritis. *Clin. Exp. Rheumatol.* **13:** 535–536.

13. Shmerling, R.H. 1994. Synovial fluid analysis. A critical reappraisal. *Rheum. Dis. Clin. North Am.* **20:** 503–512.

14. McGillicuddy, D.C., K.H. Shah, R.P. Friedberg, *et al.* 2007. How sensitive is the synovial fluid white blood cell count in diagnosing septic arthritis? *Am. J. Emerg. Med.* **25:** 749–752.

15. Shah, K., J. Spear, L.A. Nathanson, *et al.* 2007. Does the presence of crystal arthritis rule out septic arthritis? *J. Emerg. Med.* **32:** 23–26.

16. Freemont, A.J. & J. Denton. 1985. Disease distribution of synovial fluid mast cells and cytophagocytic

mononuclear cells in inflammatory arthritis. *Ann. Rheum. Dis.* **44:** 312–315.

17. Lakhanpal, S., C.Y. Li, M.A. Gertz, *et al*. 1987. Synovial fluid analysis for diagnosis of amyloid arthropathy. *Arthritis Rheum.* **30:** 419–423.

18. Zhang, W., M. Doherty, E. Pascual, *et al*. 2006. EULAR evidence based recommendations for gout: Pt. 1. Diagnosis. Report of a Task Force of the Standing Committee for International Clinical Studies Including Therapeutics (ESCISIT). *Ann. Rheum. Dis.* **65:** 1301–1311.

19. Agudelo, C.A., A. Weinberger, H.R. Schumacher, *et al*. 1979. Definitive diagnosis of gout by identification of urate crystals in asymptomatic metatarsophalangeal joints. *Arthritis Rheum.* **22:** 559–560.

20. Weinberger, A., H.R. Schumacher & C.A. Agudelo. 1979. Urate crystals in asymptomatic metatarsophalangeal joints. *Ann. Intern. Med.* **91:** 56–57.

21. Pascual, E., E. Batlle-Gualda, A. Martínez, *et al*. 1999. Synovial fluid analysis for diagnosis of intercritical gout. *Ann. Intern. Med.* **131:** 756–759.

22. Sivera, F., R. Aragon & E. Pascual. 2008. First metatarsophalangeal joint aspiration using a 29-gauge needle. *Ann. Rheum. Dis.* **67:** 273–275.

23. Pascual, E. 1991. Persistence of monosodium urate crystals, and low grade inflammation, in the synovial fluid of untreated gout. *Arthritis Rheum.* **34:** 141–145.

24. Guggi, V., L. Calame & J.C. Gerster. 2002. Contribution of digit joint aspiration to the diagnosis of rheumatic diseases. *Joint Bone Spine* **69:** 58–61.

25. Chong, Y.Y., K.R. Fong & J. Thumboo. 2007. The value of joint aspirations in the diagnosis and management of arthritis in a hospital-based rheumatology service. *Ann. Acad. Med. Singapore* **36:** 106–109.

26. Pascual, E. & M. Doherty. 2009. Aspiration of normal or asymptomatic pathological joints for diagnosis or research indications, technique and success rate. *Ann. Rheum. Dis.* **68:** 3–7.

27. Dubost, J.J., M. Soubrier & B. Sauvezie. 2000. Pyogenic arthritis in adults. *Joint Bone Spine* **67:** 11–21.

28. Schiavon, F., M. Favero, V. Carraro & L. Riato. 2008. Septic arthritis: What is the role for the rheumatologist? *Reumatismo* **6:** 1–5.

29. Weston, V.C., A.C. Jones, N. Bradbury, *et al*. 1999. Clinical features and outcome of septic arthritis in a single UK health district 1982–1991. *Ann. Rheum. Dis.* **58:** 214–219.

30. Thiele, R.G. & N. Schlesinger. 2007. Diagnosis of gout by ultrasound. *Rheumatology* **46:** 116–121.

31. Grassi, W., A. Farina, E. Filippucci & C. Cervini. 2001. Sonographically guided procedures in rheumatology. *Semin. Arthritis Rheum.* **30:** 347–353.

32. Delaunoy, I., V. Feipel, T. Appelboom & J.P. Hauzeur. 2003. Sonography detection threshold for knee effusion. *Clin. Rheumatol.* **22:** 391–392.

33. Jones, A., M. Regan, J. Ledingham, *et al*. 1993. Importance of placement of intra-articular steroid injections. *Br. Med. J.* **307:** 1329–1330.

34. Balint, P.V., D. Kane, J. Hunter, *et al*. 2002. Ultrasound guided versus conventional joint and soft tissue fluid aspiration in rheumatology practice: A pilot study. *J. Rheumatol.* **29:** 2209–2213.

35. Raza, K., C.Y. Lee, D. Pilling, *et al*. 2003. Ultrasound guidance allows accurate needle placement and aspiration from small joints in patients with early inflammatory arthritis. *Rheumatology* **42:** 976–979.

36. Farina, A., E. Filippucci & W. Grassi. 2002. Sonographic findings of synovial fluid. *Reumatismo* **54:** 261–265.

37. Grassi, W., G. Meenagh, E. Pascual & E. Filippucci. 2007. "Crystal clear"—Sonographic assessment of gout and calcium pyrophosphate deposition disease. *Semin. Arthritis Rheum.* **36:** 197–202.

38. Frediani, B., G. Filippou, P. Falsetti, *et al*. 2005. Diagnosis of calcium pyrophosphate dihydrate crystal deposition disease: Ultrasonographic criteria proposed. *Ann. Rheum. Dis.* **64:** 638–640.

Ultrasound in the Inflammatory Myopathies

Marc-André Weber

Department of Radiology, German Cancer Research Center, Heidelberg, Germany

Dermato- or polymyositis must be diagnosed or ruled out early because early immunosuppressive therapy prevents irreversible muscle degeneration. Acute poly- and dermatomyositis are accompanied by normal or increased size, low echogenicity, and elevated perfusion of affected muscles, whereas in chronic poly- and dermatomyositis, the size and perfusion of affected muscles are reduced and echogenicity is increased. Although magnetic resonance imaging is more sensitive in detecting edema-like muscular changes and thereby acute myositis, contrast-enhanced ultrasound with its capability of measuring perfusion has become a useful diagnostic tool in diagnosing acute inflammation in poly- and dermatomyositis.

Key words: **inflammatory myopathies; ultrasound; skeletal muscle**

Introduction

The idiopathic inflammatory myopathies make up the largest group of subacute, chronic, or acute acquired diseases of skeletal muscle. They have in common the presence of moderate to severe muscle weakness and an autoimmune inflammation in the muscle.[1] The idiopathic inflammatory myopathies must be distinguished from inflammatory myopathies caused by infectious agents such as bacteria, viruses, fungi, or parasitic agents. The latter are encountered in tropical countries, in immunocompromised patients, and in intravenous drug abusers, and are called pyomyositis.[2–4]

Detection of inflammatory myopathies is clinically important because unlike many other myopathies, these disorders are potentially treatable.[1] The treatment of the idiopathic autoimmune inflammatory myopathies remains largely empirical because their precise etiology, which is still unknown, includes corticosteroids, immunosuppressive agents, and intravenous immunoglobulin, all of which have

nonselective effects on the immune system.[5] On the basis of clinical, histopathological, immunological, and demographic features, they can be differentiated into three major and distinct subsets: dermatomyositis (DM), polymyositis (PM), and sporadic inclusion-body myositis (IBM).[1,5] Dermatomyositis is typified by a characteristic rash accompanied by muscle weakness and may occur in childhood or in adult life. Individuals suffering from DM also face an increased risk of cancer. Polymyositis is best defined as a subacute myopathy that evolves over weeks to months, affects primarily adults, and presents with symmetrical weakness of the proximal muscles.[1,5] The onset of symptoms is usually more acute and the rate of progression more rapid in DM than in PM. It is slowest in IBM so that particular diagnosis may not be made for several years.[5]

Differential diagnoses include endocrine disease, neurogenic disease, dystrophies, and metabolic myopathies. Classically, the clinical diagnosis of PM and DM is based on the clinical presentation, past medical history, elevation of creatine kinase (CK) activity—up to 50 times in active disease—and may rely upon invasive procedures, such as electromyography and muscle biopsy.[1] However, the serum CK level may be normal or only mildly elevated in

Address for correspondence: Dr. Marc-André Weber, Associate Professor of Radiology, German Cancer Research Center, Im Neuenheimer Feld 280, D-69120 Heidelberg, Germany. Voice: +49–6221-422580; fax: +49–6221-422462.

MRI and Ultrasound in Diagnosis and Management: Ann. N.Y. Acad. Sci. 1154: 159–170 (2009).
doi: 10.1111/j.1749-6632.2009.04390.x © 2009 New York Academy of Sciences.

DM, IBM, and in focal forms of myositis.[5] Needle electromyography typically shows increased spontaneous activity with fibrillations, complex repetitive discharges, and positive sharp waves. However, these electromyographic signs are not disease specific. They are only useful to confirm active myopathy but are not able to correctly classify it.[1,5] Only muscle biopsy can establish a definite diagnosis,[1,5] but muscle inflammation may be spotty, and a false-negative rate of up to 25% without imaging guidance has been reported.[4,6-8] Thus, guiding the muscle biopsy toward active disease by imaging techniques such as MRI or ultrasound (US) appears to be crucial for reducing the sampling error in order to rapidly diagnose DM and PM and exclude other disorders. In addition to reducing the problem of sampling error, an early diagnosis and initiation of immunosuppressive therapy prevent severe (and irreversible) muscle weakness in DM and PM,[1,5] whereas misdiagnosis may lead to irreversible muscle weakness.

Structural Ultrasound Imaging Appearance in Inflammatory Myopathies

Muscles are among the soft tissues best suited for being examined by US. In fact, it was the first imaging technique available for the evaluation of muscle disease.[9] Its availability, low cost, and ease of examination makes US superior to MRI for follow-up of lesions and searching for complications such as fibrosis, cystic hematomas, and myositis ossificans. Moreover, muscle atrophy, inflammation, avulsion injuries, and tumors are indications for US.[3,4,9] As it is very sensitive in the detection of fluid, US may also help in guiding needle aspiration to establish a correct diagnosis (e.g., in pyomyositis).[2,3]

B-Mode Ultrasound Signs of Myositis

Noninvasive diagnostic modalities such as computed tomography (CT), MRI, and tra-

ditional gray-scale US can detect muscular edema, fluid collections, fatty infiltration, atrophy, fibrosis, and calcifications. As morphologically muscle tissue can only react in a limited number of ways, morphological imaging in myositis—be it MRI or US—can describe edema-like, lipomatous, and atrophic changes in muscular tissue.[10] For diagnosis and biopsy planning, detection of muscular edema as a criterion for acute or ongoing muscle inflammation is the most important finding. Muscular edema manifests on gray-scale images as nearly anechoic, swollen muscle fibers[11,12] and increased muscle diameter (Fig. 1).[9,11,13,14] For comparison, in normal muscles, fascicles appear hypoechoic relative to the echogenic fibroadipose septa (perimysium) (Fig. 2).[4,9,11,15] Criteria of lipomatous muscular degeneration and muscle atrophy as a marker of chronicity are hyperechoic muscle due to diminution of the hypoechoic muscle bundles and fatty infiltration (Fig. 1).[9,11,15] When describing muscle echogenicity, it is important to realize that the angulation of the transducer with respect to the transverse plane influences the echogenicity.[16] Thus, muscles should always be examined in two perpendicular planes. Moreover, the degree of muscular contraction influences its echogenicity.[4,9] The examiner should guarantee a comfortable resting position for the patient during the examination, in order to avoid high muscle tone that in turn falsifies the gray-scale US findings.

Depending on the duration of the disease and the degree of inflammatory activity, the echogenicity of the affected muscles is either predominantly lower or higher than normal (respectively, acute myositis with edema or chronic myositis with fatty infiltration).[11,16,17] As early as 15 years ago, researchers using these criteria reported a US sensitivity of 83% in detecting evidence of histopathologically proven disease, which is comparable to that of electromyography.[11] Moreover, typical although not specific US patterns were proposed, such as atrophy and increased echogenicity predominantly of lower extremity muscles in PM,

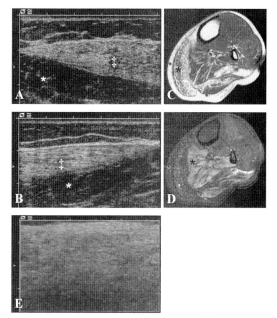

Figure 1. A 47-year-old man with a muscular channelopathy that manifests first with muscular edema and later with fatty degeneration. Transverse (**A**) and longitudinal (**B**) myosonogram (linear array, 8 MHz) of the lower left leg and corresponding T1-weighted MRI scan (**C**) and STIR image (**D**). The medial head of the gastrocnemius muscle is diffusely echogenic (double cross) with obliteration of normal anatomy and the normally hypoechoic muscle fascicles are hardly discernible. The lipomatous degeneration is well depicted on the T1-weighted MRI scan (asterisk in **C**). In contrast to the fatty infiltration within the gastrocnemius muscle, the soleus muscle is edematous, which results in strongly hypoechoic, swollen muscle fibers (asterisks). The transverse power Doppler US image of the degenerated gastrocnemius muscle after bolus injection of 10 mL Levovist® (SH U 508A, Schering AG, Berlin, Germany) at a depth of 1.5 cm (focus area) (**E**) demonstrates the maximum plateau of the microbubble replenishment. There are hardly any power Doppler signals visible owing to very low perfusion (local blood volume: ~0.8 ml, blood flow velocity: 0.5 mm/s, and blood flow: ~0.4 ml/min/100 g tissue).

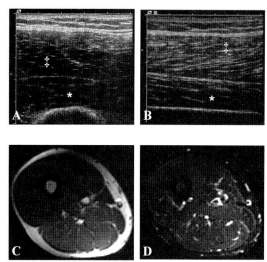

Figure 2. Normal transverse (**A**) and longitudinal (**B**) myosonogram (linear array, 8 MHz) of the right thigh of a 33-year-old healthy man (who regularly performs endurance training as a sports instructor). Below the vastus lateralis (double cross), first the vastus intermedius muscle (asterisk) and then the femur is visible. The muscle fascicles are normally hypoechoic, whereas the perimysial connective tissue appears as echogenic thin lines. The corresponding MRI of the right thigh shows normal muscles without fatty infiltration (**C**, T1-weighting) or edema-like changes (**D**, STIR).

relative absence of atrophy in DM, and severe muscle atrophy in IBM.[11]

However, since affected muscle tissue can react morphologically only in a limited number of ways,[10] edema-like, lipomatous, and atrophic changes in muscular tissue are often not disease specific (given the large vari-ability in the distribution of muscles affected within the same condition and the observation that similar changes can result from different myopathies).[10] Thus, the hope[11] that patterns of muscle involvement might prove diagnostic of specific myopathies has been dispelled.[10] Some of these disadvantages may be overcome by functional imaging techniques. Ultrasound techniques are available that permit assessment of skeletal muscle perfusion. By detecting and spatially localizing an altered microcirculation, these new techniques may make imaging more specific for both diagnosis and treatment monitoring.[18]

Perfusion Ultrasound Imaging

Perfusion is an important parameter that may be altered in various muscular diseases, such as degenerative or inflammatory myopathies.[18] Detection of perfusion in the musculoskeletal system has been a task of earlier studies. The use of power Doppler US has enabled the depiction of changes of vascularity in or adjacent to bursitis, tendinitis, arthritis, and myositis.[15,19]

Contrast-Specific Ultrasound Techniques

To quantify skeletal muscle perfusion by US, intravenous injection of an intravascular contrast agent is necessary. Typically, microbubbles of gas stabilized by lipids or proteins about 1–5 μm in size are employed. Contrast-specific US techniques can be either high- or low-mechanical index techniques. High-energy US pulses with a mechanical index above 0.5 can destroy microbubbles, thereby provoking signals [stimulated acoustic emissions (SAE)] in power Doppler sonography (Fig. 3A),[20,21] whereas in low-mechanical index techniques bubble oscillation with generation of harmonics rather than bubble destruction contributes to the image. The advantage of the latter is that the underlying tissue as well as the dynamic process of contrast enhancement can be examined in real time.[21]

As each single microbubble can be detected, independent of flow volume or velocity,[22] contrast-enhanced ultrasound (CE-US) is highly sensitive even to blood flow within capillaries and may thereby enable quantifying of perfusion. This is especially advantageous because skeletal muscle perfusion is very low at rest.[23,24] The easiest and clinically most feasible way to obtain information about muscle perfusion is to measure indirect perfusion-related parameters by acquiring a dynamic series after US contrast bolus injection, while maintaining the probe in a constant position. The perfusion curves typically show an early increase in signal intensity, a short maximum, and then a slow exponential decay.[21] Descriptive perfusion-related parameters, such as time to peak or maximum intensity can thereby be analyzed.[21]

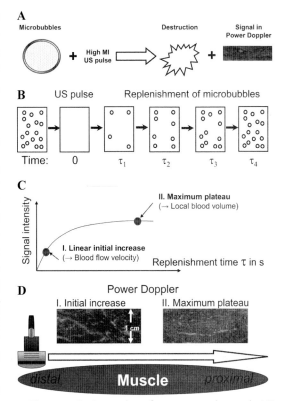

Figure 3. Principle of contrast-enhanced US analysis of skeletal muscle perfusion (modified from Weber *et al.*[18]). (**A**) Microbubbles can be destroyed by high-energy or high-mechanical index (MI) US pulses. When a microbubble bursts it causes a signal in power Doppler US. (**B**) Principle of replenishment kinetics: After administration of US contrast media, microbubbles completely fill a given region of interest (ROI). A high-energy US pulse destroys all microbubbles at time 0. Then, depending on blood flow velocity, microbubbles from outside refill the ROI at times $\tau_1 - \tau_4$. Maximum signal intensity at contrast-enhanced US (τ_4) is determined by local blood volume and concentration of microbubbles. (**C**) The power Doppler US signal has initially (τ_1) a linear increase and later (τ_4) a maximum plateau. Two measurement values (dots, initial increase and maximum plateau of the replenishment curve) are sufficient to quantify perfusion-related parameters.[20,23] (**D**) To measure these two values, the probe initially rested at the distal end and was moved after 75 s over the muscle to its proximal end. The corresponding transverse power Doppler images in a healthy volunteer demonstrate the initial increase and the maximum plateau of the microbubble replenishment.

To measure parameters directly related to tissue perfusion, such as blood flow, blood flow velocity, and volume with CE-US, a technique based on the analysis of replenishment kinetics (first introduced in heart muscle)[24] has been modified for use with skeletal muscle.[23] When all intravenously injected microbubbles in a chosen region of interest are destroyed by high-energy US pulses, replenishment kinetics describe the refilling of microbubbles from an outside region where no microbubbles have been destroyed. This principle is illustrated in Figure 3. (For a detailed description see Krix *et al.*[23] and Weber *et al.*[25]) As skeletal muscle perfusion is highly variable, in order to meet the metabolic demand of skeletal muscle care must be taken to avoid falsely high resting perfusion due to exercise prior to the measurement by guaranteeing a standardized resting period, for example, 20 min (Fig. 4).[23]

Muscles are screened using a linear transducer both in gray-scale and power Doppler mode. For power Doppler US, a transmission frequency of 7 MHz, a maximal acoustic power (mechanical index, 1.9), and a maximal pulse repetition frequency (minimal sensitivity) are used to reduce motion artifacts and to ensure that it is the signals from the microbubbles that are detected, rather than flow signals from vessels.[23] After choosing a representative US slice at the distal part of the muscle, a single bolus of contrast media is injected intravenously followed by saline solution and a continuous US video clip is acquired. Initially, the probe rests in the same position to measure the early rise in contrast agent concentration, that is, an early time point of the replenishment kinetics. When the systemic contrast agent concentration has reached a plateau, at the defined time of 75 s after contrast injection, the probe is slowly moved over the muscle to its proximal end; in these regions the microbubbles have not previously been destroyed by US (Fig. 3).[23,25,26]

It has to be emphasized that although the power Doppler mode is used to visualize SAE, that is, the presence of microbubbles, this is not power Doppler sonography in its origi-

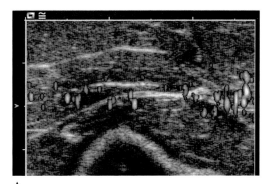

A

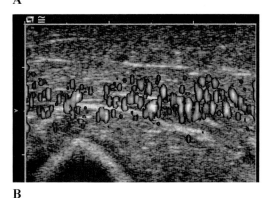

B

Figure 4. Transverse power Doppler US images of the right biceps muscle in a 19-year-old healthy volunteer after bolus injection of 10 mL Levovist® (SH U 508A, Schering AG, Berlin, Germany) at a depth of 1.5 cm (focus area) demonstrating the maximum plateau of the microbubble replenishment. (**A**) represents the situation before, and (**B**) the situation directly after 5 min of defined exercise using a 3-kg dumbbell. The contrast-enhanced power Doppler signals clearly visualize the higher microbubble concentration in the muscle tissue after exercise owing to exercise-induced hyperperfusion (results of perfusion quantification before vs. after exercise: local blood volume: 14.9 vs. ~24.8 ml, blood flow velocity: 0.06 vs. 0.96 mm/s, and blood flow: 0.9 vs. ~23.9 ml/min/100 g tissue; all within normal range[23]). Note that microbubbles are destroyed chiefly in the focus area, so that hardly any power Doppler signals are obtained from other muscular areas.

nal sense, in that it is not designed to visualize moving blood cells. On the contrary, the settings are adjusted (e.g., by using a maximal pulse repetition frequency) so that signals from moving blood cells are suppressed. The power Doppler mode is used because the transmitted signals are strong enough to cause bubble rupture and the generated SAE, "misinterpreted" as Doppler signals, are displayed on the screen (Fig. 3A). The measured color pixels, which are proportional to the microbubbles' concentration, are measured to quantify local blood volume (the blood volume within the slice obtained by the transducer), blood flow velocity, and blood flow.[23,25,26] The whole measurement takes about 2 min for one muscle and another 10 min for the calculation of the perfusion values.

Perfusion Ultrasound Imaging in the Inflammatory Myopathies

As biopsy planning is crucial in the diagnostic workup of dermatomyositis and polymyositis,[6–8] US and MRI have been proposed to better guide a biopsy to an area of active disease,[5,10,17,27,28] which requires that the muscles be screened for edema-like changes.[10] However, besides being an early sign of a myositis, edema-like changes can also occur in other conditions, including metabolic or traumatic changes, neuropathies, muscular dystrophies, myotonic dystrophy, necrotic changes such as rhabdomyolysis, diabetic muscle infarction, or even physical exercise.[4–5,12,16,27–29] By quantifying perfusion, CE-US can demonstrate a significantly increased perfusion of the affected skeletal muscles at rest in patients with histologically proven PM and DM (Fig. 5).[17,25] Edema-like changes in patients with myositis associated with increased perfusion detected by CE-US are, together, grounds for suspecting an acute or ongoing myositis.[17,25] Given the nonspecificity of edema-like changes, an increased skeletal muscle perfusion confirms the suspicion of myositis, whereas a normal perfusion argues against it (Fig. 6).

As it can demonstrate normalization of myositis-induced hyperperfusion of resting skeletal muscle after effective therapy,[25] CE-US is a valuable tool for treatment monitoring as normalization of initially elevated perfusion values indicates treatment response (Fig. 6D, E).[25] Thus this might be a more reliable criterion than manual muscle strength testing or

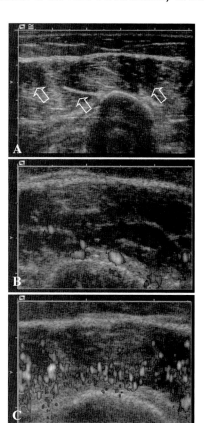

Figure 5. A 63-year-old woman with histologically confirmed severe polymyositis. The transverse gray-scale US image of the left biceps brachii muscle (**A**) clearly shows focal areas of muscular edema-like changes (open arrows). The corresponding power Doppler images without contrast agent administration show an increased microcirculation (**B**). Elevated muscular perfusion at rest is clearly demonstrated by the corresponding contrast-enhanced power Doppler image during maximum plateau phase (**C**); results of perfusion quantification: local blood volume: ~23.5 ml, blood flow velocity: 2.15 mm/s, and blood flow: ~50.4 ml/min/100 g tissue. Note the signal increase after contrast agent administration.

evaluation of serum CK concentration because a decrease in serum CK concentration, normalization of edema-like changes, and the improvement of muscle strength do not always coincide.[1,28,30]

In general, since long-standing DM or PM results in muscular degeneration with fatty infiltration and less skeletal muscle perfusion than in normal muscles,[17] the duration of symptoms and the medication history must be taken

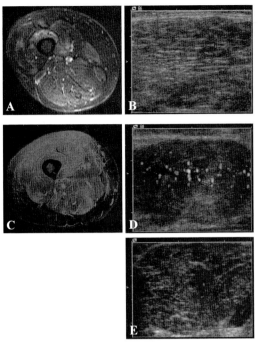

Figure 6. (A, B) A 54-year-old man with a final diagnosis of dystrophic myopathy and exclusion of myositis at histologic analysis. **(C–E)** A 45-year-old woman with histologically confirmed polymyositis. **(A)** and **(C)** MRI of the right thigh using a fat-suppressed T2-weighted STIR sequence. Focal areas of increased signal intensity are visible in the right quadriceps femoris muscles of both patients. The transverse images at a power Doppler US of 7 MHz of these muscles after bolus injection of 10 mL Levovist® at a depth of 1.5 cm **(B, D)** demonstrate the maximum plateau of the microbubble replenishment at rest in both patients. The contrast-enhanced power Doppler signals clearly visualize the higher concentration of microbubbles in muscle tissue of the woman with acute polymyositis **(D)** owing to the higher muscle perfusion. The results show that muscular edema-like changes are not specific for myositis. In this case, additional use of contrast-enhanced US helped to differentiate between the two entities. The woman was successfully treated. The contrast-enhanced power Doppler US after immunosuppressive treatment **(E,** all parameters corresponding to **D)** showed normalization of both muscular microcirculation and edema-like changes.

into account when interpreting CE-US findings (Fig. 1E). Disease duration may impact the interpretation of gray-scale US findings.[15] The presence of muscle edema with decreased echogenicity in the acute phase shifts to muscle degeneration and atrophy with increased echogenicity when the disease lasts longer.[11,15] Unfortunately, some studies dealing with imaging patterns in myositis do not normalize imaging findings to disease duration and medication usage, which then makes interpretation more difficult.

What Is the Pathophysiological Basis for Ultrasound Findings?

Apart from the stage of disease (acute or chronic), the kind and pattern of inflammation also determine the US appearance. In pyomyositis, two stages can be distinguished. The first stage is a phlegmon of muscle tissue. With early US assessment, one of two considerations is possible, namely: (i) muscular edema can be depicted appearing as hypoechoic, ill-defined areas within the muscle,[2] or (ii) inflammatory exudates assemble around the fibroadipose septa leading to a seemingly reverse image of normal with hyperechoic muscle fibers and hypoechoic fibroadipose septa.[9,14] It must be emphasized, however, that these findings are not specific for pyomyositis. Later in the course of pyomyositis, as a second stage, an intramuscular fluid accumulation is seen corresponding to a formed abscess (Fig. 7). In more than 90% of all cases, the muscular abscess is caused by *Staphylococcus aureus*.[2,3,14] With color Doppler US, hyperemia at the periphery of the abscess and an absence of flow in its center are most typical (Fig. 7).[2,3] Both the formation of an abscess (e.g., in pyomyositis)[2,4,14] and necrosis (e.g., diabetic muscle infarction)[12] appear as focal hypoechoic areas on US. On MRI these areas appear strongly hyperintense on T2-weighted images (Fig. 7C, D).

In contrast to pyomyositis caused by infectious agents, the idiopathic inflammatory myopathies are histologically characterized by autoimmune-mediated perivascular and intrafascicular inflammatory infiltrates—mainly by T cells and macrophages—and often by de- and regeneration of fibers.[16,27,31] The cellular

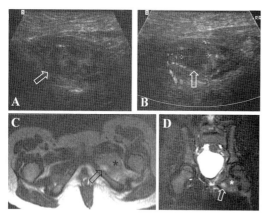

Figure 7. Transverse gray-scale (**A**) and color Doppler scans (**B**) of the left short adductor muscles in a 5-year-old girl with pyomyositis. Note the hypoechoic swollen muscle fibers owing to edema in **A** (open arrow). In (**B**) diffuse muscle hyperemia surrounding a well-demarcated hypoechoic fluid accumulation 1 cm in diameter (open arrow) representing beginning abscess formation is visible. The corresponding T2-weighted MRI scans (**C**, **D**; **D** with fat-suppression) demonstrate the muscular edema within the external obturator and short adductor muscles (asterisk) and the abscess formation (open arrow). [Courtesy of Jens Peter Schenk, MD, Department of Pediatric Radiology, University Hospital Heidelberg, Germany.]

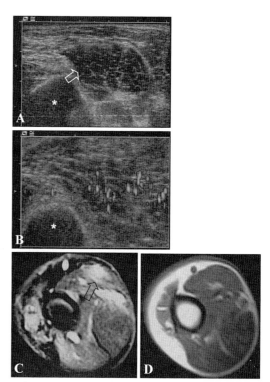

Figure 8. Confirmed acute dermatomyositis in a 65-year-old woman. (**A**) Transverse gray-scale US of the right biceps brachii muscle (open arrow). Figures 1 and 2 enable comparison of muscle edema with normal muscle. It is difficult to reliably diagnose muscular edema using only gray-scale US. However, the transverse power Doppler US image of the respective area 77 s after injection of 10 mL Levovist® clearly shows increased muscular perfusion (**B**) indicative of acute myositis (results of perfusion quantification: local blood volume: ~19.0 ml, blood flow velocity: 0.6 mm/s, and blood flow: ~11.1 ml/min/100 g tissue). The right humerus is indicated by an asterisk in **A** and in **B**. The corresponding transverse fat-suppressed T2-weighted MRI clearly demonstrates edema-like changes in the right biceps brachii, while absence of fatty infiltration or atrophy is proven by the T1-weighted MRI (**D**).

inflammatory infiltrates seen on biopsy of DM lesions are localized predominantly perivascularly or in the interfascicular septae and around rather than within the fascicles,[1] whereas in PM multifocal lymphocytic infiltrates surround and invade healthy muscle fibers. The additional presence of rimmed vacuoles and congophilic amyloid deposits within or next to the vacuoles, however, favor a diagnosis of IBM.[1] As the diagnosis of IBM is often delayed, muscle atrophy is the most common finding.[11] Chronic inflammation leads to muscular lipomatosis and the degree of muscular lipomatosis at histopathological examination correlates with increased echogenicity on US[11] and hyperintensity on T1-weighted MRI.[10]

Acute inflammatory infiltrates are associated with muscle edema,[16] which histopathologically appears as a loosely packed peri- and endomysial connective tissue and leads to decreased echogenicity of the affected muscles

on US[11] and hyperintensity on T2-weighted MRI.[10] Frequently however, the decrease in echotexture is too small to reliably diagnose edema, as occurred in two studies on histologically proven acute PM and DM, where the muscular edema was detected by US in only about 50% of cases.[11,25] In the latter study, MRI detected edema in all cases with histologically proven acute PM and DM (Fig. 8).[25]

In fact, instead of muscle edema in myositis, the term "edema-like changes" should be used, because decreased echogenicity or hyperintensity on fat-suppressed T2-weighted images may result either from an absolute increase in interstitial fluid content (i.e., pure edema also seen in other disorders), a relative decrease in intracellular space content (e.g., in necrosis, such as in diabetic infarction[12]), and/or an increased microcirculation as a result of inflammation, and/or from the inflammatory infiltrates themselves.[10,16] The fact that increased perfusion detected by CE-US in acute poly- and dermatomyositis and increased signal intensity on T2-weighted images detected by MRI are correlated[17,25] suggests that the inflammation-induced increase in microcirculation indeed plays a major role *in vivo*. Therefore, both an increased muscular perfusion and edema-like changes could be interpreted as suspicious parameters for an acute myositis.

In DM detection of increased muscle perfusion appears surprising at first glance because the pathological changes are suspected to be at least partially due to a complement-mediated microangiopathy, as well as because a reduction in capillary density has been reported.[1] However, the pathogenetic mechanisms of DM are still not clearly understood,[32] and despite a reduction in capillary density, a high degree of inflammation may account for a higher muscle perfusion *in vivo*, for example, via metabolic mediators. With CE-US, this may compensate the diminution in microvascularity, which is an *ex vivo* finding. Furthermore, since perfusion is not solely dependent on the tissue's capillary density, a microvascular bed injury might be only one factor influencing skeletal muscle perfusion in DM. The remaining portion of the large variability has to be attributed to factors affecting *in vivo* flow, such as recruitment dynamics and rheology, which are affected by cellular and humoral immune responses, cytokines, and other metabolic disturbances observed in myositis. These, by nature, elude all *ex vivo* biopsy studies.[17,26,33]

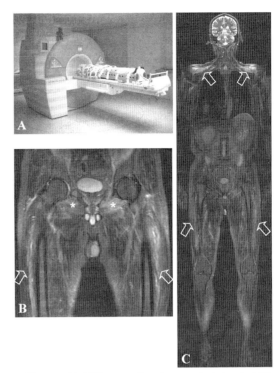

Figure 9. When performing a whole-body MRI, the patient is completely covered with coils (**A**). In this 56-year-old man with histologically confirmed dermatomyositis, symmetrical edema-like changes are visible on the coronal STIR MRIs (**B, C; B** is part of the whole-body image) in the shoulder girdle and the thighs (open arrows), as well as in the external obturator muscles (asterisks).

Future Needs of Ultrasonography Imaging in the Inflammatory Myopathies

Elsewhere in this volume, the potential of MRI in the workup of inflammatory myopathies was presented. By being more sensitive to the presence of edema-like changes than US and by offering good tissue differentiation,[16] MRI using fat-suppressed T2-weighted techniques, such as short tau inversion recovery (STIR) sequences, is very efficient in diagnosing and managing inflammatory myopathies. Moreover, with the advent of whole-body MRI,[6,17] screening of all muscles for edema-like changes has become possible within the space of 35 min (Fig. 9) in an examiner-independent manner, which is not possible even with extended-field-of-view US scans. For instance, Reimers *et al.*[11] reported that their systematic US examination including documentation and analysis of 16 skeletal muscles for each subject lasted 1–1.5 h.[11] So the questions remain as to the role of US in this setting and which imaging modality should be used. MRI has some limitations in terms of costs, availability, patient discomfort (especially in whole-body MRI, see Fig. 9A), and exclusion of certain patients with in-dwelling metals such as pacemakers. Ultrasound can be used at bedside, at rest, and during contraction, and in different clinical settings, including the emergency departments and intensive care units. The inherent disadvantage of US, however, is its observer dependence. Therefore, some patients appear more suitable for MRI and others for US, such as those unable to undergo MRI, children, and all who need frequent serial assessments.

But should there really be a competitive or rather a complementary situation? Given the higher spatial and temporal resolution of US as compared with MRI and the establishment of contrast-specific low-mechanical index techniques that enable the assessment of skeletal muscle morphology, as well as macro- and microcirculation simultaneously (Fig. 10), perfusion CE-US might have a greater role than perfusion MRI approaches such as arterial spin-labeling perfusion MRI.[18,34] At the German Cancer Research Center, the following imaging approach is currently favored for patients with symmetrical, proximal limb weakness and raised serum skeletal muscle enzyme levels to rapidly exclude or diagnose a possible dermato- or polymyositis: Whole-body MRI is done to detect edema-like changes. If none are observed, an acute dermato- or polymyositis appears unlikely. If edema-like changes are detected, perfusion US is performed on those areas to detect an elevated perfusion typical of acute dermato- or polymyositis. Biopsies are targeted to muscles with edema-like changes and elevated perfusion. If the perfu-

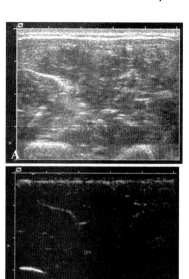

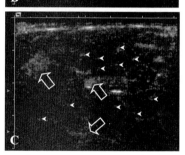

Figure 10. Transverse gray-scale US image (linear array, 8 MHz) of the right forearm flexor muscles in a 20-year-old healthy volunteer (**A**). Corresponding low-mechanical index contrast pulse sequencing (CPS) technique (linear array, 7 MHz) without contrast media application and without prior exercise (**B**). (**C**) shows the CPS-US image with the same presets and at exactly the same localization directly after exhausting isotonic exercise, while a total of 4.8 mL SonoVue® (sulfur hexafluoride, Bracco International, Amsterdam, the Netherlands) was continuously injected intravenously. Exercise consisted of clenching the fist with 50% of maximal voluntary contraction force using a handgrip dynamometer until exhaustion. In (**C**), the increased echogenicity within the muscle tissue is caused by multiple signals from microbubbles in the capillaries (some are indicated by closed arrows). The increased circulation within larger vessels is also depicted by the signals from microbubbles (open arrows).

sion within muscles, which show edema-like changes, is normal, myopathies other than acute dermato- or polymyositis seem more likely.[18]

Take Home Points

- Acute poly- and dermatomyositis are accompanied by normal or increased size, decreased echogenicity, and elevated perfusion of affected muscles.
- Chronic poly- and dermatomyositis are accompanied by reduced size, increased echogenicity, and reduced perfusion of affected muscles.
- Although MRI is more sensitive in detecting edema-like muscular changes (and thereby acute myositis) than B-mode US, the possibility of measuring perfusion with CE-US has rendered this a more useful diagnostic tool.
- Abscess formation is not a feature of dermato-or polymyositis but of pyomyositis.

Acknowledgment

I thank my ultrasound teacher at German Cancer Research Center Heidelberg, Stefan Delorme, MD, for thoroughly reviewing this chapter and his valuable comments.

Conflicts of Interest

The authors declare no conflicts of interest.

References

1. Dalakas, M.C. & R. Hohlfeld. 2003. Polymyositis and dermatomyositis. *Lancet* **362:** 971–982.
2. Bureau, N.J., R.K. Chhem & E. Cardinal. 1999. Musculoskeletal infections: US manifestations. *Radiographics* **19:** 1585–1592.
3. Chau, C.L.F. & J.F. Griffith. 2005. Musculoskeletal infections: Ultrasound appearances. *Clin. Radiol.* **60:** 149–159.
4. Kuo, G.P. & J.A. Carrino. 2007. Skeletal muscle imaging and inflammatory myopathies. *Curr. Opin. Rheumatol.* **19:** 530–535.
5. Mastaglia, F.L. *et al.* 2003. Inflammatory myopathies: Clinical, diagnostic and therapeutic aspects. *Muscle Nerve* **27:** 407–425.
6. O'Connell, M.J. *et al.* 2002. Whole-body MR imaging in the diagnosis of polymyositis. *AJR Am. J. Roentgenol.* **179:** 967–971.
7. Park, J.H. & N.J. Olsen. 2001. Utility of magnetic resonance imaging in the evaluation of patients with inflammatory myopathies. *Curr. Rheumatol. Rep.* **3:** 334–345.
8. Schweitzer, M.E. & J. Fort. 1995. Cost-effectiveness of MR imaging in evaluating polymyositis. *AJR Am. J. Roentgenol.* **165:** 1469–1471.
9. Peetrons, P. 2002. Ultrasound of muscles. *Eur. Radiol.* **12:** 35–43.
10. Lovitt, S. *et al.* 2004. MRI in myopathy. *Neurol. Clin.* **22:** 509–538.
11. Reimers, C.D. *et al.* 1993. Muscular ultrasound in idiopathic inflammatory myopathies of adults. *J. Neurol. Sci.* **116:** 82–92.
12. Chason, D.P. *et al.* 1996. Diabetic muscle infarction: Radiologic evaluation. *Skeletal Radiol.* **25:** 127–132.
13. Stonecipher, M.R. *et al.* 1994. Dermatomyositis with normal muscle enzyme concentrations. A single-blind study of the diagnostic value of magnetic resonance imaging and ultrasound. *Arch. Dermatol.* **130:** 1294–1299.
14. Trusen, A. *et al.* 2003. Ultrasound and MRI features of pyomyositis in children. *Eur. Radiol.* **13:** 1050–1055.
15. Meng, C. *et al.* 2001. Combined use of power Doppler and gray-scale sonography: A new technique for the assessment of inflammatory myopathy. *J. Rheumatol.* **28:** 1271–1282.
16. Reimers, C.D. & M. Finkenstaedt. 1997. Muscle imaging in inflammatory myopathies. *Curr. Opin. Rheumatol.* **9:** 475–485.
17. Weber, M.A. *et al.* 2006. Contrast-enhanced ultrasound in dermatomyositis and polymyositis. *J. Neurol.* **253:** 1625–1632.
18. Weber, M.A., M. Krix & S. Delorme. 2007. Quantitative evaluation of muscle perfusion with CEUS and with MR. *Eur. Radiol.* **17:** 2663–2674.
19. Newman, J.S. & R.S. Adler. 1998. Power Doppler sonography: Applications in musculoskeletal imaging. *Sem. Musculoskeletal Radiol.* **2:** 331–340.
20. Krix, M. *et al.* 2003. A multivessel model describing replenishment kinetics of ultrasound contrast agent for quantification of tissue perfusion. *Ultrasound Med. Biol.* **29:** 1421–1430.
21. Delorme, S. & M. Krix. 2006. Contrast-enhanced ultrasound for examining tumor biology. *Cancer Imaging* **6:** 148–152.
22. Calliada, F. *et al.* 1998. Ultrasound contrast agents: Basic principles. *Eur. J. Radiol.* **27**(Suppl. 2): S157–S160.
23. Krix, M. *et al.* 2005. Assessment of skeletal muscle perfusion using contrast-enhanced ultrasonography. *J. Ultrasound Med.* **24:** 431–441.
24. Wei, K. *et al.* 1998. Quantification of myocardial blood flow with ultrasound-induced destruction of

microbubbles administered as a constant venous infusion. *Circulation* **97:** 473–483.

25. Weber, M.A. *et al.* 2006. Pathologic skeletal muscle perfusion in patients with myositis: Detection with quantitative contrast-enhanced US—initial results. *Radiology* **238:** 640–649.

26. Weber, M.A. *et al.* 2006. Relationship of skeletal muscle perfusion measured by contrast-enhanced ultrasonography to histologic microvascular density. *J. Ultrasound Med.* **25:** 583–591.

27. Garcia, J. 2000. MRI in inflammatory myopathies. *Skeletal Radiol.* **29:** 425–438.

28. Maillard, S.M. *et al.* 2004. Quantitative assessment of MRI T2 relaxation time of thigh muscles in juvenile dermatomyositis. *Rheumatology (Oxford)* **43:** 603–608.

29. May, D.A. *et al.* 2000. Abnormal signal intensity in skeletal muscle at MR imaging: Patterns, pearls, and pitfalls. *Radiographics* **20:** S295–S315.

30. Lane, R.J.M. *et al.* 1989. Clinical, biochemical and histological responses to treatment in polymyositis: A prospective study. *J. R. Soc. Med.* **82:** 333–338.

31. Lundberg, I.E. 2001. The physiology of inflammatory myopathies: An overview. *Acta Physiol. Scand.* **171:** 207–213.

32. Greenberg, S.A. & A.A. Amato. 2004. Uncertainties in the pathogenesis of adult dermatomyositis. *Curr. Opin. Neurol.* **17:** 359–364.

33. Lundberg, I.E. & M. Dastmalchi. 2002. Possible pathogenic mechanisms in inflammatory myopathies. *Rheum. Dis. Clin. North Am.* **28:** 799–822.

34. Raynaud, J.S. *et al.* 2001. Determination of skeletal muscle perfusion using arterial spin labeling NMRI: Validation by comparison with venous occlusion plethysmography. *Magn. Reson. Med.* **46:** 305–311.

Ultrasound in the Diagnosis of Noninflammatory Musculoskeletal Conditions

Mandana Hashefi

Division of Rheumatology, George Washington University, Washington, DC, USA

Sonography is an attractive tool for the diagnosis of musculoskeletal conditions. The clinician can evaluate the anatomic segment during active and/or passive flexion and extension maneuvers, and its real-time capability allows imaging in positions that trigger symptoms. Scanning the contralateral asymptomatic extremity can be used as a reference for normal anatomy in a given patient. A common application of ultrasound is for the assessment of rotator cuff tendons. It can also be used to assess soft tissue infections, nerve pathology, and various sports-related injuries.

Key words: ultrasound; musculoskeletal; tendon; ligament; joint; cellulitis; effusion; foreign body; fracture; abscess

Introduction

The development of compact real-time ultrasound systems in the 1980s and the subsequent availability of broadband high-frequency (7- to 15-MHz) linear array transducers in the 1990s have revolutionized the bedside assessment of musculoskeletal disorders. Other recent advances such as power Doppler sonography and extended field-of-view function have further facilitated the progressive bedside utility of sonography. Musculoskeletal sonography is now a widely accepted and available tool in Europe and other parts of the world, where it is the technique of choice for many clinical indications. It is, however, relatively underused in the United States because of the wide availability of MRI and the small number of training programs offering instruction and experience in musculoskeletal sonography.

Synovitis of the knee was the earliest musculoskeletal disorder assessed by ultrasound (US)

in the clinic,[1] and ultrasonographic assessment of synovitis of the small joints of the hands, in patients with rheumatoid arthritis followed a decade later.[2]

Ultrasound energy is carried by waves, which have different average propagation speeds in different tissues. For example, the average ultrasound propagation speed in the synovium of a knee with arthritis has been shown to be 1548 m/s or approximately 3500 mi/h.[3]

The principle of ultrasonography is based on generation of US pulses by a transducer. The pulses are then sent into the patient, where they produce echoes at organ boundaries and within tissues. Sound waves travel in a similar way to light waves, so the denser the material (e.g., bone cortex), the more reflective it is and the whiter it appears on the screen. Water is the least reflective body material and the sound waves travel straight through it, so water shows as black. Echoes return to the transducer, where they are detected and displayed on the monitor. The US unit processes the echoes and shows them as visible dots, which form the anatomic image. The brightness of the image corresponds to the echo strength, producing what is known as the gray-scale image.

Address for correspondence: Mandana Hashefi, The George Washington University —Medicine/ Rheumatology, 2150 Pennsylvania Ave., NW, Washington DC 20037. Voice: 202/741-2488; fax: 202/741-2490. mhashefi@mfa.gwu.edu

MRI and Ultrasound in Diagnosis and Management: Ann. N.Y. Acad. Sci. 1154: 171–203 (2009).
doi: 10.1111/j.1749-6632.2009.04391.x © 2009 New York Academy of Sciences.

The most common scanning format in diagnostic musculoskeletal ultrasonography is the linear array scan, where rectangular elements are arranged in a line.[4] Linear array transducers, as opposed to sector scanners, provide optimal images. In this situation the sound beam is oriented perpendicular to the structures of interest (such as tendons) throughout the imaging field. Sector scanners (used in abdominal and obstetric ultrasonography) generate a wedge-shaped image and have several disadvantages, including narrow near field of view, poor resolution in the near field, and obliquity of the sound beam when tendons are examined in their longitudinal axis. Newer US techniques include color and power Doppler imaging, which provide color maps of the tissues. The strength of the color is related to the amount of blood, making it useful in assessing the degree of vascularity in the setting of tissue inflammation. To further increase the sensitivity of power Doppler, intravenous bubble contrast agents can be utilized.

Ultrasound is an attractive tool for the diagnosis of musculoskeletal conditions for several reasons. To begin with, the clinician can evaluate the anatomic segment during active and/or passive flexion and extension maneuvers.[5] In addition, the real-time capability of sonography allows imaging in positions that trigger symptoms, which can be done by using a standoff pad: while the examiner slides the tissue or joint to be examined between the pad and the skin, the other hand keeps the transducer in place over the region evaluated. Finally, scanning the contralateral asymptomatic extremity can be used as a reference for normal anatomy in a given patient.

The ability to obtain the true longest measurements of lesions in three dimensions is a significant advantage of sonography, as these longest diameters are not necessarily aligned with the standard MRI axial, sagittal, and coronal planes. Patient comfort is another important consideration that makes US a preferred procedure for those with claustrophobia or pacemakers as well as infants and the elderly.

Figure 1. Needle aspiration of brachial cleft cyst. The needle is seen as it enters from upper right of the screen. (Courtesy of Dr. Keith Boniface.)

Real-time sonography is ideal for guiding needle biopsy of soft tissue masses, cysts, and abscesses (Figs. 1 and 2).

The greatest value of US is at the bedside, where the clinician can interpret the images in the light of the clinical history and the physical examination. One limitation of sonography is the issue of operator dependency. Specifically, the quality and consistency of sonographic studies are a direct function of the expertise of the examiner. Other drawbacks are the physician hands-on time required for a thorough examination and the relatively long course of the operator learning curve.

In an attempt to standardize the quality of musculoskeletal US education, national and international (e.g., EULAR) societies have established training guidelines . Although there is no substitute for practical experience, knowledge of the basic laws of physics relevant to sound

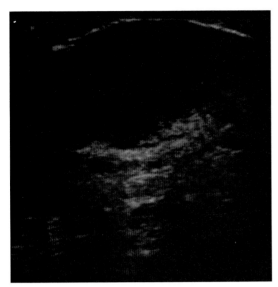

Figure 2. Submental abscess. (Courtesy of Dr. Keith Boniface.)

waves and a detailed knowledge of anatomy are mandatory. EULAR guidelines for musculoskeletal US imaging emphasize the need for careful documentation of the images. Images may be recorded on paper, films, video cassettes, laser-printed X-ray acetates, optical discs, or digital storage systems.

In this chapter we discuss the uses of ultrasonography in the evaluation of noninflammatory musculoskeletal conditions.

Background

In general, most structures examined during musculoskeletal ultrasonography are superficial; hence, high-frequency (>7- to 12-MHz) linear array transducers are usually the most appropriate choice.[6] For example, high- frequency (7.5- to 20-MHz) linear transducers are more suitable for demonstrating structures such as tendons, ligaments, and small joints, whereas low-frequency transducers (3.5- to 5- MHz) are better for larger or more deeply situated joints such as the shoulder and hip. Although higher-frequency transducers provide better spatial resolution, they have a shallower depth of penetration when compared to lower-

frequency models. Another factor is the "footprint" of the transducer, defined as the surface area of the transducer in contact with the skin. For example, transducers with a large footprint are often inadequate to fully visualize small joints such as the metacarpophalangeals and cannot be maneuvered adequately.

The brightness of images, called echogenicity, depends on the degree of reflection of the US waves. Echogenicity of a tissue depends not only on the characteristics of the tissue but on the transducer frequency as well. The terms used to describe such characteristics include hyperechoic (white signal), isoechoic, hypoechoic, and anechoic (black) echogenicity. Table 1 summarizes the echogenic features of different musculoskeletal structures.

Ultrasound remains the most sensitive imaging technique for determining the extent of tendon tears, and the evaluation of tendon abnormality is the most common clinical indication for musculoskeletal sonography. Tendons should have a fibrillar pattern of parallel hyperechoic lines in the longitudinal plane and a hyperechoic round-to-ovoid shape in the transverse plane.[7] The parallel fascicles of collagen fibers produce hyperechoic lines, whereas the interfascicular ground substance produces anechoic lines in between the collagen fibers (Figs. 3 and 4).[7]

One of the characteristic US features of tendons and ligaments is anisotropy, defined as change in the echogenicity of the structure depending on the angle of the US beam, which can be useful in identifying the scanned structure as either a tendon or a ligament. For example, the tendon appears hyperechoic when the beam is perpendicular to it and hypoechoic when the beam is oblique. Care must be taken not to misinterpret anisotropy as a partial tear or other pathology.[8]

Many tendons are embedded in a synovial sheath. Examples of sheathed tendons include the long head of the biceps brachii muscle at the shoulder and the digital extensor and flexor tendons at the wrist. The finger flexor tendons are also sheathed starting at the

TABLE 1. Echogenic Properties of Musculoskeletal Structures

Cartilage	Hyaline cartilage is anechoic and black. Degenerated cartilage may have increased echogenicity and have an irregular surface.
Fibrocartilage (glenohumeral labrum and knee meniscus)	Hyperechoic (white).
Bursae	Hypoechoic or anechoic depending on the structures in the bursae. Ultrasound may not detect a small amount of fluid present in normal bursa.
Tendons	Fine internal fibrillar pattern. Hyperechoic if localized perpendicular to the probe. Hypoechogenicity of tendons is an artifact (anisotropy) due to scattering of the beam that is not perpendicular to the tendon surface.
Ligaments	Fibrillar pattern like that of tendons, but fibers may run in different directions.
Bone surface	Bright and hyperechoic with posterior acoustic shadowing (black).
Bone erosions	Regular or irregular discontinuities of the cortical surface.
Synovium	Medium echogenicity (i.e., between that of cartilage and bone). Normal synovium has no color Doppler or power Doppler signals.
Synovial fluid	Normal synovial fluid is anechoic, displaceable, compressible and does not demonstrate a power Doppler signal.
Joint capsule	The joint capsule is the anatomical structure that forms the boundary between the hypoechoic synovium, anechoic synovial fluid, or anechoic cartilage and the midechoic periarticular soft tissues.
Nerves	Similar but more dotted, less echogenic and less fibrillar than tendons.
Muscles	Mainly hypoechoic but sometimes mid- or hyperechoic, according to the transducer orientation. Fine intramuscular hyperechoic lines represent the epi- and perimysium; thicker hyperechoic lines represent septae and fascia.
Connective tissue and SQ fat	Midechoic and slightly irregular.
Fat	Slightly less echoic than the surrounding connective tissue.

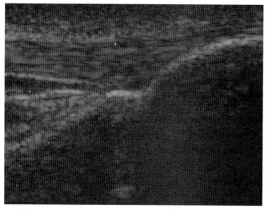

Figure 3. Normal patellar tendon insertion to tibia. (Courtesy of Dr. Keith Boniface.)

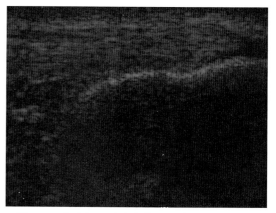

Figure 4. Normal Achilles tendon insertion into calcaneous. (Courtesy of Dr. Keith Boniface.)

metacarpophalangeal (MCP) joints down to their respective insertions. Similarly, the flexor and extensor tendons around the ankle joint are all sheathed. Unsheathed tendons, including the rotator cuff tendons (which are adjacent to the synovium-lined shoulder joint and the subacromial bursa) and the Achilles tendon (adjacent to the retrocalcaneal bursa) may become involved in the inflammatory process as innocent bystanders. The use of US in imaging of inflammatory conditions is discussed elsewhere in this volume.

Ultrasound features of tendon degeneration include irregularities of fibrillar pattern, such as thickening, fragmentation, focal hypoechoic areas, and calcifications. Chronic tendinosis in tendons with a synovial sheath results in widening of the tendon sheath, loss of normal fibrillar echotexture, and loss of definition of tendon margins. The presence of clusters of punctate and/or soft echoes within a widened tendon sheath may sometimes be of uncertain significance. Echoes inside the sheath can be generated by crystals, fibrous material, pus, blood clots, or debris. These echoes appear to be floating within the fluid collection. The distinction between synovial proliferation and proteinaceous material can be achieved by dynamic maneuvers such as local pressure by the transducer or active or passive movements of the tendon. If the soft echoes are due to synovial hypertrophy, no substantial change is detected in the sonographic pattern. On the other hand, if the echoes are due to proteinaceous material, dynamic examination induces some changes in these clusters.[9]

Loss of the typical fibrillar echotexture is the most sensitive early marker of tendon damage and can be seen in both inflammatory and degenerative disorders. Typical sonographic features of tendon damage include a focal area of fibrillar interruptions, blurring of the tendon texture, and areas of lower echogenicity. In tendons without a synovial sheath, pathology manifests as focal or diffused thickening of the tendon, with loss of fibrillar echotexture and patches of hypoechogenicity.

Tendon ruptures can range from partial to complete (or massive) and appear as fragmented fibrils. It is difficult to distinguish between tendon degeneration and intrasubstance tears in the absence of hematoma, especially since the two conditions are not mutually exclusive. Hematoma is characterized by anechoic (or hypoechoic) areas or heterogeneous abnormal mixed echogenicity with a mass effect. Complete tears of the tendon are characterized by retraction of torn edges, with hypoechoic hematoma or granulation tissue. Passive movement to accentuate the tendon interruption is a useful maneuver during imaging of a suspected tear. In tendons with a synovial sheath, fluid can collect in the space between the retracted ends of the tendon. Partial-thickness tears present with a combination of intact and retracted ruptured portions of the tendon, often accompanied by hematoma.[10]

An essential part of US examination of tendons is dynamically moving the joint or extremity to assess tendon movement and anatomical integrity. For example, the snapping phenomenon that accompanies trigger finger and the bulging of the supraspinatus tendon on the anterolateral edge of the acromion as a result of shoulder impingement can be elicited during dynamic imaging.

Ligaments appear similar to tendons but they have a more compact fibrillar, hyperechoic pattern.[1] Normal peripheral nerves typically appear as echogenic fascicular structures and tend to be slightly less echogenic than tendons or ligaments.[11] Evaluation of muscle injury and trauma as well as partial or complete muscle tears is another utility of ultrasonography. Dynamic imaging with contraction of the affected muscle enables assessment and measurement of the degree of retraction. Split-screen images provide an internal control and allow for comparison of the symptomatic side with the normal side, increasing the ability to detect muscle atrophy and other architectural abnormalities. Other noninflammatory conditions diagnosed with ultrasonography include radiographically occult fractures, which can be seen as a "step

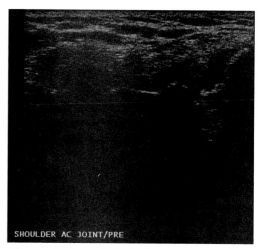

Figure 6. Acromioclavicular joint osteoarthritis with hypertrophic osteophyte.

Figure 5. Distal tibia cortical fracture. (Courtesy of Dr. Keith Boniface.)

off" cortical disruption (Fig. 5), and visualization of hypertrophic osteophytes in osteoarthritis (Fig. 6).

Site-Specific Standard Scans and Their Applications

In this section we review the possible indications as well as the standard scans recommended for evaluation of noninflammatory musculoskeletal conditions, based on the location of the symptoms. An excellent review of the technical aspects including patient positioning and standard scans recommended by a panel of European experts is available in print and on the official EULAR website. There is also an excellent collection of images available online to aid clinicians in establishing standardized images and techniques.[12,13]

Ultrasonography for Evaluation of Shoulder Symptoms

A variety of conditions involving the shoulders can be evaluated at bedside with the use of US, which is performed with the patient sitting and the elbow joint maintained at a 90° flex-

ion. In the neutral position, the patient's hand is supinated and resting on his/her thigh. Dynamic positioning to assess different structures is discussed below. To verify that the structure is a tendon, the associated muscle can be contracted, demonstrating the sliding movement of the tendon fibrils in longitudinal view along with contraction of the muscle bundles in both transverse and longitudinal views.

One of the common applications of musculoskeletal US in both Europe and the United States is for evaluation of shoulder tendons and specifically evaluation of the rotator cuff tendons. From the standpoint of cost, there is an economic incentive for using ultrasonography for imaging rotator cuff tears because it can be done at less than one-third the cost and one-quarter the time required for MRI of the shoulder. Moreover, it has a sensitivity of 67–100% and a specificity of 85–100% for the diagnosis of full-thickness rotator cuff tears.[14,15]

Middleton *et al.*[16] analyzed interpretation errors with sonography in 106 patients. They divided the errors into four categories: errors from failure to recognize normal anatomy, errors caused by soft tissue abnormalities (calcific tendinitis), errors caused by bony abnormalities, and errors caused by technical limitations of the study. They found that errors in

recognition of normal anatomy can be overcome with experience and with comparison to
normal, contralateral anatomy. It was noted
that errors in interpretation of fractures and
glenohumeral subluxation could have been
avoided by review of the radiographs before
sonography. An important technical limitation
is the inability to image the rotator cuff beneath the acromion. Passive maneuvers during
ultrasonography often allows otherwise hidden
parts of the rotator cuff to be seen.

Ultrasound may be the best diagnostic test
for assessment of the rotator cuff after shoulder
surgery. Its sensitivity in detecting postoperative
rotator cuff tears has been reported to be 100%,
with a specificity of 90%, and an overall accuracy of 98%.[17] In contrast, shoulder arthrography is unreliable because of the high number of
false positives from the lack of watertight clo-
sure and the possibility of false negatives from
postoperative shoulder adhesions.[18]

Harryman *et al.*[19] used ultrasonography to
evaluate 105 operative repairs of the rotator
cuff in 89 patients at an average of 5 years
postoperatively. The shoulders in which the re-
paired cuff was intact at follow-up had better
function and a greater range of active flexion
compared with shoulders that had a recurrent
tear. Crass *et al.*[20] reported that the criteria for
retear after a rotator cuff tear must be different from those used in detecting new tears in a
nonoperated cuff. They noted that the finding
of a defect or gap was the only accurate sign of
a recurrent rotator cuff tear. Gaenslen *et al.*[21]
reported a sensitivity of 91% for MRI in the
detection of failed repairs of the rotator cuff.
Ultrasonography may be indicated in patients
when imaging of the postoperative rotator cuff
is needed.

STANDARD SCANS FOR EVALUATION OF THE
SHOULDER

1. *Anterior transverse scan in neutral position:*
   - Best for visualizing the bicipital groove
     and for the biceps tendon transverse
     view.

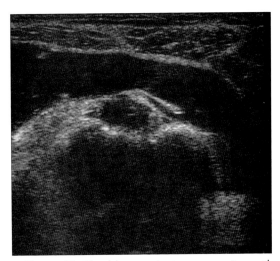

Figure 7. Shoulder anterior transverse view with
hypoechoic effusion in the bicipital groove surrounding the bicipital tendon as well as subdeltoid bursa
effusion.

   - Can detect effusion (hypoechoic/black)
     halo around the hyperechoic, ovoid, or
     round tendon bundle (Fig. 7).
   - May detect other pathology such as subdel-
     toid bursitis and shoulder effusion (ventral
     transverse scan of the shoulder).
   - Dislocation or absence of the biceps ten-
     don (as in complete tendon tear) can be
     demonstrated using the split-screen im-
     ages, comparing findings with the con-
     tralateral shoulder.

2. *Anterior transverse scan in maximal internal rota-
   tion:*
   - Visualizes humeral head cortex with its
     hyaline cartilage, supraspinatus tendon,
     and overlying deltoid muscle.
   - Calcific tendinitis of the supraspinatus ten-
     don can be seen as linear calcification at
     the superior margin of supraspinatus ten-
     don with posterior acoustic shadowing.

3. *Anterior longitudinal scan:*
   - Is used for evaluation of the biceps ten-
     don and subdeltoid bursa in different
     planes.
   - Can detect longitudinal tear, complete ten-
     don rupture with distal retraction of the
     bulk of biceps.

- Hypertrophy and proliferation of tendon sheath and effusion superimposed on inflammatory conditions may be imaged.

4. *Anterior longitudinal scan in maximal internal rotation:*
   - This view allows imaging of the hyaline cartilage (as a hypoechoic layer) overlying the bright signal of humeral head.
   - The characteristic beaklike supraspinatus tendon insertion into the humeral greater tubercle is best seen in this view.
   - This is the best view for detecting supraspinatus tendon partial or complete tear, manifesting as an irregular hypoechoic or anechoic region without a fibrillar tendon pattern (and an absence of anisotropy).
   - Even in normal individuals a thin hypoechoic line, characterizing a normal amount of effusion in the subacromial bursa, can sometimes be visualized in this view.
   - The deltoid muscle and subcutaneous fat can be interrogated as well.
   - Humeral head cortical pathology such as irregular contour, bony erosions, osteophytes, Hill–Sachs lesion (i.e., posterolateral humeral head fracture when it strikes the inferior glenoid rim during anterior dislocation of the shoulder) can also be detected.

5. *Lateral longitudinal scan in neutral position:*
   - This view shows the humerus with supraspinatus tendon attachment as well as part of the acromion. Also noted is the deltoid muscle.
   - In a complete supraspinatus tear, the supraspinatus tendon attachment to humerus disappears and there is superior migration of the humeral head in relation to the acromial cortex.

6. *Lateral longitudinal scan in the maximal internal rotation:*
   - Can again demonstrate acromion, humeral head, and supraspinatus tendon.
   - Subdeltoid bursitis can be noted in this view as well, with the presence of hypoanechoic (black) effusion in the bursa.

7. *Posterior transverse scan:*
   - This view shows the posterior aspect of the glenohumeral joint (for deeper penetration, transducers with lower frequency should be used).
   - The integrity of the infraspinatus tendon can be assessed in this view.

8. *Axillary longitudinal scan with elevated arm:*
   - Visualizes the axillary recess.
   - One of the best views for detecting synovial proliferation and effusion.

9. *Acromioclavicular joint scan:*
   - Dislocation.
   - Synovial proliferation/effusion.

The sequence for rotator cuff interrogation includes:

1. *Biceps tendon:* Forearm resting in a supinated position on the thigh.
2. *Subscapularis tendon:* Arm externally rotated.
3. *Supraspinatus:* The hand in a back pocket, palm toward the gluteal muscles, and the elbow directed posteriorly.
4. *Infraspinatus, teres minor, and posterior glenohumeral joint:* The arm across the chest and the hand on the opposite shoulder.

Ultrasonography for Evaluation of the Elbow

The ideal position for evaluation of the elbow is for the patient to be sitting with: (i) full extension of the elbow joint and supination of the lower arm (ventral scans); (ii) flexion of the elbow joint in a 90° angle (dorsal scans). Hand can be placed on the hip or on the thigh of the patient with moderate internal rotation of the humerus.

STANDARD SCANS FOR THE EVALUATION OF THE ELBOW

1. *Anterior humeroradial longitudinal scan (lateral/radial aspect):*
   - This view shows the humeroradial joint space with the round cortex of distal

humerus and the more flattened radial head cortical outline.

- A joint effusion manifests as hypoanechoic joint space widening. The homogeneously anechoic content is the hallmark of an exudative inflammation.
- Cortical irregularities.
- Loose joint body.

2. *Anterior humeroulnar longitudinal scan (medial/ulnar aspect):*

- This view shows the humeroulnar joint space with the round cortex of distal humerus and the more flattened ulnar head cortical outline.
- Joint effusion manifests as hypoanechoic joint space widening.
- Cortical irregularities.
- A loose joint body can also be visualized.

3. *Anterior transverse scan:*

- The anterior transverse scan at the distal humeral epiphysis can detect abnormalities in its articular cartilage and overlying muscles.

4. *Posterior longitudinal scan:*

- This view can be used to detect gouty tophi, osteophytes with cortical proliferation and irregularity, effusion, and olecranon bursitis.
- Effusions can be seen at the olecranon fossa, located between the distal humeral epiphysis and the olecranon process of ulna, underlying the distal triceps muscle fibers.
- After an intra-articular injection, US allows the detection of triamcinolone, which appears as hyperechoic drops.

5. *Posterior transverse scan:*

- This view visualizes the humerus with its articular cartilage and the triceps muscle.

6. *Lateral longitudinal scan in 90° flexion:*

- This view shows the humerus and its attachment with the common extensor tendon. The radius is seen distally.
- In this view, lateral epicondylitis is seen as marked focal thickening and loss of the typical "fibrillar" echotexture of the common extensor tendon.

7. Additional views: Cubital tunnel for ulnar nerve: (a) To assure full probe contact to the curvilinear bony structures in the elbow, US should be done with small-field-of-view transducers. With larger transducers, a thin and flexible standoff pads or even a thicker layer of gel with minimal pressure can help with the scanning. (b) The patient is examined while supine with the arm abducted. (c) The transverse plane is preferred in order to follow the course of the nerve. (d) In longitudinal scans, the nerve may be mistaken for echoes from the triceps and flexor carpi ulnaris muscles, which course along the same plane. (See also the use of ultrasonography for evaluation of peripheral nerves pathology, which is discussed below).

Ultrasonography for Evaluation of the Wrist

Patient is in a sitting position, with the hand on top of the thigh or on an examining table. Dynamic examination with active flexion/extension of the fingers.

STANDARD SCANS OF THE WRIST

1. *Volar transverse scan:* On transverse scan the median nerve appears as an oval-to-round structure with internal punctate echoes. The flexor tendon's echotexture is characterized by clearly evident echoic dots reflecting end-on collagen bundles. (See also the section on median nerve entrapment in carpal tunnel below.)

2. *Volar longitudinal scan:* On longitudinal scan the median nerve appears as a hypoechoic structure with parallel but discontinuous linear echoes. Flexor tendons have a typical fibrillar structure, lying deep to the median nerve.

3. *Dorsal transverse scan (radial):* This scan visualizes the second and third compartments of extensor tendons: (a) extensor carpi radialis longus tendon; (b) extensor carpi

radialis brevis tendon; (c) extensor pollicis longus tendon. Tendinitis manifests as marked hypoanechoic widening of the tendon sheath.

4. *Dorsal transverse scan (median):* This scan shows the third, fourth, and fifth compartments of extensor tendons: (a) extensor pollicis longus tendon; (b) extensor digitorum and extensor indicis tendons; (c) extensor digiti minimi tendon.

5. *Dorsal longitudinal scan (radial):* In this view the most proximal bony cortex is that of the radius. Adjacent but more distal is the lunate cortex. The capitate cortex lies more distal and deeper. Joint effusion collects deep to the extensor tendons in this view as anechoic signal.

6. *Dorsal transverse scan (median):* Typical fibrillar echotexture of the extensor digitorum tendon is well noted in this view.

7. *Lateral/ radial transverse scan:* Shows the first compartment of extensor tendons: (a) abductor pollicis longus tendon; (b) extensor pollicis brevis tendon. Tenosynovitis of these tendons (deQuervain's tenosynovitis) manifests as hypoanechoic widening of these tendon sheaths. Application of power Doppler shows the radial artery located in close proximity.

8. *Lateral longitudinal scan:* In this view the radial artery lies under the first compartment of extensor tendons between the radius and trapezius bones.

9. *Medial transverse scan:* This view shows the sixth compartment of extensor tendons, which contains the extensor carpi ulnaris tendon.

10. *Medial longitudinal scan:* The extensor carpi ulnaris tendon overlying the hyperechoic cortex of ulna can be scanned in this view.

Ultrasonography for Evaluation of the Hand

STANDARD SCANS OF THE HAND

1. *Dorsal longitudinal scan*
2. *Dorsal transverse scan*
3. *Palmar longitudinal scan*
4. *Palmar transverse scan*
5. *Thenar longitudinal scan*
6. *Thenar transverse scan*
7. *Lateral longitudinal scan*

These views can help demonstrate erosions (depressed loss of cortical continuity), osteophytes (fluffy lifting of the otherwise smooth hyperechoic bony cortex), effusion, Heberden's and Bouchard's nodes (both are isoechoic hypertrophy of periarticular tissue with echogenicity similar to subcutaneous soft tissue). One can also see homogeneous hypoanechoic monosodium urate (MSU) deposits in otherwise echogenic subcutaneous tissue.

Ultrasonography for Evaluation of the Hip

Patient is positioned supine with the hip in a neutral position.

STANDARD SCANS OF THE HIP

1. *Anterior longitudinal scan:* Can visualize fluid in the joint capsule (Fig. 8) as well as ileopsoas bursitis (Fig. 9) as an anechoic collection of effusion superficial to the actetabulofemoral joint.

2. *Anterior transverse scan.*

3. *Lateral longitudinal scan:* Can diagnose hypoechoic effusion overlying the trochanteric tuberosity.

Ultrasonography for Evaluation of the Knee

Positioning of the patient:

• Supine position for ventral and lateral scans.
• Prone position for dorsal scans.
• Knee joint in neutral position and/or 30° flexion.
• Maximal flexion for imaging of the sulcus intercondylaris.
• Dynamic examination of the recessus suprapatellaris with relaxed and contracted quadriceps femoris muscle.

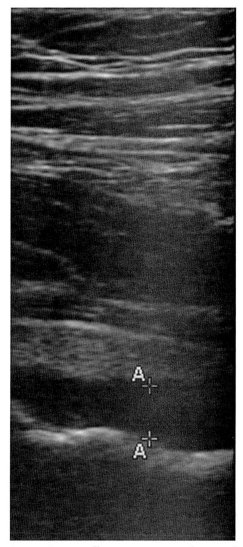

Figure 8. Hip effusion. (Courtesy of Dr. Keith Boniface.)

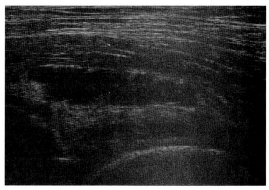

Figure 9. Longitudinal view of iliopsoas bursitis. (Courtesy of Dr. Wolfgang A. Schmidt.)

STANDARD SCANS OF THE KNEE

1. *Suprapatellar longitudinal scan:* Demonstrates the suprapatellar bursa and the quadriceps tendon.
2. *Suprapatellar transverse scan in neutral position.*
3. *Suprapatellar transverse scan in maximal flexion:* Can demonstrate the homogeneous anechogenicity of the hyaline cartilage and the sharply defined outer and inner margins of the femoral articular cartilage.
4. *Infrapatellar longitudinal scan:* Can visualize the femur with its articular cartilage, tibial tuberosity, inferior patellar apex, patellar tendon, and Hoffa's fat pad.
5. *Infrapatellar transverse scan:* Images the articular cartilage, Hoffa's fat pad, and patellar tendon.
6. *Medial longitudinal scan:* Visualizes the medial collateral ligament integrity. In patients with osteoarthritis there can be medial joint space loss and a degenerate medial meniscus emerging from between the femur and the tibia, which may be both painful and noncompressible when pressure is applied by the probe. Calcification of the medial meniscus presents as a brightly hyperechoic area seen at the edge of the medial joint space. The medial collateral ligament may stretch over the top of the meniscus.
7. *Lateral longitudinal scan:* Images the fibular collateral ligament.
8. *Posterior medial longitudinal scan:* Can demonstrate a popliteal cyst as a hypoanechoic distention of the semimembranosus gastrocnemius bursa in the popliteal fossa with hypoechoic or anechoic effusion.
9. *Posterior lateral longitudinal scan.*
10. *Posterior transverse scan:* Shows the femoral condyles with their articular cartilage as well as the popliteal fossa.

Ultrasonography for Evaluation of the Ankle

Position of the patient is supine for ventral and lateral scans and prone for the dorsal scan.

STANDARD SCANS OF THE ANKLE

1. *Anterior longitudinal scan:* Demonstrates the tibiotalar joint space.
2. *Anterior transverse scan:* Shows the talus with its articular cartilage.
3. *Perimalleolar medial longitudinal scan:* Can image the medial malleolus, the talus, and the tibialis posterior tendon.
4. *Perimalleolar medial transverse scan:* Visualizes the following structures from medial to lateral: the medial malleolus, tibialis posterior tendon, flexor digitorum longus tendon (adjacent and lateral to tibialis posterior), vessels, and flexor hallucis longus tendon.
5. *Perimalleolar lateral longitudinal scan:* images the peroneal tendons overlying the fibular lateral malleolus.
6. *Perimalleolar lateral transverse scan:* Images the peroneal tendon cross section.
7. *Posterior longitudinal scan:* Demonstrates the Achilles tendon, calcaneal bone, and retrocalcaneal fat pad. Anechoic distension of the retrocalcaneal bursa can be seen in acute bursitis. Calcaneal erosions and retrocalcaneal hypoanechoic fluid collection within the retrocalcaneal bursa can be seen in enthesopathy (e.g., in the setting of seronegative spondyloarthropathies). Ultrasound detects diffuse thickening and loss of the normal fibrillar echotexture of the Achilles tendon in Achilles tendonitis.
8. *Posterior transverse scan:* Demonstrates the Achilles tendon, retrocalcaneal fat pad, and, if present, calcaneal erosions and retrocalcaneal bursitis.

There are several limiting factors in the examination of lower extremity structures, including lower extremity edema and poor penetration of the sound waves to the deeper pre-Achilles fat pad, the bursae subtendinea, and the tricipitis surae muscle if there is a pathologically enlarged Achilles tendon. In such cases, MRI examination would provide better anatomical detail. Moreover, use of lower-

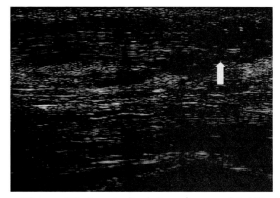

Figure 10. Longitudinal view of ruptured Achilles tendon (arrow). (Courtesy of Dr. Wolfgang A. Schmidt.)

frequency transducers offers deeper penetration of the US waves and may better image deeper structures underlying the edematous subcutaneous tissue.

In sports and traumatic injuries, knowledge of conditions that may occur simultaneously is quite useful. For example, in tears of the peroneus brevis tendon, ruptures of the lateral collateral ligaments, stripping of the superior peroneal retinaculum, peroneal longus subluxations, and low lying muscle bellies of the peroneus brevis and peroneus quartus may occur concomitantly.

The Achilles tendon can be examined by positioning the patient prone with feet hanging over the table edge. The Achilles tendon is a confluence of the individual tendons of the gastrocnemius and the soleus muscles. The anteroposterior diameter of Achilles tendon is less than 6.9 mm in normal males and less than 5.2 mm in normal females. The muscle fibers at the musculotendinous junction appear linear and hypoechoic and have to be distinguished from a tear. The hypoechoic Kager's fat lies dorsal to the tendon. The flexor hallucis longus muscle lies in deeper planes. Most tendon ruptures occur in a hypovascular region, about 6 cm proximal to the calcaneal insertion, which is where the fibers twist (Fig. 10). The tendon tear is seen as an anechoic blood- or fluid-filled defect that disrupts the echogenic tendon fibers. Retraction of the proximal and distal edges may be demonstrated with dorsiflexion and plantar flexion maneuvers. However, chronic tears may lose the tendon fluid interface and even the disrupted tendon fibers may be quite difficult to image.

Tendonitis is diagnosed when the distance between the tendon bundles is increased and there is a 2-mm increase in anteroposterior diameter of the affected tendon as compared to the normal contralateral side. The Achilles tendon does not have a tendon sheath, but in cases of tendonitis and tendon tear, fluid may be found in the adjacent bursae and there may also be increased echogenicity in the adjacent fat pad. Xanthomas of the Achilles tendon may be present in patients with familial hypercholesterolemia and appear as a speckled or reticulated pattern within the tendon.[22]

Ultrasonography for Evaluation of the Feet

Positioning of the patient is supine for the dorsal scans and prone for plantar scans.

STANDARD SCANS OF THE FEET

1. *Plantar longitudinal scan:* In this view the calcaneal bone and the plantar fascia are visualized. In plantar fasciitis the fascial thickness is greater than 6 mm, whereas in healthy subjects it is fewer than 5 mm.
2. *Plantar transverse scan:* In plantar fasciitis the US examination shows a diffuse thickening and a decreased echogenicity of the plantar fascia.
3. *Dorsal longitudinal scan:* (a) at the MTP joint, prominent osteophytes can be seen in this view; (b) IP joint changes can be visualized.
4. *Dorsal transverse scan:* Visualizes structures such as ganglion cysts.
5. *Lateral longitudinal scan:* (a) first MTP joint; (b) fifth MTP joint.

The posterior tibial muscle tendon junction rises several centimeters above the medial malleolus. It then turns under the malleolus to fan out in its insertion on the navicular, cuneiforms, and bases of the second through the fourth metatarsal bones. The normal supramalleolar tendon is hyperechoic and oval shaped, having an anteroposterior diameter from 4 to 6 mm. A thin hypoechoic tendon sheath surrounds the tendon and may contain a thin layer of fluid.

Posterior tibial tendon tears are usually longitudinal. With cross-sectional tears, in transverse scanning, the supramalleolar groove will appear empty. In longitudinal images, the ruptured ends may have a wavy fibrillar appearance that results from the absence of tendon tension. In chronic and late-stage injuries, fluid may be absent and the retracted tendon ends may be sonographically invisible.[23] Of note is that the flexor digitorum longus may simulate a normal posterior tibial tendon in the longitudinal scan.

The peroneus longus tendon rises from the tibia and fibula heads plus the intermuscular septum. The peroneus brevis tendon originates from the lower fibula and intermuscular septum somewhat anteriorly to the peroneus longus. Both tendons are bound in their common synovial sheath by a fibrous superior and inferior retinacula. The peroneal tendons lie in a tunnel that is formed by the malleolus in front, the superior peroneal retinaculum posterolaterally, and the posterior talofibular and calcaneofibular ligaments medially. Distal to the malleolus, the peroneus brevis and longus tendons diverge and have separate tendon sheaths. Small amounts of fluid can be seen in asymptomatic patients. A large volume or proximally located fluid is considered abnormal. Hypertrophy of the peroneus longus may be noted in conjunction with hypertrophy of the peroneal tubercle and appears with the normal striated echo pattern and increase in size.

The peroneal tendons usually tear in a longitudinal plane. Lateral malleolar bursitis or a lateral malleolar ganglion cyst must not be mistaken for peroneal tendon pathology. The anterior tibiofibular ligament is seen sonographically as an echogenic band between the tibia and fibula. Also seen anteriorly are the anterior tibiotalar recess and the echo-poor hyaline cartilage covering the talar dome. A lateral scan of the malleolus will image the echogenic anterior tibiofibular and calcaneofibular ligaments.

Posterior Transverse Approach

The posterior tibiofibular ligament is short and horizontal and best seen with posterior transverse scans. In tenosynovitis, the peritendon anechoic areas disappear with compression by the transducer, indicating displaceable fluid. However the hypoanechoic pannus (thickened) synovial membrane is not compressible and remains fairly unchanged with compression. Ganglia and their possible communication with a joint or tendon sheath can also be evaluated. Ganglia commonly found around the ankle and dorsum of the foot are typically anechoic. The communicating neck of the ganglion can be seen as it enters the adjacent joint space. Aspiration may be performed under US guidance.

The tibiotalar joint is imaged in the longitudinal plane, with the foot in plantar flexion. Posttraumatic fluid collections are echo-free and usually resolve within a month following injury. Calcific debris within the fluid produces bright echoes with posterior acoustic shadowing. Free air or gaseous media within the synovial effusion will also cast a sonic shadow with bright echoes. At times, small loose bodies may be readily identified in the effusion by pressing alternately on the lateral and medial joint recesses.

Ultrasonography can be used in diagnosis of plantar fasciitis. The normal plantar fascia is homogeneously echogenic and measures between 2 and 4 mm in both normal males and females. The plantar fascia is scanned transversely for overall integrity and geometry. It is then imaged longitudinally to show the total length of the fascia and its insertion site. Plantar fasciitis manifests as thickening of the fascia, most commonly noted about 2 cm from the insertion point into the calcaneus. There may also be focal or diffuse hypoechoic transformation of the fascia. Edema near the insertion site as well as *de novo* fluid collection can sometimes be identified. Plantar fibromas appear as hypoechoic nodules with a heterogeneous echo pattern.

Ultrasound in the Evaluation of Osteoarthritis

Pain is the predominant feature of clinical knee osteoarthritis (OA). The source of OA-related pain remains vague and is attributed to the synovial tissue or subchondral bone, or both.[24] The pain and functional impairment associated with a clinical "flare-up" of OA are associated with inflammation of synovial tissue.[25] On MRI there is an association between pain and synovial thickening and effusions.

Assessment of disease activity (synovitis) in knee OA by a visual analog scale (VAS) is not sufficient. New methods of digital synovial vascular quantification have been developed. Contrast-enhanced musculoskeletal ultrasonography (CE-MUS) has recently been used for detecting synovitis in patients with knee OA and compared with power Doppler sonography (PDS) and contrast-enhanced MRI.[26] US- PDS appears to be more sensitive than B-mode and CE-MUS is more sensitive than US-PDS and CE-MRI in detecting synovitis in patients with painful knee OA. Moreover, CE-MRI is more sensitive in detecting inflammatory changes in the superior recess than noncontrasted MRI. Using CE-MUS and performing time/intensity analyses has further been shown to be a good model for evaluation of an inflammatory process in the superior recess.

CPPD calcifications are hyperechoic deposits that present one of the following patterns[27]:

• Thin hyperechoic bands, parallel to the surface of the hyaline cartilage (frequently observed in the knee).[28,29]

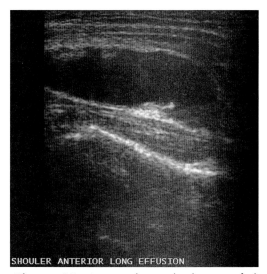

SHOULER ANTERIOR LONG EFFUSION

Figure 11. Anterior longitudinal view of the shoulder demonstrating synovial effusion with hyperechoic nodular or oval deposits localized in subdeltoid bursa effusion—polarized microscopy positive for CPPD crystals.

- A punctate pattern composed of several thin hyperechoic spots, more common in fibrous cartilage and in tendons.
- Homogeneous hyperechoic nodular or oval deposits localized in bursae (Fig. 11) and articular recesses(frequently mobile)

Calcifications have a sparkling appearance and create posterior shadowing only when they reach dimensions greater than 10 mm. In contrast, calcifications that present a hypoechoic appearance with posterior shadowing (2–3 mm in diameter) may reflect crystalline deposits of another nature, such as hydroxyapatite crystal deposition disease.[30]

Ultrasound in Diagnosis and Management of Musculoskeletal Infections

Ultrasound may help to (i) differentiate acute or chronic infection from tumors or noninfective inflammatory conditions with similar clinical presentations; (ii) localize the site and extent of infection (e.g., subcutaneous, muscle, bursa, tendon sheath, joint); (iii) ascertain the form of infection (e.g., cellulitis, preabscess, abscess); (iv) identify precipitating factors (e.g., foreign bodies, fistulation); and (v) provide guidance for diagnostic or therapeutic aspiration, drainage, or biopsy.[31,32] Split-screen comparison with the unaffected side will assist in detecting subtle architectural changes in cellulitis, pyomyositis, and other soft tissue infections. Ultrasound can be useful in diagnosis and management of the conditions described in what follows.

Septic Arthritis

Septic arthritis and septic bursitis are probably the most commonly encountered rheumatologic emergencies, with an annual incidence of approximately 2–10 per 100,000 in the general population and up to 70 per 100,000 in patients with rheumatoid arthritis or a prosthetic joint.[33]

Other risk factors include intravenous drug abuse, immunocompromised host, an age of more than 80 years, and diabetes.[34] Septic arthritis presents with joint pain with fever, chills, and rigor. Mortality rates are low for gonococcal arthritis but can be as high as 50% in patients with *Staphylococcus aureus* septic arthritis.[35] Early diagnosis and appropriate treatment are the main determinants of outcome.

The knee joint is involved in 50% and the shoulder in 10–15% of the cases of septic arthritis.[36] Successful arthrocentesis of the shoulder may be difficult. One study looking at the success rate of shoulder arthrocentesis done by orthopedic surgeons (via an anterior approach) showed that only 26% of attempted, landmark-guided, anterior glenohumeral joint injections succeeded. The success rate was even lower for the posterior approach.[37]

Real-time sonographic guidance of arthrocentesis is particularly useful when the exact location of the fluid collection is undetermined. For example, septic bursitis can sometimes be clinically difficult to distinguish from septic arthritis.[38] Joint fluid in septic arthritis may be hypoechoic and clearly demarcated from joint synovium and capsule or hyperechoic and less clearly demarcated from joint synovium or capsule. Here, an appreciation of normal anatomy is crucial.

The anterior joint capsule of the normal pediatric hip consists of anterior and posterior layers, mainly composed of fibrous tissue with only a thin synovial membrane. In children, the distance between the cortex of the femoral neck and the outer margin of the hip capsule should not be greater than 5 mm or more than 2 mm thicker than the contralateral normal side.[39] In adults, a thickness of 9 mm or more than 2 mm thicker than the contralateral normal hip is considered abnormal.[40] A normal US examination has a strong negative predictive value for septic arthritis.[41]

Although power Doppler imaging in the context of animal studies has shown increased synovial vascularity in about 50% of septic arthritis cases, in clinical practice, demonstrable synovial hypervascularity was shown in only 1 out of 11 patients.[42] Contrast-enhanced imaging may improve the sensitivity of US in this respect. For joints with nondistensible capsules (sacroiliac, sternoclavicular, and acromioclavicular joints), the absence of a visible joint effusion is not sufficient to exclude septic arthritis. MRI (or CT) examination together with guided joint aspiration should be undertaken.

Infective Bursitis

Bursitis usually results from chronic mechanical stress or trauma and consequent sterile inflammation of the bursal wall. However, *S. aureus* can infect superficial bursae, such as the olecranon or prepatella bursa. Ultrasound reveals peribursal edema, bursal wall thickening, and distension by fluid or gelatinous material of mixed echogenicity. Occasionally internal debris and calcification may be apparent. Power Doppler may show bursal wall hyperemia. Ultrasonography cannot distinguish infected bursa from noninfective bursitis, and bursal aspiration for culture is recommended

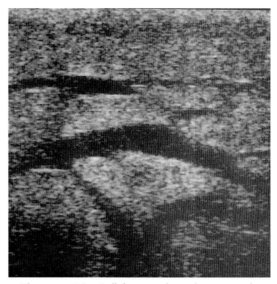

Figure 12. Cellulitis with edema tracking through tissue planes. (Courtesy of Dr. Keith Boniface.)

to exclude an infective element. Rice bodies (aggregates of fibrin) have been described as a feature of tuberculous bursitis.[43]

Cellulitis

The US appearance of cellulitis ranges from diffuse swelling and increased echogenicity of the skin and subcutaneous tissues to a superficial cobblestone appearance (Figs. 12 and 13), depending on the amount of perifascial fluid, the degree of subcutaneous edema, and the orientation of the interlobular fat septa. However, gray-scale US cannot differentiate cellulitis from subcutaneous edema due to noninfectious causes such as venous insufficiency or cardiac failure. In this setting application of power Doppler and the demonstration of hyperemia are helpful in determining an inflammatory element. Cellulitis may occur in conjunction with superficial thrombophlebitis and may lead to abscess formation.[32]

Necrotizing Fasciitis

Necrotizing fasciitis usually affects the lower extremities and can have up to 50% mortality

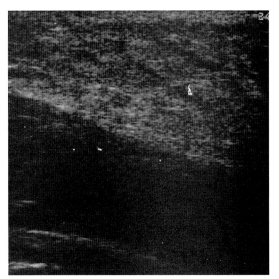

Figure 13. Cellulitis with underlying normal deltoid—gain is turned way down. (Courtesy of Dr. Keith Boniface.)

if left untreated. Pain may be out of proportion to the degree of overlying cellulitis. It may also result in dusky cutaneous discoloration with purpuric patches.[44] Group A *streptococci* are the most common offending organisms, resulting in inflammation and necrosis of the subcutaneous tissues and the underlying fascia. Necrosis is due in part to microcirculation thrombosis and ischemia.[45]

The US appearance has been described as thickened distorted fascia with perifascial hypoechoic fluid collection, as well as some swelling of the subcutaneous tissues and muscle. Ultrasound-guided aspiration of perifascial fluid can help isolate the pathogen.[46] Successful treatment requires early recognition, aggressive antibiotic therapy, and adequate surgical debridement.

Infectious Tenosynovitis

Acute suppurative tenosynovitis is caused mainly by *S. aureus* and *S. pyogenes*, usually involves the flexor tendons of hands and wrists, and results from a penetrating trauma. The radial and ulnar bursa on the volar aspect of the wrist and carpus communicate with the flexor tendon sheaths of the thumb and little finger, respectively.

Ultrasound can demonstrate variable thickening of the tendon and tendon sheath. Power Doppler may demonstrate hyperemia in the tendon sheath and occasionally within the substance of the tendon. Tendon sheath thickening is usually hypoechoic and as such may resemble viscous fluid. Power Doppler is helpful in differentiating chronic synovial sheath thickening from a synovial sheath effusion. It is felt that surgery may potentially be less beneficial in patients without visible tendon sheath effusion. Infection can occasionally spread from the tendon sheath into the peritendinous tissues.

Mycobacteria Tuberculosis Tenosynovitis

Rice bodies can be seen in both typical and atypical mycobacterial tuberculous tenosynovitis. MRI may be more sensitive for detecting small rice bodies than US.[44] Ultrasound-guided aspiration of tendon sheath fluid is helpful in differentiating infectious from noninfectious causes of tenosynovitis. Ultrasound can also be used for guiding percutaneous biopsy of a thickened tendon sheath.

Pyomyositis

Pyomyositis is bacterial infection of muscle, which usually affects the larger muscles of the lower limbs. Some 90% of the cases are due to *S. aureus*, and symptoms include fever, myalgia, and localized muscle tenderness. Ultrasound of pyomyositis shows diffuse muscle hyperechogenicity with or without localized hypoechogenicity (due to severe muscle edema or early necrosis). Power Doppler shows diffuse hyperemia. If untreated, muscle abscess formation will follow, requiring surgical or percutaneous drainage.

Abscess

Abscesses are usually round, but can also be tubular or geographical (Fig. 14). Abscess

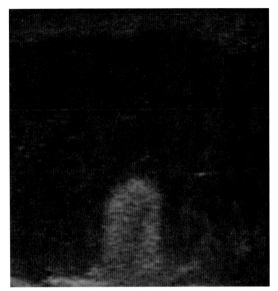

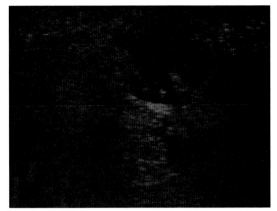

Figure 15. Groin abscess with posterior acoustic enhancement. (Courtesy of Dr. Keith Boniface.)

Figure 14. Abdominal wall abscess. (Courtesy of Dr. Keith Boniface.)

echogenicity can vary from hypoechoic to isoechoic or hyperechoic. Posterior acoustic enhancement (hyperechoic shadow) is characteristic (Fig. 15). Debris or gas loculations can be seen inside the abscess cavity. Internal septae are a feature of more chronic, low-grade infection. Power Doppler frequently demonstrates hyperemia of the abscess wall and surrounding tissues. Aspiration or catheter drainage can be performed under US guidance.

Osteomyelitis

Osteomyelitis is usually caused by *S. aureus* in young patients and by Gram-negative bacteria in the elderly. Plain radiographic features can be delayed by up to 2 weeks and include osteolysis or periosteal new bone formation. Ultrasound examination may show features of osteomyelitis several days earlier than radiographs.[47] The earliest US sign of acute osteomyelitis is juxtacortical soft tissue swelling and early periosteal thickening, followed by increased periosteal thickening. Subperiosteal exudate can be seen in up to two-thirds of cases, and rarely subperiosteal abscesses may occur as well. Cortical erosions are later findings.[48]

However, the sensitivity and specificity of US examination at diagnosing osteomyelitis are not likely to be as high as MRI or nuclear medicine studies. Therefore, if there is clinical suspicion of osteomyelitis, either MRI or phosphonate bone scintigraphy should be considered.

Emergency Musculoskeletal Sonography in Diagnosis of Skeletal Fractures and Sports Injuries

The bone–soft tissue interface has very high acoustic impedance with a high reflectance that can be used to visualize breaks in contour, including fractures. Ultrasonography has been used in the diagnosis of scaphoid fracture since as early as 1982,[49] but its reliability has been challenged by other studies.[50] High-spatial-resolution US of the scaphoid bones can be performed from the palmar, lateral, and dorsal directions in the longitudinal and transverse planes. Ultrasound findings indicative of a scaphoid fracture are cortical discontinuity and/or periosteal elevation, with an accuracy of 87% versus 73% for conventional radiography.[51]

Ultrasound can be a useful modality for early diagnosis and management of sports injuries. Avulsion injuries of the apophysis are a problem in young athletes. A correct diagnosis is necessary for establishing the appropriate treatment and the rehabilitation program. However, it is often difficult to distinguish between a simple muscle strain and an avulsion fracture. The X-ray examination is helpful only when an ossification center of the apophysis exists. Ultrasonography is considered the suitable diagnostic tool for these cases.

Proposed criteria for the sonographic diagnosis of apophyseal avulsion injuries include (i) a hypoechogenic zone (edema), (ii) increased distance to the apophysis (lysis), (iii) dislocation of the apophysis (avulsion), and (iv) mobility of the apophysis on dynamic examination (correlating with the instability of the apophyseal avulsion. In comparison to X-ray examination, ultrasonography has the advantages of no radiation exposure, early detection even without an ossification center, and dynamic examination.[52]

Ultrasonography is an acceptable screening examination for recurrent scapulohumeral dislocation and can be used prior to other investigative techniques such as double- contrast CT or MRI. Ultrasonography has shown a sensitivity of 95.6%, specificity of 92.8%, and diagnostic accuracy of 95%, when used against CT arthrogram as the true standard.[53] Ultrasound is better than lateral radiography for diagnosing sternal fractures; however, conventional radiography remains the standard means of demonstrating the grade of displacement.[54]

Studies looking at the value of US in the diagnosis of fractures in children have shown that US is most reliable for the detection of simple femoral and humeral diaphyseal fractures and fractures of the forearm. It is less dependable for compound injuries and fractures adjacent to joints, lesions of the small bones of the hand and foot, nondisplaced epiphyseal fractures (Salter–Harris type 1) or those with a fracture line of less than 1 mm.[55]

Central slip ruptures of the extensor mechanisms of a digit often are missed at the initial presentation. The patient may return with a boutonniere deformity 2 to 3 weeks later. Diagnostic US is a very accurate noninvasive study that can identify central slip injuries in the extensor mechanism of the finger. Clinically suspected cases of boutonniere injury can be scanned by high-frequency US to confirm the diagnosis and allow either early initiation of splinting or eliminate the need for prolonged splinting.[56]

Quantitative Ultrasound

Osteoporosis is a systemic skeletal disease characterized by low bone mass and microarchitectural deterioration of bone tissue, with a consequent increase in bone fragility and susceptibility to fracture. It affects approximately 200 million people worldwide.

In most countries dual-energy X-ray absorptiometry (DXA) is the most widely used method for diagnosing osteoporosis. The test involves positioning the body site of interest in the path of an X-ray beam and measuring the beam attenuation, which is related to bone mineral content. Bone mineral density (BMD) is calculated as the ratio of bone content to the scanned area.[57] The World Health Organization's (WHO) operational definition for osteoporosisis a BMD that is 2.5 SDs (T-score) or more below the mean for young healthy adult women; the WHO's operational definition of osteopenia is a T-score between –1 and –2.5.[58]

Quantitative ultrasound (QUS) measurement [broadband US attenuation (BUA) and velocity] has been looked at as an alternative to photon absorptiometry techniques in the assessment of osteoporosis. The consensus is that US seems to provide structural information in addition to density.

Calcaneal quantitative US for bone assessment typically involves placing US transducers on either side of the calcaneus; one acts as a wave transmitter and the other as the receiver.[59]

These devices assess three main types of parameters: broadband US attenuation, speed or velocity of sound, and quantitative US index stiffness. Broadband US attenuation measures the frequency-dependent attenuation of the US signal that occurs as energy is removed from the wave, primarily by absorption and scattering in the bone and soft tissue. Speed and velocity of sound measure the distance the US signal travels per unit time. Quantitative US index and stiffness are composite parameters derived from broadband US attenuation and speed of sound or velocity of sound.[60] Ultrasound parameter values are typically lower in osteoporotic bone than in healthy bone.[61]

There are numerous calcaneal quantitative US devices in use, but there are no universal guidelines establishing normal versus abnormal measurement values. In addition, studies have reported correlation coefficient values between 0.44 and 0.93 for measurements of the same parameters by different quantitative US devices.[62] Several large prospective studies have shown that calcaneal quantitative US can predict future fracture risk nearly as well as DXA.[63–65]

Quantitative US also has several potential advantages over DXA: it is less expensive, is portable, and does not involve ionizing radiation. Moreover, unlike DXA, quantitative US may be able to assess bone quality in addition to BMD. However, there are two prohibitive issues limiting the use of quantitative US as a first-line diagnostic tool in clinical practice. First is the lack of consensus diagnostic criteria for osteoporosis using this technique. The WHO's operational definition for osteoporosis was derived in the context of DXA and has typically been applied to DXA. Hence, this definition is not necessarily applicable to quantitative US. Second, current guidelines for therapy of osteoporosis in individuals with no prior history of fractures is based on DXA findings. Therefore, until more standardized guidelines for assessment of fracture risk and efficacy of treatment based on quantitative US findings are established, the clinical utility of this test for improving osteoporosis outcomes depends on its degree of correlation with DXA results.[66] In several larger studies the correlation coefficients between calcaneal quantitative US measurements and DXA BMD at the spine or the hip have ranged between 0.27 and 0.7.

Some researchers have suggested that quantitative US could be used as a prescreening test to reduce the number of patients who require additional DXA testing. It has also been suggested that several different calcaneal quantitative US cutoff thresholds, including quantitative US index T-scores of 0, –1, and –1.5 to determine which patients should be considered for additional testing with DXA.[67,68]

Ultrasound has been shown to correlate better with certain types of hip fracture (intertrochanteric or cervical) than BMD. It also provides comparable diagnostic sensitivity to spine BMD in vertebral fractures. Some authors suggest combining the results of both US and DXA BMD to further improve hip fracture prediction.[69] However, a recent meta-analysis found that the sensitivity and specificity of calcaneal quantitative US at commonly used cutoff thresholds seems to be too low to conclusively rule out or rule in DXA-determined osteoporosis for persons with pretest probabilities within the range typically encountered in clinical practice.[70] Therefore, pending availability of more fracture risk data based on quantitative US results, DXA remains the standard screening tool for identifying individuals most likely to benefit from osteoporosis therapy.

Ultrasonography for Diagnosis of Peripheral Nerve Pathology

Sonography can be used as the primary technique for imaging peripheral nerve pathology owing to its availability, low cost, comfort to the patient, lack of contraindications, and the capacity to provide imaging of the entire length of the major peripheral nerves of both limbs.

Peripheral Nerve Mass Lesions

Fornage[71] published the first review of imaging findings of peripheral nerves using sonography in 1988. He used high-resolution real-time ultrasonography to evaluate peripheral nerves of the extremities in healthy subjects and in 11 patients with a mass developing from a peripheral nerve lesion.

Pathologic findings included nine cases of benign tumors. These tumors consisted of four schwannomas, three neurofibromas, two traumatic neuromas (that included one case of neurilemmitis and one of tuberculoid leprosy). All lesions were hypoechoic. Three of the four schwannomas had well-defined contours, and two were associated with a typical distal sound enhancement. Inflammatory conditions were characterized by a hypoechoic, thickened nerve.

The normal median and ulnar, sciatic, and external popliteal nerves all have echogenic fibrillar echotexture. A 5- to 12-MHz linear array transducer is used to scan the entire peripheral nerve in both the transverse and the longitudinal plane. Normal peripheral nerves have a typical sonographic appearance, showing multiple longitudinal hypoechoic bands representing fascicular bundles. These bundles are separated by discontinuous bands of increased echogenicity, corresponding to the surrounding epineurium.

Numerous neurogenic tumors can affect the musculoskeletal system, including traumatic neuroma, Morton's neuroma, neural fibrolipoma, nerve sheath ganglion, neurilemoma, neurofibroma, and malignant peripheral nerve sheath tumors (PNSTs).[72,73] The diagnosis of neurogenic tumors can be suggested from their imaging appearances, including lesion shape and intrinsic imaging characteristics.

It is also important to establish lesion location along a typical nerve distribution (e.g., plantar digital nerve in Morton's neuroma, median nerve in neural fibrolipoma, large nerve trunk in benign and malignant PNSTs. A nerve sheath ganglion has a cystic appearance and commonly occurs about the knee. Sonography is unreliable in distinguishing between schwannomas and neurofibromas; both appear as discrete homogeneous ovoid hypoechoic masses, with a healthy nerve at the proximal and distal aspects of the mass. The presence of cystic degeneration favors schwannoma rather than neurofibroma.[72–74] Traumatic neuromas are commonly related to an amputation stump.

Because of their fibrous capsule, they are usually well defined and hypoechoic with attenuation characteristics similar to muscle. Traumatic neuromas and neurofibromas are less sharply delineated.

Morton's neuroma is a misnomer because it is a benign mass of perineural fibrosis involving a plantar digital nerve lying between two metatarsal heads, which probably develop owing to friction of the nerve against the transverse intermetatarsal ligament. Morton's neuromas may be multiple and bilateral and most commonly occur between the heads of the third and fourth metatarsals. On sonography, an ovoid hypoechoic compressible mass is visible in the intermetatarsal space. Sonographically, there may also be some effusion in the intermetatarsal bursae, located at the first three web spaces. (See also intermetatarsal nerve entrapments below.)[75]

Sonography of neural fibrolipomas shows thickened alternating hyperechoic and hypoechoic bands, reflecting the fibrofatty infiltrate. Fibrolipomas can be seen in association with macrodactyly in children. The syndrome is termed "macrodystrophia lipomatosa" and usually affects the second or third digit of the hand or foot. There is extensive fatty infiltration of the nerve and the whole digit, with accompanying osseous overgrowth.[76]

Nerve Entrapments

Peripheral nerves are vulnerable to compression as they pass through fibro-osseous tunnels. Nerve compression can result from a variety of extrinsic causes, including congenital, traumatic, and infiltrative processes; synovitis; ganglia; tumors; and other acquired disorders. Neural compression leads to ischemia and venous congestion. Chronic nerve compression may cause fibrosis and loss of nerve function with atrophy of the innervated musculature. In the upper limb, osteofibrous tunnels amenable to US examination include the carpal tunnel for the median nerve and the cubital and Guyon tunnels for the ulnar nerve. In the lower limb, these tunnels include the fibular neck for the common peroneal nerve, the tarsal tunnel for the posterior tibial nerve, and the intermetatarsal spaces for the interdigital nerves.

Diagnosis can be made based on clinical manifestations and nerve conduction studies. However, in atypical cases, sonography can show causative extrinsic abnormalities at the site of compression, with associated changes in nerve contour and echotexture.[77,80] A cascade of events after compression includes demyelination, endoneurial edema, inflammation, damming of axoplasmic flow, fibrosis, distal axonal degeneration, growth of new axons, remyelination, and thickening of the perineurium and endothelium.[78]

Median Nerve Entrapment in Carpal Tunnel[79]

The carpal tunnel is confined by the carpal bones and a roof consisting of the unextensible flexor retinaculum (transverse carpal ligament). It contains the median nerve, eight tendons of the flexor digitorum superficialis and profundus, and the tendon of the flexor pollicis longus. The retinaculum is approximately 3–4 cm wide and is attached to the scaphoid and pisiform tuberosities (proximal carpal tunnel) and to the trapezium tubercle and hamate hook (distal carpal tunnel). The radial side of the retinaculum splits into two vertical layers, which surround the flexor carpi radialis tendon and continue to the midportion of the palm forming palmar aponeurosis.

Sonographically, the median nerve is hypoechoic with bright central reflectors and lies under a thin, hyperechoic flexor retinaculum. It is superficial and parallel to the hyperechoic structures of the second and third flexor tendons. It is also medial to the flexor pollicis longus tendon. The median nerve angles away from the transducer upon entering the tunnel. The normal median nerve is elliptical and gradually flattens as it courses distally. The bony structures imaged in the longitudinal view of the carpal tunnel include the lunate

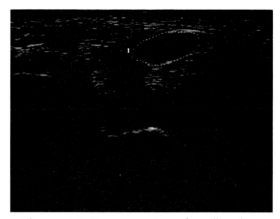

Figure 16. Transverse view of swollen, hypoechoic median nerve (22 mm^2) in secondary carpal tunnel syndrome. (Courtesy of Dr. Wolfgang A. Schmidt.)

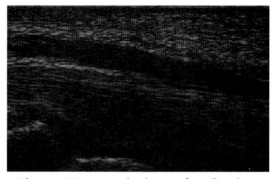

Figure 17. Longitudinal view of swollen, hypoechoic median nerve in carpal tunnel syndrome. (Courtesy of Dr. Wolfgang A. Schmidt.)

and distal radius cortex. Longitudinal US scans done while flexing the fingers or clenching a fist demonstrate passive shifting of the median nerve along the underlying flexor tendons.

Ultrasound criteria for median nerve compression include: (i) nerve swelling (thicker and more hypoechoic) at the distal radius or occasionally in the proximal tunnel, (ii) palmar bowing of the flexor retinaculum, and (iii) nerve flattening in the distal tunnel.[80] The best diagnostic criterion is reported to be a nerve cross-sectional area greater than 0.09 cm^2 at the level of the proximal tunnel (Figs. 16 and 17).[77] The increase in cross-sectional diameter correlates well with the severity of electromyographic findings or the functional outcome after surgery.[81] Several studies have noted that maximum swelling occurs at the level of the pisiform.[82,84]

Reduced transverse sliding of the nerve beneath the retinaculum during flexion and extension of the index finger may also be noted. A few studies have compared ultrasonography to MRI for the diagnosis of carpal tunnel syndrome (CTS), and have shown that US is capable of producing results at least equal to those of MRI.[82] However, MRI appears to be superior to US in identification of subtle cases and has better sensitivity than color and power Doppler US in showing changes caused by nerve edema and blood perfusion abnormalities.[83,84]

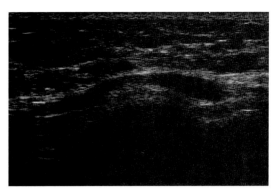

Figure 18. Longitudinal view of swollen, hypoechoic ulnar nerve in cubital tunnel syndrome. (Courtesy of Dr. Wolfgang A. Schmidt.)

Ulnar Nerve Entrapment in Cubital Tunnel

Anteromedial transverse sonogram of the cubital tunnel region can show the ulnar nerve between the medial epicondyle of the humerus and the olecranon process of the ulna, and bridged by the cubital tunnel retinaculum (or Osborne fascia). The nerve position can be confirmed on the longitudinal axis. The ulnar nerve enters the hiatus between the ulnar and humeral heads of the flexor carpi ulnaris muscle. The cubital tunnel changes from ovoid to elliptical during elbow flexion and extension. The cubital tunnel changes in shape (from slightly ovoid to elliptical) and volume because of the eccentric origin of the retinaculum.

During normal flexion of the elbow, the ulnar nerve curves over the medial epicondyle, resulting in traction-related flattening and elongation of the nerve. Also there is up to a 55% decrease in cross-sectional area and a sixfold increase in interstitial pressure in the cubital tunnel due to increased tension of the retinaculum and bulging of the medial collateral ligament.[85] These factors may predispose the nerve to extrinsic compression at this level. The cubital tunnel retinaculum consists of thin fascia and is usually not visualized.

The ulnar nerve is an ovoid or bifid structure located close to the hyperechoic osseous cortex of the epicondyle. Owing to its curvilinear course, the nerve tends to appear less echogenic at the elbow, owing to anisotropy. Color Doppler imaging can help differentiate the nerve from the adjacent ulnar recurrent artery and veins. Compression of the ulnar nerve usually occurs proximally at the condylar groove and distally at the edge of the aponeurosis of the flexor carpi ulnaris.

Other conditions that may result in ulnar nerve compression include bone spurs in the condylar groove, heterotopic ossification in the cubital tunnel area, thickening of the medial collateral ligament on the floor of the tunnel, the anomalous anconeus epitrochlearis muscle, intra-articular loose bodies, ganglion cysts, or deformities from previous elbow fractures (cubitus valgus). High-resolution US demonstrates abrupt narrowing and displacement of the nerve within the tunnel. The nerve may appear swollen with loss of the fascicular pattern proximal to this level (Figs. 18 and 19). The cross-sectional area of the nerve at the epicondyle is significantly larger than in healthy subjects and also larger than the cross-sectional area of the normal contralateral nerve.[86] After surgical decompression or translocation, US may detect scarring along the course of the nerve in patients with recurrent symptoms.

Guyon Tunnel

The Guyon tunnel houses the ulnar nerve, the ulnar artery, and the ulnar vein. The ulnar nerve descends the forearm between the flexor

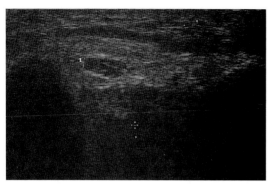

Figure 19. Transverse view of swollen, hypoe-choic ulnar nerve (14 mm²) in cubital tunnel syndrome. (Courtesy of Dr. Wolfgang A. Schmidt.)

digitorum profundus and flexor carpi ulnaris muscles. It then pierces the deep fascia and enters the wrist through the Guyon tunnel. The walls of this canal consist of the pisiform medially and the hook of the hamate laterally; the floor is formed by the flexor retinaculum, and the roof by the palmar carpal ligament and the palmaris brevis muscle. In the distal canal, the ulnar nerve bifurcates into a superficial sensory branch and a deep motor branch, which supplies the hypothenar muscles and then passes across the palm, distributing to other intrinsic hand muscles.

High-frequency (>10 MHz) US can demonstrate the ulnar nerve at the pisiform level as a thin, rounded structure medial to the artery. Its sensory branch continues to run in proximity to the ulnar artery, whereas the motor branch courses more deeply, adjacent to the medial surface of the hamate hook.

Ulnar neuropathies at the Guyon canal are uncommon. Chronic repeated external pressure by tools, handles of canes, or crutches is the usual cause of nerve entrapment.[87] On transverse scans, US enables detection of space-occupying lesions within the Guyon tunnel, such as ganglion cysts related to the pisotriquetral joint space, anomalous muscles (accessory abductor digiti minimi, anomalous hypothenar adductor), pseudoaneurysms of the ulnar artery, and fracture residuals, which can cause compression of the nerve.

Nerve Entrapment at the Fibular Neck[92]

At the apex of the popliteal fossa, the sciatic nerve divides into two branches: the larger tibial nerve and the smaller common peroneal nerve. The tibial nerve continues the line of the sciatic nerve, but the common peroneal nerve descends obliquely through the popliteal fossa and winds around the fibular neck. It then divides into two branches, the superficial and the deep peroneal nerve, which have both sensory and motor fibers. The superficial peroneal nerve supplies the evertor muscles (peroneus longus and brevis) in the lateral compartment of the leg. The deep peroneal nerve supplies the extensors and dorsiflexors of the foot and toes (tibialis anterior, extensor hallucis longus, extensor digitorum longus, and brevis). A complete lesion of the common peroneal nerve leads to a characteristic foot drop and slapping gait, with sensory loss extended over the anterolateral surface of the lower leg and the dorsum of the foot.

The linear array transducers with a 10- to 15-MHz frequency range are able to demonstrate the common peroneal nerve through the lateral portion of the popliteal fossa down to the fibular neck. The posterior margin of the biceps femoris tendon and the echogenic profile of the fibular head can be useful landmarks for identifying the nerve. However, in obese patients, subcutaneous fat can obscure the thin image of the nerve.

Entrapment of the common peroneal nerve typically occurs in the restricted space between the bone and the fascia as the nerve winds around the back of the fibular neck.[88] In many instances, lesions probably result from pressure on the nerve at the fibular neck during sleep or from habitual leg crossing. Nerve compression can also result from space-occupying lesions, such as ganglion cysts, soft tissue tumors, osseous masses, or a large fabella. Other causes include fracture, dislocation, application of skeletal traction, or a tight cast or bandage around the knee. Nerve sheath ganglia typically involve the common peroneal nerve blindfolding in the space between the epineurium and the nerve fascicles. Ultrasonography shows a spindle-shaped cystic structure within the nerve sheath. The hypoechoic cyst causes focal enlargement of the nerve bundle, and the entering and exiting nerve may be thickened with loss of fascicular structure, thus producing a tapering appearance of the cystic mass.[89] Internal septations may be seen as well.

Tarsal Tunnel Syndrome

The tibial nerve is the continuation of the medial trunk of the sciatic nerve. It passes deep to the flexor retinaculum in the space between the medial malleolus and the medial wall of the calcaneus. The retinaculum consists of a thin fascia and forms the roof of the tarsal tunnel, which contains the tibial nerve, three tendons (tibialis posterior, flexor digitorum longus, and flexor hallucis longus), and the posterior tibial artery and veins. Posteroinferior to the medial malleolus, the tibial nerve divides into the medial and lateral plantar nerves and a calcaneal sensory branch. The plantar nerves supply the intrinsic foot muscles, except for the extensor digitorum brevis, which is innervated by the deep peroneal nerve.

Proximal tarsal tunnel syndrome consists of entrapment of the tibial nerve in the retromalleolar region, whereas distal tarsal tunnel syndrome involves the smaller divisions of the tibial nerve. In cases of standard tarsal tunnel syndrome, it should be assumed that the pathologic condition exists in both these zones; however, localized nerve disease involving only one of these nerves may occur.[90] External compression resulting from ill-fitting footwear or tight plaster casts is probably the most common cause. However, space-occupying lesions of the medial ankle, such as flexor tenosynovitis, ganglia related to the talocalcaneal joint, fascial septa, an anomalous tendon or muscle (flexor digitorum accessorius longus), or fracture residuals may also constrict the nerve.[91] Although typical symptoms include numbness or pain in the foot and ankle and paresthesia

in the sole of the foot, the clinical and electromyographic diagnosis of tarsal tunnel syndrome is often not straightforward, especially when there is no soft tissue swelling on the medial ankle. The tibial nerve lies posterior to the flexor digitorum longus tendon and superficial to the flexor hallucis longus tendon, close to the posterior tibial vessels. Identification of these vessels with color Doppler imaging may provide a useful landmark for visualizing the nerve. In cases of space-occupying lesions within the tunnel, US can provide exact information on the nature and extent of the constriction. Local fusiform thickening of the nerve, possibly associated with disappearance of the fascicular pattern, or a size discrepancy between the medial and lateral branches may also be demonstrated.

The neurovascular bundles of the tarsal tunnel contents are fixed by fibrous septae. Traction disorders or compression from mass lesions results in sensory symptoms. Ultrasonography may show a ganglion as an echo-free, focal, well-circumscribed cystic region, whereas free fluid will conform to the anatomy of the adjacent tarsal tunnel. Peripheral nerve sheath tumors and neurilemmomas are usually hypoechoic and lie in the plane of the nerve structure. Hemangiomas have various echo patterns and are thus not easily diagnosed. Doppler flows may be high or low in these masses. Dilated or varicose veins have a wormlike appearance. Doppler flow shows a blue color (i.e., flow away from the transducer) and compression results in venous reflux. Fibrous scars are typically echo-poor. Hypertrophy of the abductor hallucis muscle or accessory abductor hallucis muscle appears as typical echogenic linear muscle striations and will pose no diagnostic difficulty. Tenosynovitis with effusion or synovial hypertrophy may also be detected. Various posttraumatic causes may be noted depending on the type of pathology involved. Although most disorders of the tarsal tunnel are identifiable by US, pathologies of the sinus tarsi, especially of the bifurcated ligament, can only be studied by MRI.

Intermetatarsal Nerve Entrapments[92]

The medial and lateral plantar nerves divide into interdigital nerves near the bases of the metatarsals. These nerves supply motor branches to the muscles of the sole and cutaneous branches to the toes. The interdigital nerves pass deep to the transverse intermetatarsal ligament, which connects the metatarsal heads and maintains the transverse arch of the foot. Recurrent local impingement of the nerve underneath this ligament, with subsequent nerve structure degeneration and perineural fibrosis, is the most commonly accepted cause of Morton's neuroma (interdigital neuritis).[92] Other possible causes include ischemia and compression of the interdigital nerve by an inflamed and enlarged intermetatarsal bursa.[93] The main symptoms of Morton's neuroma are pain in the forefoot with numbness and paresthesia in the adjacent toes. The symptoms are typically exacerbated by stressing of the metatarsophalangeal joints, with dorsiflexion of the toes or with walking in narrow shoes.

Ultrasonography evaluation can be performed by placing the probe on the dorsal or plantar aspect of the foot. For the dorsal approach, the toes are plantar flexed and manual pressure in the affected web space is applied on the plantar side. For the plantar approach, the toes are dorsiflexed and finger pressure is exerted in the web spaces on the dorsal side. The quality of sonograms obtained by placing the probe on the dorsal surface is somewhat higher, probably owing to the thinner skin and the absence of keratosis.

Owing to the relatively small size of normal interdigital nerves (approximately 2 mm in diameter), US examination of these nerves is difficult. Doppler imaging can aid in localization of the nerve by demonstrating the adjacent intermetatarsal artery and vein. Morton's neuromas most frequently occur within the second or third interspace and are located at the level of or slightly proximal to the metatarsal heads. They appear as fusiform or ovoid hypoechoic masses elongated along the major axis of the metatarsals. Beyond the tumor, the entering and exiting nerve may be slightly thickened and is therefore more easily identified on longitudinal US scans than is the case with normal subjects. Power Doppler US may be helpful in identifying these lesions on the basis of their increased vascularity.[94] Intense tenderness elicited by pressure with the transducer over the suspected neuroma supports the diagnosis.

In the appropriate clinical setting, US has a reported sensitivity of 95–100%[95] for detection of Morton's neuromas, with a specificity of 83% and accuracy of 95%.[96] Similar results have been reported for MRI, which has demonstrated a sensitivity of 87%, specificity of 100%, and accuracy of 89%.[97] Small lesions (<5 mm in diameter) can be difficult to identify with US, which may explain the higher sensitivity of MRI in some series.

Nerve Dislocation

The ulnar nerve normally lies in the cubital tunnel as it courses behind the posterior aspect of the elbow. During elbow flexion, sonography can be used to scan dynamically, showing ulnar nerve dislocation as the nerve becomes displaced around and anterior to the tip of the medial epicondyle. Sonography can also differentiate ulnar nerve dislocation from other causes of medial elbow pain and ulnar nerve neuropathy, such as cubital tunnel syndrome and snapping triceps syndrome.[98]

Ultrasonography in Diagnosis of Noninflammatory Muscle Conditions

Evaluation of Muscle Injury

Muscle fibers are arranged in parallel hypoechoic bundles surrounded by echogenic fibroadipose septa in a pennate configuration. Ultrasound can be used in several capacities: (i) to determine the extent of injury; (ii) to determine the stage of healing (limited athletic activity being safe when the lesion has filled with hyperechoic tissue and near normal muscle architecture with peripheral organization is seen); and (iii) assessment of the magnitude of scar formation. (Fibrotic scars are seen as hyperechoic zones within the muscle and often occur when the lesion was large or when sporting activities were resumed too early.)[99] The best time for ultrasonographic evaluation of muscle injuries is between 2 and 48 h after the traumatic event, which is when the hematoma best outlines a potential tear.[100]

Sonography is capable of detecting a wide spectrum of muscle damage caused by excessive fiber elongation. Minimal elongation injuries (grade 1) have no demonstrable fiber discontinuity with or without diffuse hyperechoic echo texture and swelling of the muscle. Partial (grade 2) and complete (grade 3) tears are noted as hypoechoic or anechoic fluid-filled gaps. Differentiation between elongation with and without tears is critical because the fiber tear requires at least 4 weeks of inactivity, whereas the nondisrupted lesions recover within a period of 1–2 weeks.

Sonography is a reliable method to diagnose and stage tears involving the myotendinous junction of the medial gastrocnemius and plantaris muscles ("tennis leg"). This type of injury occurs most frequently during amateur sports practice, owing to powerful contraction of the gastrocnemius muscle with concomitant extension of the knee. This leads to excessive tensile force and disruption of the myotendinous junction, characterized by detachment of the medial gastrocnemius muscle fibers from the distal aponeurosis. Rarely, the plantaris muscle may be involved. Clinical symptoms may overlap with those caused by ruptured Baker's cyst and deep venous thrombosis, which can be promptly differentiated with sonographic examination.[101]

Muscle Changes Resulting from Nerve Pathology

Denervating neuromuscular disorders typically result in soft tissue and muscle atro-phy, which is associated with loss of muscle bulk and fatty infiltration. Causes include acute brachial neuritis and quadrilateral space syndrome. Pseudohypertrophy represents a combination of true muscle hypertrophy and an increase in intramuscular connective tissue and fat. Pseudohypertrophy frequently occurs in the calf muscles, and this phenomenon is seen in some dystrophic muscle conditions, hemihypertrophy syndromes, and chronic neuropathies. True muscle hypertrophy results from a pure increase in muscle bulk, without fatty infiltration. This is a paradoxical response to nerve injury and, although rare, is associated with chronic nerve irritation.[102]

Muscular Dystrophies

Ultrasound imaging has proved to be a useful, noninvasive screening tool for examining children with neuromuscular disease. Ultrasound can show striking changes in children with muscular dystrophies, including an increase in the intensity of echo reflected from the muscle substance, with corresponding loss of bone echo. Spinal muscular atrophies and neuropathies have also shown an increase in muscle echo along with atrophy of the muscle and increase in depth of subcutaneous tissue. Various congenital myopathies have demonstrated US changes as well. However, infants with hypotonia from nonneuromuscular causes have had normal scans. The severity of change on the scan did not correlate to functional disability as some children had good function yet strikingly abnormal scans. However, the degree of change on the scan did correlate with the degree of disruption of muscle architecture on biopsy.[103]

Pseudohypertrophy of calf muscles can be detected with a longitudinal 5- to 12-MHz sonogram showing increased echogenicity within gastrocnemius and soleus muscles of the calf. Increased muscular echogenicity and bulk, caused by fatty infiltration, confirms pseudohypertrophy on sonography.

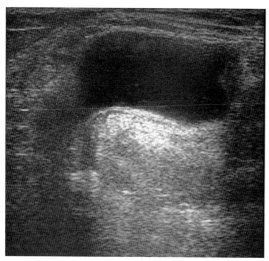

Figure 20. Knee posterior transverse view demonstrating a popliteal cyst.

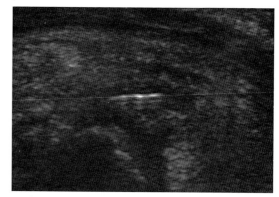

Figure 21. Foreign body in foot—needle with reverberation artifact. (Courtesy of Dr. Keith Boniface.)

Fluid Collections

Ultrasound can detect periarticular cystic structures as well-defined anechoic structures with posterior acoustic enhancement. Successful diagnosis and aspiration of glenoid paralabral cysts have been described.[104]

Ganglion cysts of the wrist can be differentiated from a fluid-filled dorsal radiocarpal recess using dynamic imaging. A joint recess typically collapses to some degree upon wrist motion and with transducer pressure, whereas a ganglion cyst tends to remain distended.[105] In the knee, meniscal and popliteal cysts can be promptly diagnosed as well (Fig. 20).

Subcutaneous fluid collections have internal mobile septations and are usually anechoic and compressible. Intra- and intermuscular hematomas exhibit variable sonographic characteristics related to the time elapsed since the traumatic event. In the first hours after trauma, the hematoma can still be diffuse, not collected, and appear as either hyperechogenicity of the muscle or as abnormal distance between the muscle bundles with poor definition of the fibroadipose septa. After 2 h, hematomas are usually hypoechoic or anechoic and may outline the torn margins of the affected muscle. If the aponeurosis is torn, the hematoma can

spread outside of the muscle boundaries and not be seen. Organization occurs in the ensuing 3–4 weeks, and progressive filling with fibrinous septations may occur.

Ultrasound for Evaluation of Soft Tissue Foreign Bodies

Ultrasound imaging can diagnose inflammation and infection due to foreign bodies and may identify fistulous tracts. It may also be used to guide the removal of non- radio-opaque objects such as wooden splinters, toothpicks, pieces of plastic, fishbones, glass fragments, and cactus spines.

Only 15% of wooden fragments are seen on plain film X-rays, whereas US can demonstrate wooden fragments as small as 2.5 mm with 87% sensitivity and 90% specificity.[106] Sutures, plastic, and small glass pieces are not well visualized radiographically. These materials can be identified either by their bright reflections or by the associated acoustic shadowing that occurs when sound transmission is blocked. Metal objects have a specific comet tail artifact that is recognizable as a series of bright echoes trailing the initial bright echo (Fig. 21). Ultrasound can also be used to assist percutaneous removal of foreign bodies.

The associated inflammatory response may be seen as an anechoic fluid collection or hypoechoic area that typically forms a halo around the foreign body. Foreign bodies may become more apparent later in the course if surrounded by hypoechoic reparative granulation tissue. Postinflammatory, post traumatic, and bursal calcifications cast acoustic shadows.

Other Diagnostic Applications of Musculoskeletal Ultrasonography

Osteogenesis imperfecta (OI) type II was diagnosed accurately in an at-risk fetus at 16 weeks gestation by real-time sonography. The most important findings were shortening, deformity, and possibly fracture in the long bones, particularly the femurs.[107] Others have reported successful ultrasonographic diagnosis of fracture-separation of the distal humeral epiphysis in a neonate. The distal humeral epiphysis in neonates is cartilaginous and radiolucent. Ultrasound was noted to provide a clear delineation of the injury in otherwise difficult to diagnose radiographic cases.[108]

Ultrasonography can effectively assess the extraosseous component of malignant and aggressive benign lesions and those tumors arising from the surface of the bone. Periosteal reaction, cortical destruction, pathological fracture, matrix mineralization, fluid–fluid levels and involvement of the neurovascular bundle are all identified. Although ultrasonography does not offer any superiority over plain radiography or MRI in diagnosis and local staging, it is very useful in guiding percutaneous needle biopsy.[109]

Doppler sonography has not been helpful for diagnosis of complex regional pain syndrome (RSDS) and can only assess the hemodynamic stage of the disease. One study revealed loss of normal triphasic arterial waveforms in some of the cases of stage I disease, but many cases of stage I disease and all cases of stage II disease had normal findings.[110]

Acknowledgments

I hereby acknowledge Dr. Keith Boniface, Department of Emergency Medicine, George Washington University, Washington, DC, and Dr. Wolfgang A. Schmidt, Medical Center for Rheumatology, Berlin-Buch, for their contributions to the images in this chapter. Their generosity is greatly appreciated.

References

1. Cooperberg, P.L., I. Tsang, L. Truelove, *et al*. 1978. Gray scale ultrasound in the evaluation of rheumatoid arthritis of the knee. *Radiology* **126:** 759.

2. De Flaviis, L., P. Scaglione, R. Nessi, *et al*. 1988. Ultrasonography of the hand in rheumatoid arthritis. *Acta Radiol.* **29:** 457.

3. Alasaarela, E.M., E.L. Alasaarela & O. Rasanen. 1994. Ultrasound propagation speed in arthritic synovial tissue. *Ultrasound Med. Biol.* **20:** 975–979.

4. Kremkau, F.W. 1998. *Diagnostic Ultrasound: Principles and Instruments*. W.B. Saunders. Philadelphia.

5. Fornage, B.D. 1988. Ultrasonography of muscles and tendons. In *Examination Technique and Atlas of Normal Anatomy of the Extremities*. Springer-Verlag. New York.

6. Jacobson, J.A. & M.T. van Holsbeeck. 1998. Musculoskeletal ultrasonography. *Orthop. Clin. North Am.* **29:** 135–167.

7. Martinoli, C., L.E. Derchi, C. Pastorino, *et al*. 1993. Analysis of echotexture of tendons with US. *Radiology* **186:** 839–843.

8. Crass, J.R., G.L. de Vegte & L.A. Harkavy. 1988. Tendon echogenicity: ex vivo study. *Radiology* **167:** 499–501.

9. Grassi, F., E. Filippucci, A. Farina, *et al*. 2000. Sonographic imaging of tendons. *Arthritis Rheum.* **43:** 969–976.

10. Lew, H.L., C.P. Chen, T.G. Wang, *et al*. 2007. Introduction to musculoskeletal diagnostic ultrasound: Examination of the upper limb. *Am. J. Phys. Med. Rehab.* **86:** 310–321.

11. Silvestri, E., C. Martinoli, L.E. Derchi, *et al*. 1995. Echotexture of peripheral nerves: Correlation between US and histologic findings and criteria to differentiate tendons. *Radiology* **197:** 291–296.

12. Backhaus, M., G.-R. Burmester, T. Gerber, *et al*. 2001. Guidelines for musculoskeletal ultrasound in rheumatology. *Ann. Rheum. Dis.* **60:** 641–649.

13. EULAR Working Group for Musculoskeletal Ultrasound: M. Backhaus, P. Balint, G. Bruyn, A. Farina, E. Filippucci, T. Gerber, W. Grassi, J. Koski, K. Machold, B. Manger, S. Mariacher-Gehler, E.N. Sánchez, W. Schmidt, W.A. Swen & R. Wakefield. Guidelines for Musculoskeletal Ultrasound in Rheumatology. www.doctor33.it/eular/ultrasound/Guidelines.htm

14. Brenneke, S.L. & C.J. Morgan. 1992. Evaluation of ultrasonography as a diagnostic technique in the assessment of rotator cuff tendon tears. *Am. J. Sports Med.* **20:** 287–289.

15. Teefey, S.A., S.A. Hasan, W.D. Middleton, *et al.* 2000. Ultrasonography of the rotator cuff: A comparison of ultrasonographic and arthroscopic findings in one hundred consecutive cases. *J. Bone Joint Surg.* **82A:** 498–504.

16. Middleton, W.D., W.R. Reinus, G.L. Melson, *et al.* 1986. Pitfalls of rotator cuff sonography. *Am. J. Radiol.* **146:** 555–560.

17. Mack, L.A., D.A. Nyberg, F.R. Matsen, *et al.* 1988. Sonographic evaluation of the postoperative shoulder. *AJR Am. J. Roentgenol.* **150:** 1089–1093.

18. van Holsbeeck, M.T. & J.H. Introcaso. 2001. Sonography of the shoulder. In *Musculoskeletal Ultrasound*, 2nd ed. L. Bralow, Ed.: 463–516. Mosby, Inc. St Louis.

19. Harryman, D.T., L.A. Mack, K.Y. Wang, *et al.* 1991. Repairs of the rotator cuff. Correlation of functional results with integrity of the rotator cuff. *J. Bone Joint Surg.* **73A:** 982–989.

20. Crass, J.R., E.V. Craig & S.B. Feinberg. 1986. Sonography of the postoperative rotator cuff. *Am. J. Radiol.* **146:** 561–564.

21. Gaenslen, E.S., C.C. Satterlee & G.W. Hinson. 1996. Magnetic resonance imaging for evaluation of failed repairs of the rotator cuff. *J. Bone Joint Surg.* **78A:** 1391–1396.

22. Bureau, N. & G. Roederer. 1996. *Achilles tendon xanthoma: Ultrasound vs. MRI*. Presented at Sixth Annual Conference on Musculoskeletal Ultrasound, Montreal.

23. Hsu, T., C. Wang, T. Wang, *et al.* 1997. Ultrasonographic examination of the posterior tibial tendon. *Foot Ankle Int.* **18:** 34.

24. Creamer, P., M. Hunt & P. Dieppe. 1996. Pain mechanisms in osteoarthritis of the knee: Effect of intra-articular anaesthetic. *J. Rheumatol.* **23:** 1031–1036.

25. D'Agostino, M.A., P. Conaghan, M. Le Bars, *et al.* 2005. EULAR report on the use of ultrasonography in painful knee osteoarthritis: Pt. 1. Prevalence of inflammation in osteoarthritis. *Ann. Rheum. Dis.* **64:** 1703–1709.

26. Song, I.H., G.R. Burmester, M. Backhaus, *et al.* 2008. Knee osteoarthritis. Efficacy of a new method of contrast-enhanced musculoskeletal ultrasonography in detection of synovitis in patients with knee osteoarthritis in comparison with magnetic resonance imaging. *Ann. Rheum. Dis.* **67:** 19–25.

27. Frediani, B., G. Filippou, P. Falsetti, *et al.* 2005. Diagnosis of calcium pyrophosphate dihydrate crystal deposition disease: Ultrasonographic criteria proposed. *Ann. Rheum. Dis.* **64:** 638–640.

28. Coari, G., A. Iagnocco & A. Zoppini. 1995. Chondrocalcinosis: Sonographic study of the knee. *Clin. Rheumatol.*. **14:** 511–514.

29. Foldes, K. 2002. Knee chondrocalcinosis. An ultrasonographic study of the hyaline cartilage. *J. Clin. Imag.* **26:** 194–196.

30. Garcia, G.M., G. McCord & R. Kumar. 2003. Hydroxyapatite crystal deposition disease. *Sem. Musculoskeletal Radiol.* **7:** 187–193.

31. Chau, C.L.F. & J.F. Griffith. 2005. Musculoskeletal infections: Ultrasound appearances. *Clin. Rad.* **60:** 149–159.

32. Cardinal, N.J., B. Bureau & R.K. Chhem. 2001. Role of ultrasound in musculoskeletal infections. *Radiol. Clin. North Am.* **39:** 191–201.

33. García-De La Torre, I. 2003. Advances in the management of septic arthritis. *Rheum. Dis. Clin. North Am.* **29:** 61–75.

34. Ho, G., Jr, 2002. Septic arthritis update. *Bull. Rheum. Dis.* **51:** 1–10.

35. Epstein, J.H., B. Zimmermann and G. Ho Jr. 1986. Polyarticular septic arthritis. *J. Rheumatol.* **13:** 1105–1107.

36. Lossos, I.S., O. Yossepowitch, L. Kandel, *et al.* 1998. Septic arthritis of the glenohumeral joint: A report of 11 cases and review of the literature. *Medicine (Baltimore)* **77:** 177–187.

37. Sethi, P.M., S. Kingston & N. Elattrache. 2005. Accuracy of anterior intra-articular injection of the glenohumeral joint. *Arthroscopy* **21:** 77–80.

38. Costantino, T.G., B. Roemer & E.H. Leber. 2007. Ultrasound in emergency medicine. Septic arthritis and bursitis: Emergency ultrasound can facilitate diagnosis. *J. Emerg. Med.* **32:** 295–297.

39. Robben, S.G., M.H. Lequin & A.F. Diepstraten. 1999. Anterior joint capsule of the normal hip and in children with transient synovitis: US study with anatomic and histologic correlation. *Radiology* **210:** 499–507.

40. Cardinal, E., R.K. Chhem & B. Aubin. 1999. Adult hip. In *Guidelines and Gamuts in Musculoskeletal Ultrasound*, 1st ed. R.K. Chhem & E. Cardinal, Eds.: 125–160. Wiley-Liss. New York.

41. Zawin, J.K., F.A. Hoffer, F.F. Rand, *et al.* 1993. Joint effusion in children with an irritable hip: US diagnosis and aspiration. *Radiology* **187:** 459–463.

42. Strouse, P.J., M.A. DiPietro & R.S. Adler. 1998. Pediatric hip effusions: Evaluation with power Doppler sonography. *Radiology* **206:** 731–735.

43. Chau, C.L., J.F. Griffith, P.T. Chan, *et al.* 2003. Rice-body formation in atypical mycobacterial tenosynovitis and bursitis: Findings on sonography and MR imaging. *AJR Am. J. Roentgenol.* **180:** 1455–1459.

44. Canoso, J.J. & M. Barza. 1993. Soft tissue infections. *Rheum. Dis. Clin. North Am.* **19:** 293–309.

45. Umbert, I.J., R.K. Winkelmann, G.F. Oliver, & M.S. Peters. 1989. Necrotizing fasciitis: A clinical, microbiologic, and histopathologic study of 14 patients. *J. Am. Acad. Dermatol.* **20:** 774.

46. Chao, H.C., M.S. Kong & T.Y. Lin. 1999. Diagnosis of necrotizing fasciitis in children. *J. Ultrasound Med.* **18:** 277–281.

47. Riebel, T.W., R. Nasir & O. Nazarenko. 1996. The value of sonography in the detection of osteomyelitis. *Pediatr. Radiol.* **26:** 291–297.

48. Larcos, G., V.F. Antico, W. Cormick, *et al.* 1994. How useful is ultrasonography in suspected acute osteomyelitis? *J. Ultrasound Med.* **13:** 707–709.

49. Bedford, A.F. *et al.* 1982. Ultrasonic assessment of fractures and its use in the diagnosis of the suspected scaphoid fracture. *Injury* **14:** 180–182.

50. DaCruz, D.J., R.H. Taylor, B. Savage, *et al.* 1988. Ultrasound assessment of the suspected scaphoid fracture. *Arch. Emerg. Med.* **5:** 97–100.

51. Herneth, A.M., A. Siegmeth, T.R. Bader, *et al.* 2001. Scaphoid fractures: Evaluation with high-spatial-resolution US initial results. *Radiology* **220:** 231–235.

52. Lazovic, D., D. Wegner, U. Peters, *et al.* 1996. Ultrasound for diagnosis of apophyseal injuries. *Knee Surg. Sport Tr. A.* **3:** 234–237.

53. Pancione, L., G. Gatti & B. Mecozzi. 1997. Diagnosis of Hill-Sachs lesion of the shoulder. Comparison between ultrasonography and arthro-CT. *Acta Radiologica* **38**(4, Pt. 1): 523–526.

54. Engin, G., E. Yekeler, R. Guloglu, *et al.* 2000. US versus conventional radiography in the diagnosis of sternal fractures. *Acta Radiol.* **41:** 296–299.

55. Hubner, U., W. Schlicht, S. Outzen, *et al.* 2000. Ultrasound in the diagnosis of fractures in children. *J. Bone Joint Surg. [Br.]* **82:** 1170–1173.

56. Westerheide, E., J.M. Failla, M. van Holsbeeck, *et al.* 2004. Ultrasound visualization of central slip injuries of the finger extensor mechanism. *J. Hand Surg.* **29:** 400–405.

57. Faulkner, K.G. 2001. Update on bone density measurement. *Rheum. Dis. Clin. North Am.* **27:** 81–99.

58. World Health Organization. 1994. Assessment of fracture risk and its application to screening for post-menopausal osteoporosis. Report of a WHO study group. *W H O Tech. Rep. Ser.* **843:** 1–129.

59. Prins, S.H., H.L. Jørgensen, L.V. Jørgensen, *et al.* 1998. The role of quantitative ultrasound in the assessment of bone: A review. *Clin. Physiol.* **18:** 3–17.

60. Hans, D., T. Fuerst & F. Duboeuf. 1997. Quantitative ultrasound bone measurement. *Eur. Radiol.* **7**(Suppl. 2): S43–S50.

61. Danese, R.D. & A.A. Licata. 2001. Ultrasound of the skeleton: Review of its clinical applications and pitfalls. *Curr. Rheumatol. Rep.* **3:** 245–248.

62. Njeh, C.F., D. Hans, J. Li, *et al.* 2000. Comparison of six calcaneal quantitative ultrasound devices: Precision and hip fracture discrimination. *Osteoporos. Int.* **11:** 1051–1062.

63. Bauer, D.C., C.C. Glüer, J.A. Cauley, *et al.* 1997. Broadband ultrasound attenuation predicts fractures strongly and independently of densitometry in older women. A prospective study. Study of Osteoporotic Fractures Research Group. *Arch. Intern. Med.* **157:** 629–634.

64. Hans, D., P. Dargent-Molina, A.M. Schott, *et al.* 1996. Ultrasonographic heel measurements to predict hip fracture in elderly women: The EPIDOS prospective study. *Lancet* **348:** 511–514.

65. Khaw, K.T., J. Reeve, R. Luben, *et al.* 2004. Prediction of total and hip fracture risk in men and women by quantitative ultrasound of the calcaneus: EPIC-Norfolk prospective population study. *Lancet* **363:** 197–202.

66. Ultrasonography of peripheral sites for selecting patients for pharmacologic treatment for osteoporosis. 2000. *TEC Bull. (Online)* **19:** 25–28.

67. Sim, M.F., *et al.* 2005. Cost effectiveness analysis of using quantitative ultrasound as a selective prescreen for bone densitometry. *Technol. Health Care* **13:** 75–85.

68. Hans, D., F. Hartl & M.A. Krieg. 2003. Device-specific weighted T-score for two quantitative ultrasounds: Operational propositions for the management of osteoporosis for 65 years and older women in Switzerland. *Osteoporos. Int.* **14:** 251–258.

69. Njeh, C.F., C.M. Boivin & C.M. Langton. 1997. The role of ultrasound in the assessment of osteoporosis: A review. *Osteoporos. Int.* **7:** 7–22.

70. Nayak, S., M.D. Stone, C.J. Phillips, *et al.* 2006. Meta-analysis: Accuracy of quantitative ultrasound for identifying patients with osteoporosis. *Ann. Intern. Med.* **144:** 832–841.

71. Fornage, B.D. 1988. Peripheral nerves of the extremities: Imaging with ultrasound. *Radiology* **167:** 179–182.

72. Murphey, M.D., W.S. Smith, S.E. Smith, *et al.* 1999. Imaging of musculoskeletal neurogenic tumors: Radiologic–pathologic correlation. *Radiographics* **19:** 1253–1280.

73. Stuart, R.M., E.S.C. Koh & W.H. Breidah. 2004. Sonography of peripheral nerve pathology. *AJR Am. J. Roentgenol.* **182:** 123–129.

74. Martinoli, C., S. Bianchi & L.E. Derchi. 1999. Tendon and nerve sonography. *Radiol. Clin. North Am.* **37:** 691–711.

75. Zanetti, M., J.K. Strehle, H. Zollinger, *et al.* 1997. Morton neuroma and fluid in the intermetatarsal bursae on MR images of 70 asymptomatic volunteers. *Radiology* **203:** 516–520.

76. Goldman, A.B. & J.J. Kaye. 1977. Macrodystrophia lipomatosa: Radiographic diagnosis. *AJR Am. J. Roentgenol.* **128:** 101–105.

77. Duncan, I., P. Sullivan & F. Lomas. 1999. Sonography in the diagnosis of carpal tunnel syndrome. *AJR Am. J. Roentgenol.* **173:** 681–684.

78. Rempel, D., L. Dahlin & G. Lundborg. 1999. Pathophysiology of nerve compression syndromes response of peripheral nerves to loading. *J. Bone Joint Surg.* **81A:** 1600–1610.

79. Martinoli, C., S. Bianchi & N. Gandolfo. 2000. US of nerve entrapments in osteofibrous tunnels of the upper and lower limbs. *Radiographics* **20:** S199 – S217.

80. Buchberger, W., W. Judmaier, G. Birbamer, *et al.* 1992. Carpal tunnel syndrome: Diagnosis with high-resolution sonography. *AJR Am. J. Roentgenol.* **159:** 793–798.

81. Lee, D., M.T. van Holsbeeck, P.K. Janevski, *et al.* 1999. Diagnosis of carpal tunnel syndrome: Ultrasound versus electromyography. *Radiol. Clin. North Am.* **37:** 859–872.

82. Buchberger, W., G. Schon, K. Strasser, *et al.* 1991. High-resolution ultrasonography of the carpal tunnel. *J. Ultrasound Med.* **10:** 531–537.

83. Sugimoto, H., N. Miyaji & T. Ohsawa. 1994. Carpal tunnel syndrome: Evaluation of median nerve circulation with dynamic contrast-enhanced MR imaging. *Radiology* **190:** 459–466.

84. Martinoli, C., L.E. Derchi, M. Bertolotto, *et al.* 2000. US and MR imaging of peripheral nerves in leprosy. *Skeletal Radiol.* **29:** 142–150.

85. Gelberman, R.H., K. Yamaguchi, S.B. Hollstien, *et al.* 1998. Changes in interstitial pressure and cross-sectional area of the cubital tunnel and of the ulnar nerve with flexion of the elbow. *J. Bone Joint Surg. [Am.]* **80:** 492–501.

86. Chiou, H.J., Y.H. Chou, S.P. Cheng, *et al.* 1998. Cubital tunnel syndrome: Diagnosis by high-resolution ultrasonography. *J. Ultrasound Med.* **17:** 643–648.

87. Stewart, J.D. 1993. Compression and entrapment neuropathies. In *Peripheral Neuropathy,* 3rd ed. P.J. Dyck, P.K. Thomas, ed.: 1354–1379. W. B. Saunders. Philadelphia.

88. Loredo, R., J. Hodler & R. Pedowitz, *et al.* 1998. MRI of the common peroneal nerve: Normal anatomy and evaluation of masses associated with nerve entrapment. *J. Comput. Assist. Tomogr.* **22:** 925–931.

89. Martinoli, C., S. Bianchi & L.E. Derchi. 1999. Tendon and nerve sonography. *Radiol. Clin. North Am.* **37:** 691–711.

90. Shon, L.C. 1994. Nerve entrapment, neuropathy, and nerve dysfunction in athletes. *Orthop. Clin. North Am.* **25:** 47–59.

91. Nagaoka, M. & K. Satou. 1999. Tarsal tunnel syndrome caused by ganglia. *J. Bone Joint Surg. [Br.]* **81:** 607–610.

92. Alexander, I.J., K.A. Johnson & J.W. Parr. 1987. Morton's neuroma: A review of recent concepts. *Orthopedics* **10:** 103–106.

93. Awerbuch, M.S., E. Shepard & B. Vernon-Roberts. 1982. Morton's metatarsalgia due to intermetatarsophalangeal bursitis as an early manifestation of rheumatoid arthritis. *Clin. Orthop.* **167:** 214–221.

94. Murphey, M.D., W.S. Smith, S.E. Smith, *et al.* 1999. Imaging of musculoskeletal neurogenic tumors: Radiologic-pathologic correlation. *Radiographics* **19:** 1253–1280

95. Redd, R.A., V.J. Peters, S.F. Emery, *et al.* 1989. Morton neuroma: Sonographic evaluation. *Radiology* **171:** 415–417.

96. Sobiesk, G.A., S.J. Wertheime, R. Schulz, *et al.* 1997. Sonographic evaluation of interdigital neuromas. *J. Foot Ankle Surg.* **36:** 364–366.

97. Zanetti, M., T. Ledermann, H. Zollinger, *et al.* 1997. Efficacy of MR imaging in patients suspected of having Morton's neuroma. *AJR Am. J. Roentgenol.* **168:** 529–532.

98. Jacobson, J.A., P.J.L. Jebson & A.W. Jeffers. 2001. Ulnar nerve dislocation and snapping triceps syndrome: Diagnosis with dynamic sonography—report of three cases. *Radiology* **220:** 601–605.

99. van Holsbeeck, M.T. & J.H. Introcaso. 2001. Sonography of muscle. In *Musculoskeletal Ultrasound,* 2nd ed. M.T. van Holsbeeck & J.H. Introcaso, Eds.: 23–75. Mosby. St. Louis.

100. Peetrons, P. 2002. Ultrasound of muscles. *Eur. Radiol.* **12:** 35–43.

101. Bianchi, S., C. Martinoli, I.F. Abdelwahab, *et al.* 1998. Sonographic evaluation of tears of the gastrocnemius medial head ("tennis leg"). *J. Ultrasound Med.* **17:** 157–162.

102. Reimers, C.D., B. Schlotter, B.M. Eicke, *et al.* 1996. Calf enlargement in neuromuscular diseases: A quantitative ultrasound study in 350 patients and review of the literature. *J. Neurol. Sci.* **143:** 46–56.

103. Heckmatt, J.Z., S. Leeman & V. Dubowitz. 1982. Ultrasound imaging in the diagnosis of muscle disease. *J. Pediatr.* **101:** 656–660.

104. Hashimoto, B.E., A.S. Hayes & J.D. Ager. 1994. Sonographic diagnosis and treatment of ganglion cysts causing suprascapular nerve entrapment. *J. Ultrasound Med.* **13:** 671–674.

105. Jacobson, J.A. 2002. Ultrasound in sports medicine. *Radiol. Clin. North Am.* **40:** 363–386.

106. Jacobson, J.A., A. Powell, J.G. Craig, *et al.* 1998. Wooden foreign bodies in soft tissue: Detection at US. *Radiology* **206:** 45–48.

107. Ghosh, A., J.S. Woo, C.W. Wan, *et al.* 1984. Simple ultrasonic diagnosis of osteogenesis imperfecta type II in early second trimester. *Prenat. Diagn.* **4:** 235–240.

108. Ziv, N., A. Litwin, K. Katz, *et al.* 1996. Definitive diagnosis of fracture-separation of the distal humeral epiphysis in neonates by ultrasonography. *Pediatr. Radiol.* **26:** 493–496.

109. Saifuddin, A., S.J. Burnett & R. Mitchell. 1998. Pictorial review: Ultrasonography of primary bone tumors. *Clin. Radiol.* **53:** 239–246.

110. Pekindil, G., Y. Pekindil & A. Sarikaya. 2003. Doppler sonographic assessment of posttraumatic reflex sympathetic dystrophy. *J. Ultrasound Med.* **22:** 395–402.

Section IV. Research Aspects

Quantifying Disease Activity and Damage by Imaging in Rheumatoid Arthritis and Osteoarthritis

Olga Kubassova,[a] Mikael Boesen,[b] Philipp Peloschek,[d] Georg Langs,[d,e] Marco A. Cimmino,[c] Henning Bliddal,[b] and Søren Torp-Pedersen[b]

[a] Image Analysis Ltd., University of Leeds, Leeds, West Yorkshire, United Kingdom

[b] The Parker Institute, Frederiksberg Hospital, Frederiksberg, Copenhagen, Denmark

[c] Clinica Reumatologica, DI.M.I., Universita di Genova, Genoa, Italy

[d] CIR Lab, Medical University of Vienna, Department of Radiology, Vienna, Austria

[e] INRIA–Saclay, Ecole Centrale de Paris, MAS Laboratory, GALEN Group, Châtenay-Malabry, France

Traditional imaging, represented by radiographs, provides a very concise description of anatomical pathology of bony structures. Both degenerative and inflammatory joint diseases are characterized by progressive joint destruction, and valid, reproducible measures of disease impact are available. Much effort has been expended to develop scoring systems for joint destruction in both osteoarthritis and rheumatoid arthritis, and the most common internationally accepted semiobjective scores are presented. The anatomical pathology mirrors the past activity of the disease, and advanced imaging gives an impression of the actual disease processes, which subsequently lead to the damage. Such information is required to facilitate the development of efficient therapy against arthritis. Newer technology, exemplified by MRI and ultrasound Doppler, supplements images of structural change with functional data of ongoing disease activity. This chapter focuses on the possibilities for quantification of images in MRI and ultrasound, in which postcontrast enhancement and Doppler information, respectively, are of special interest for the evaluation of the inflammatory changes of arthritis. To save time and eliminate human bias, automation is mandatory. In ultrasound, semiautomatic evaluations are coming that allow for a real-time, reproducible estimate of disease activity. With MRI fully automated algorithms have been developed for processing of data of bony structures, cartilage, and soft tissue, and are currently being implemented into everyday clinical practice.

Key words: quantifying damage; quantifying disease activity; rheumatoid arthritis; osteoarthritis; scoring systems; automatic scoring; computer-aided scoring

Introduction

Chronic joint diseases such as rheumatoid arthritis (RA) and osteoarthritis (OA) affect millions of people around the world and can lead to severe disability with major socioeconomic impact. Despite extensive research into both disease etiology and intervention strategies, there are no effective medical treatments for OA, and even with recent advances in RA research, only a minority of patients fully benefit from therapy.

Development of new, more effective treatments is hampered by the lack of valid scoring and grading methods, which would permit evaluation of disease activity and the effect of

Address for correspondence: Olga Kubassova, Image Analysis Ltd, 5–7 Cromer Terrace, University of Leeds, Leeds, LS2 9JT, West Yorkshire, UK. olga@imageanalysis.org.uk

MRI and Ultrasound in Diagnosis and Management: Ann. N.Y. Acad. Sci. 1154: 207–238 (2009).
doi: 10.1111/j.1749-6632.2009.04392.x © 2009 New York Academy of Sciences.

treatment at early stages of the disease. Scoring schemes currently employed in everyday clinical routine and clinical trials often suffer from a lack of sensitivity and reproducibility caused by the use of manual measurements combined with semiquantitative scores. These drawbacks make them subjective to the reader's experience and are time-consuming, which limits their applicability and value in daily practice.

Accurate quantification of disease progression is a decisive factor during treatment. In recent years, a large number of semimanual and computer-aided methods for quantitative analysis that take advantage of the new imaging technologies and focus on automation of the existing scoring schemes have surfaced.[1,2] These new computer-aided systems permit quantification of disease progression or a patient's condition in a fast, objective manner and potentially open the way to significant advances in imaging technology, image analysis methodology, and new treatments.

In this chapter, we give an overview of the traditional scoring systems, developed mainly for radiographic data, and emerging innovative computer-aided schemes for MRI and ultrasound (US) imaging modalities. These techniques are illustrated with data acquired from patients suffering from musculoskeletal diseases such as RA and OA.

Osteoarthritis

Osteoarthritis is a common noninflammatory joint disorder that affects approximately 70% of the population over the age of 65 years (70% refers to the anatomical/radiological features). Symptomatic OA has a lower prevalence of about 50%. Disease evolution is slow, occurring over several years or decades. The development of OA follows a complex pathway with gradually evolving disease symptoms, such as changes in water content, degradation of cartilage matrix components, collagen fibers, and glycosaminoglycans (GAG).[3,4] At present, the process is irreversible owing to the poor innate

repair potential of the hyaline cartilage tissue, whatever the underlying etiology.

Until recently, the assessment of damage determined by radiological progression has been considered the basis for studies on the disease modification for OA[5] and RA.[6–8] However, the assessment of progression with such methods is rather insensitive to change, even with meticulous description of the anatomical status of the joint. Although radiographs remain the usual means of assessing osteoarthritic changes in the knee (by joint space narrowing and the presence of osteophytes), the correlation between osteoarthritic findings on radiographs and clinical features is poor. In OA, where the cartilage repair is poor, radiography shows the damage only indirectly by joint space narrowing, which is not detected in the early stages of the disease. Moreover, when using this technique, exposure to ionizing radiation must be considered.

The need for early disease detection and for more sensitive methods for monitoring treatment has led to new imaging modalities such as MRI and US becoming techniques of choice for the detection of preerosive changes. No international agreement has been reached regarding a common definition of OA, but it is generally accepted that the disease process involves cartilage destruction, bony changes in the subchondral zone, and loss of function. Classification of this multifaceted joint disorder has to embrace the great disparity and is often the result of a consensus.

Kellgren and Lawrence Scoring System

In 1957, Kellgren and Lawrence were the first to systematically use radiographic changes to assess the severity of OA.[9] They developed the four-grade Kellgren–Lawrence (KL) scoring system, which uses characteristic radiographic features of OA, including changes in subchondral bone. KL grades of severity of OA of the knee in the original system are as follows:

- Grade 1: Doubtful narrowing of joint space and possible osteophytic lipping.

- Grade 2: Definite osteophytes and possible narrowing of joint space.
- Grade 3: Moderate multiple osteophytes, definite narrowing of joint space, and some sclerosis and possible deformity of bone ends.
- Grade 4: Large osteophytes, marked narrowing of joint space, severe sclerosis, and definite deformity of bone ends.

Recent overall grading of OA tends to consider joint space narrowing as the most important feature of the radiographic changes.[10] Subchondral changes in bone mineral density in gonarthrosis assessed *in vivo* by photon absorption may be a sensitive method, but it only shows one of the features of OA and has been abandoned owing to radiation exposure.[11]

Modifications of the original scoring system[12–14] were suggested in a recently published meta-analysis paper by Schiphof *et al.*[15] The authors argued that major OA studies disagree on the definition and grading of the disease, even among themselves, and urged researchers to reach a consensus on a single valid and feasible classification system.

Scoring MRI Data

MRI is regarded as the most powerful soft tissue and joint imaging modality.[16–19] It offers unparalleled discrimination among articular soft tissues by direct and topographic visualization of all components of the joint simultaneously.[20,21] MRI permits evaluation of the joint as a whole organ[22] and performs direct chondral imaging. This potentially allows evaluation of regional thickness as well as of the water content and cartilage matrix compositions throughout the joint.[19,23–27]

MRI in OA can reliably image pathology such as osteophytes, bone marrow edema, sub- and periarticular cysts, meniscal tears, ligament abnormalities, synovial thickening, joint effusion, and intra-articular loose bodies and has been shown to be useful in imaging cartilage abnormalities.[19,22,28–32] The utility of MRI in OA studies has been limited by the lack of techniques that can provide rapid quantitative assessment of multiple tissues. Most of the existing qualitative and semiquantitative scoring methods for articular cartilage grade the severity of cartilage involvement on a scale from 0 to 3 or 0 to 4, based on subjective evaluations by one or more readers. These systems commonly differentiate between less than 50% depth, more than 50% depth, and full-thickness cartilage lesions.[18,33,34] Such evaluations are time-consuming and might be very much influenced by the experience of a reader. It has been demonstrated that the same person, when confronted with the same radiological images for the second time, provides significantly different results.[7]

A scoring system developed by Peterfy *et al.*,[22] known as whole-organ MRI scoring (WORMS), was devised to grade OA based on various features, including cartilage signal and morphology, subchondral bone marrow abnormalities, subarticular cysts, subarticular bone attrition, marginal osteophytes, medial and lateral meniscal integrity, anterior and posterior cruciate ligament integrity, medial and lateral collateral ligament integrity, synovitis/effusion, intra-articular loose bodies, and periarticular cysts/bursitis. Each feature is evaluated in distinct regions of the knee using an eight-point scale. The authors report high interobserver agreement. Intraclass correlation coefficients between two trained readers are more than 0.98 for cartilage abnormalities and more than 0.80 for most features, excluding bone attrition and synovitis.[35]

An alternative compartment-based scoring system, known as knee osteoarthritis scoring system (KOSS), was published by Kornaat *et al.*[36] Several features, such as the depth of the femorotibial and patellofemoral cartilage; the surface extent of diffuse, focal, or osteochondral cartilage defects, osteophytes, subchondral cysts; and bone marrow edema are evaluated on a scale from 0 to 3, corresponding to minimal, moderate, and severe damage. Intra- and interobserver (two observers) reproducibility of 0.76–0.96 and 0.63–0.915, respectively, are reported. Limitations of these scoring systems were discussed by Conaghan *et al.*[37] and Eckstein *et al.*[19,38] and include mainly criticism concerning several subscales, in particular those for cartilage signal, morphology, and osteophytes. Note that evaluations provided by these scoring systems may be limited owing to the nonuniform dimensionality and absence of unifying scaling of the items (especially in "early" OA cohorts, where only the lower end of scales may be used), which raises concerns about the responsiveness of the instruments to detecting minimally significant change.

Recently, a new quantitative system, Boston–Leeds osteoarthritis knee score (BLOKS), has been developed.[39] The authors present a scoring scheme that involves grading of cartilage integrity, attrition, bone marrow lesions and cysts, osteophytes, ligaments, meniscal health, and synovitis, as well as meniscal displacement, collateral ligament contour, osteophyte signal, synovitis separate from effusion, subchondral plate signal and thickness, limb alignment, and muscle quality.

It should be recognized that in the absence of data concerning the importance of certain pathological features as well as standardized definitions of the features, these qualitative scoring systems tend to be broadly inclusive. In order to perform such evaluations, the readers are often required to undergo initial training, and even then the inter- and intrastudy evaluation and reproducibility of the results are not perfect. The inclusion of more and more features decelerate evaluation time and might lead to even larger diversity in results.

Mathematical descriptions of cartilage surface topography or cartilage volume allow for more detailed analysis of the geometric topography of the joint surfaces.[40–43] This is particularly useful in the context of computer modeling in joint biomechanics and surgery.[40,44,45] Several quantitative measures of cartilage morphology have been proposed that are based on automated segmentation and measurement

of parameters such as cartilage volume, thickness, and surface area; total subchondral bone (or bone interface) area; denuded subchondral bone area; cartilaginous subchondral bone area; cartilage surface curvature (joint incongruity); surface roughness; and lesion size and depth.[46]

It is challenging to deliver perfect segmentation results, especially when measurements have to be performed in areas where cartilage has been lost and thus is not visible. In this case, a user might get undersegmented results. If, for example, osteophytes are not excluded from the segmentation results, premorbid bone interface area is often overestimated. So far, fully automated segmentation of cartilage has not been 100% successful and various semi-automated segmentation techniques have been proposed to tackle this problem. Some of them are very basic, such as region growing[47–50] and edge detection,[51] whereas others are more sophisticated and are based on active shape models,[52] B-spline snakes (active contours),[53–56] and watershed segmentation.[57]

Automated techniques for patient motion correction[58–61] allow for matching of bone structures in the data sets acquired within a particular time interval or upon the follow-up examinations. Of course, such an analysis should always take into account a local mismatch of cartilage thickness after the joints have been repositioned. Reconstruction of the joint structure from MRI normally preserves three-dimensional anatomical information, so the influence of the misplacements is not that significant. This represents a potential advantage for multicenter clinical trials, which require robust acquisition techniques.[19]

Despite the research in medical imaging, to date most of the studies in clinical practice rely on manual segmentation. Many argue that a skilled user will spend the same amount of time on manual segmentation as on correction of the results obtained with machine vision systems.[19] However, even accepting the assumption that the time spent is the same, the emphasis has to be put on the objectivity of the results. In the majority of cases, with a computed-aided system, the error can be estimated prior to the evaluation and thus accounted for, whereas the human reader might generate somewhat unpredictable errors. Moreover, reproducibility of reliably designed computed-aided systems is much higher, so such techniques will generate results that reflect pathological changes with statistical confidence.

Molecular Imaging and dGEMRIC

In the last decade, several techniques were suggested for quantification of the cartilage matrix.[19,27,62] Research in this field is driven by technological development and the fact that early OA changes occur within the molecular composition of the cartilage before structural damage is visible using arthroscopy or conventional imaging modalities such as X-ray and MRI. Overall *in vivo* assessment of the accuracy of these imaging markers is not a trivial matter as the "gold standard" (histology) is not readily available.

T2 mapping, which is a promising modality for measuring cartilage composition,[19,62–64] is a sensitive technique that reflects many aspects of cartilage composition, including hydration, molecular structure, and molecular concentration.[19,64,65] Its clinical value is still being debated and owing to the limited available data, it remains to be seen if the technique can differentiate unhealthy from healthy controls and identify changes in a patient's condition on followup examinations. Stahl *et al.*[66] reported that T2 measures (in a longitudinal study) could differentiate OA patients from control groups but showed no change over the course of 1 year. More importantly, T2 values show little difference between the two groups.[63,67]

Another promising technique is the delayed gadolinium-enhanced MRI of cartilage (dGEMRIC) method using either intravenous[68] (indirect) or intra-articular (direct)[69,70] delayed MR arthrography and T1 relaxation mapping.[19,27,62] The proteoglycan component of cartilage matrix has GAG side chains with abundant negatively charged carboxyl and sulfate groups, and when a negatively charged MRI contrast agent, such as a gadolinium diethylenetriamine pentaacetic acid (Gd-DTPA) is allowed to penetrate into the cartilage volume passively over time, it will distribute in lower concentration in the areas with higher GAG. The Gd-DTPA distribution in cartilage is reflected in the MRI parameter of T1, so T1 relaxation imaging in the presence of Gd-DTPA can be used as an index of GAG concentration.[68,71] This may lead to a better understanding of the early manifestations of cartilage disease and provide important information regarding early treatment response.

An *in vitro* study[68] has shown that delayed Gd-DTPA-enhanced MRI can be used to follow GAG replenishment over time in degraded cartilage. Several *in vivo* studies confirmed the clinical feasibility of the technique on 1.5-T scanners, relating the dGEMRIC index to physiological and pathological processes.[72–76] Thus dGEMRIC can be used to indirectly image the GAG content within the cartilage.[77–80] One of the problems with dGEMRIC is the relatively long time that patients have to spend in the MRI scanner, as the imaging has to be done twice: before and 90–120 min after Gd-DTPA application. In addition, the joint coverage using the conventional two-dimensional inversion recovery fast spin-echo technique is limited within a reasonable scan time (fewer than 30 min), making the T1 relaxation measures clinical unacceptable. Finally, the large doses of Gd-DTPA required for the intravenous approach makes this a rather costly procedure.

In order to perform quantitative analysis of the relaxation time maps, the cartilage volume has to be presegmented from the surrounding tissues and the time series derived from the pixels located within the volumes approximated with the modeling equation.[77,78] Further analysis can be done either by taking average signal intensities from the outlined region of interest and reporting the mean value or by plotting parameters for each individual time series on a relaxation map.

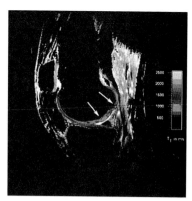 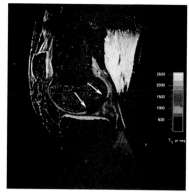

Figure 1. Sagittal image of the knee, 3D-dGEMRIC using 3 T. Color-coded cartilage transplant precontrast image. *Left:* The three-dimensional dual-flip-angle dGEMRIC technique was applied in the case of a patient 22 months after cartilage transplantation. There are slightly higher T_1 values in the cartilage transplant region compared with normal cartilage (white arrows mark the borders of the transplant): *Right:* Color-coded cartilage transplant postcontrast. The contrast enhancement of cartilage transplant after intravenous administration of contrast agent reflects a smaller amount of GAG in the transplanted area compared to the normal surrounding hyaline cartilage. [Images are courtesy of Prof. S. Trattning *et al.* [86]]

It can be expected that the signal-to-noise and contrast-to-noise ratios in the relaxation-weighted images will not always produce good definition between the cartilage and the surrounding tissues.[81,82] Moreover, the varying size of the imaging matrix and slice plane in the follow-up studies influence the reproducibility of the quantitative measurements and might introduce a major bias in evaluation of a patient's condition. To overcome these limitations clinical applications of the method are currently being tested on 3-T MRI scanners, using a three-dimensional sequence that has shown promising preliminary results in regard to reduction in imaging time, along with an increased signal-to-noise ratio and joint coverage.[83–86] Figure 1 illustrates a sagittal image of the knee acquired using 3D-dGEMRIC and 3-T scanning equipment.

Assessment of the GAG variation in both morphologically intact and damaged cartilage may yield information about early cartilage degeneration and possible repair. The *in vivo* assessment of the technique has yet to be determined, as no "gold standard" such as a histological reference is readily available and the correlation with clinical markers and out-comes is not fully understood. Future studies especially with the increasing availability of 3-T magnets should permit assessment of this promising biomarker of early cartilage breakdown.

Scoring Ultrasound Data

Ultrasound systems with transducer frequencies above 12 MHz provide sectional imaging with axial and lateral resolution below 200 μm. This makes US well suited for the evaluation of the soft tissues surrounding most joints. Furthermore, with Doppler techniques, inflammatory hyperemia may be detected and quantified. Unfortunately, US performance is not uniform from joint to joint or even from one part of a joint to another. For example, all aspects of the distal femoral articular cartilage may be investigated with US compared to almost none of the corresponding tibial cartilage. Ultrasound is not able to measure joint space narrowing and has no role in the evaluation of pathology below the bone surface. On the other hand, US is well suited for the detection of secondary osteoarthritic pathologies such as osteophytes, synovial hypertrophy, and synovitis.

The superior resolution of US is somewhat counteracted by its poor spatial orientation. With conventional free-hand technique it is not possible to select and compare identical scan planes over time. However, even though US is not able to detect or grade all aspects of OA, it may still be able to play a role in the detection and grading of the disease. Qvistgaard *et al.*[87] developed a scoring system for hip OA based upon grading of the following OA-induced pathologies:

- Shape of the femoral head (round, flattened, destroyed).
- Osteophytes: (none, questionable, minor, major).
- Synovial contour on the femoral neck (concave, flat, convex).
- Intra-articular fluid collection (absent, possible, definite).

For examination of the hip joint, a semiquantitative scoring system was employed. The parameters were defined as follows:

- *Osteophyte score* described the femoral osteophytes as 0, no occurrence; 1, slight degree (irregularity on the cartilage–bone transition is just visible); 2, medium degree (well-defined osteophytes, shelf formation or irregularities on the femoral neck); and 3, severe degree (involvement of the whole femoral neck including shelf formation).
- *Femoral head score* described the curvature of the visible part as 0, round; 1, slightly flattened (still visible curvature but with an abnormally large radius); 2, very flattened (no visible curvature of the caput); and 3, no obvious contour (the femoral head cannot be defined for osteophytes/erosions).
- *Synovial profile* was defined from the course of the anterior surface of the capsule on the anterior surface of the femoral neck (technically including effusion, synovium, and capsule): 0 corresponds to concave (follows the bone surface); 1, flat; and 2, convex.
- *Joint effusion* was defined as a hypoechoic coherent region present inside the synovium delimitation: 0, none; 1, perhaps present; and 2, present.

Figure 2 illustrates examples of the osteophyte score.

The overall assessment of the hip by an investigator was also standardized semiquantitatively as follows: (i) Global US evaluation of OA: 0, normal; 1, slight; 2, moderate; and 3, severe. (ii) Global US evaluation of synovitis: 0, none; 1, moderate; and 2, severe. Intraobserver agreement was good to excellent and interobserver agreement was fair to good.

The knee may be better suited for OA grading than the hip because the knee joint is located more superficially and can be accessed from all sides. As with the hip, US does not readily provide information about the cartilage. However, either the presence or the absence of osteophytes, meniscal bulging, synovial hypertrophy, and perfusion as well as joint fluid can be accurately determined with US. Hence grading of the knee joint is possible.

Ultrasound is at present far from validated in diagnosis and grading of OA. It may be that it will prove to be a valuable tool and may even be enhanced with improved spatial orientation through image fusion with CT-MRI or 3D-US techniques. Parallel to the application of conventional US imaging in OA detection as outlined above, research has focused on tissue characterization with US. Studies have suggested that qualitative and quantitative US imaging could sensitively detect articular surface fibrillation, degeneration of the articular surface, and changes in the subchondral bone during development of OA.[79,88–93]

Qualitatively, fibrillation is assessed visually as a decrease in sharpness and echogenicity or as an increase in the irregularity of the cartilage surface.[89,93,94] Quantitative US analysis of the cartilage–bone interface is challenging, as absorption and scattering in the overlying cartilage tissue and incomplete US transmission through the cartilage surface may significantly affect the results.[92] Recently, an US roughness index was used as a parameter for the

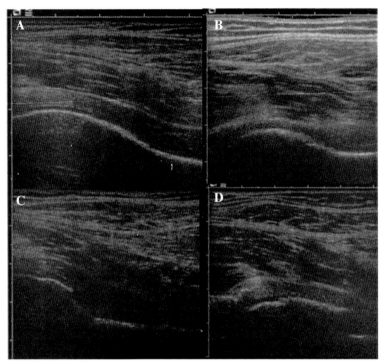

Figure 2. Examples of osteophyte score: (**A**) Score 0, no visible osteophyte. (**B**) Score 1, irregularity on the cartilage–bone transition is just visible. (**C**) Score 2, well-defined osteophytes, shelf formation, or irregularities on the femoral neck. There is one large osteophyte with shelf formation, which is an US discontinuity between the distal border of the osteophyte and the femoral neck. (**D**) Score 3, involvement of the whole femoral neck, including shelf formation. There is one large osteophyte with shelf formation. The femoral head is seen between the two vertical arrows. [With permission from Qvistgaard *et al.*[87]]

quantification of cartilage surface roughness.[92] The experiments were performed with normal, experimentally degraded articular surfaces and *in vivo* in bovine cartilage samples with spontaneously developed tissue degeneration using the histological degenerative grade of the cartilage as a reference. The authors concluded that the combination of US measurement of the cartilage surface roughness and US reflection at the cartilage–bone interface complement each other and may together enable more sensitive analyses.[92]

The reversibility and sensitivity of the new quantitative methods are still being debated. The major benefit of quantitative US measurements is the possibility of evaluation of degenerative changes, such as increased roughness of the cartilage surface during early stages of the disease, even before degeneration can be seen visually. It is expected that novel diagnostic systems and computer science algorithms will ultimately provide the clinician with new information about the natural history and optimal treatment of OA at an early stage. However, there is not yet a reliable method for detecting microscopic changes in early OA.

Summary

Merging all acquired data and symptoms into an acceptable grading system that can be used on a daily basis is a daunting challenge. For example, there is variability in joint involvement and disease activity as well as low correlation among results produced by different imaging modalities. Furthermore, different anatomical sites may respond differently to the same therapy. To date, virtually all symptoms and visual findings have been employed in the evaluation, but no scoring system has gained general acceptance.

Qualitative means for evaluation of superficial deterioration of the cartilage, such as arthroscopic inspection of cartilage surface and manual probing, may be used for diagnosis of joint injuries and monitoring of the success of surgical cartilage repair. Nevertheless, it is obvious to many researchers and practitioners that cartilage location, depth, size, and shape vary from study to study and probing is not always adequate for evaluating such anatomy quantitatively. Obviously the invasiveness of the technique limits its applicability.

Various quantitative imaging methods for grading the degenerative changes and injuries of articular cartilage at the time of surgery or arthroscopy with direct observation of the cartilage surface have been proposed.[95,96] These include optical coherence tomography,[97] electromechanical evaluation,[98] mechanical indentation,[99] US evaluation,[100] and US indentation.[101,102] X-ray and scoring of the radiographs remain the usual practice for assessing osteoarthritic changes. Recent studies have shown that the correlation between osteoarthritic findings on radiographs and clinical features is poor and new modalities such as MRI and US have to be used in order to arrive at adequate diagnoses. MRI, with its excellent soft tissue contrast, is the best noninvasive technique currently available for the assessment of cartilage injury, but its applicability is limited by the cost of the examination and the lack of efficient scoring methods.

Recent advances in imaging technologies and computer science have generated interest in the development of automated measurements of the histological cartilage changes in OA. These scoring methods attempt to characterize OA by measuring the surface erosion and irregularities, deep fissures, and alterations in the staining of the matrix. Some systems have been developed for quantitative assessment of the cartilage repair process,[88,89,94] but most of these approaches are still under development and in need of thorough clinical evaluation.

Rheumatoid Arthritis

Rheumatoid arthritis (RA) is a painful chronic inflammatory joint disease that, owing to its joint-related symptoms as well as general malaise and fatigue, has an enormous impact on all aspects of one's life.[103] In two-thirds of cases, RA begins with symmetric arthralgia and arthritis in the small joints of the hands and feet, which can lead to severe skeletal changes and destruction of the affected joints.[104]

Generally, an RA diagnosis includes a case history, clinical signs, laboratory abnormalities, and an X-ray examination. The classification criteria for RA along with therapeutic recommendations were published by the American College of Rheumatology (ACR) in 1988.[105] These criteria have facilitated RA research by ensuring a uniform patient group for comparing experiences and treatment results among countries and clinical treatment centers, but they are not diagnostic.

Evaluation of RA is a challenging task because many factors, such as the number of affected joints, the presence of rheumatoid factor (RF), functional status, the presence and size of bone erosions, and the condition of bone marrow edema can potentially be useful for assessing a patient's condition or disease progression. The multiplicity and heterogeneity of the disease make it difficult to assess the relative or absolute importance of each factor and its possible value for RA diagnosis. Many researchers have attempted to design comprehensive evaluation systems that will permit assessment of disease activity, progress of the patient's condition, and the effect of treatment.

Joint Assessment

Clinical assessment of joint swelling and tenderness may be done in a qualitative or quantitative way. The former implies evaluation of the presence or absence of swelling and joint damage and the latter of grading of disease activity in respect to a particular scale. The qualitative form of assessment allows for higher reliability in measuring disease activity[106] and the former for higher interobserver agreement.[107,108] When successive joint assessment is performed by the same assessor, the intraobserver variation is lower.[109]

According to ACR recommendations, RA activity can be established by evaluating 68 joints for tenderness and 66 for swelling. Fuchs *et al.*[110] suggested a reduced 28-joint count, which allows for the evaluation of the easily accessible joints commonly affected in RA and has been shown to correlate to the 66/68-joint count when assessing changes in relation to therapy.[111] This 28-joint count, however, omits foot joints, where RA often starts, with a consequent decrease in sensitivity. The tender and swollen joint assessment is supplemented by several other measures of disease activity related to the functional status, pain assessment, and joint damage.

Symmons *et al.*[112] developed a measure of overall RA status using a number of destroyed large joints as a measure of articular damage. Cranney *et al.*[113] suggested a deformity index based on measuring limited joint motion and deformity, which was adapted from the joint alignment and motion scale[114] and the Escola Paulista de Medicina range-of-motion scale (EPM-ROM).[115] Another scoring system for assessment of irreversible long-term articular damage in RA was developed by Zijlstra *et al.*,[116] who suggested quantifying damage based on the examination of 35 large and small joints using a three-point scale. On this scale, 0 corresponds to no irreversible damage, 1 to partial damage, and 2 to severe damage, ankylosis, or prosthesis. Note, that inter- and intraobserver variability and discriminate validity of these scores have never been formally evaluated.

Functional status may be evaluated by health assessment questionnaires,[117,118] which have been shown to correlate well with isokinetic muscle strength.[119,120] Pain assessment can be quantified using a 100-mm visual analogue scale.[121] The severity and duration of morning stiffness, recorded in minutes, can be considered as another measure of the arthritis.

More objective measures of clinical status and disease activity include laboratory tests. Specific RA-related biochemical changes such as RF and, more recently, anticyclic citrullinated peptide antibodies, which have been found to be diagnostic and to some extent prognostic, although they are only of limited value for monitoring disease activity.

Radiographic Scoring Methods

Conventional X-ray remains the gold standard for imaging for joint damage progression, as estimated by joint space narrowing (JSN) and erosions.[105] Other potential findings include juxta-articular osteoporosis, bone cysts, and in late stages of the disease joint subluxation, malalignment, and ankylosis. Many studies have shown that the presence of radiographic erosion remains one of the hallmarks of RA, although erosions may be present in only about 40% of patients at the time of clinical diagnosis. Several scoring methods for assessing RA radiographic damage have been proposed. The most common approaches are modifications of the Sharp score or the Larsen index.

In 1971, *Sharp et al.* proposed a scoring method for joint assessment in the hands and wrists. The method was modified in 1985 and the later version is now the standard.[122,123] The method evaluates 17 areas for erosion and 18 areas for JSN in each hand and wrist. Presence of an erosion scores one point, with a maximum of five points for each area, reflecting loss of more than 50% of either articular bone. The total erosion scores range from 0 to 170. For JSN, one point is scored for focal joint narrowing, two points for diffuse narrowing of less than 50% of the original space, and three points if the reduction is more than half of the original joint space. The score for JSN ranges from 0 to 144. Ankylosis is scored as four. Subluxation is not scored.

In 1983, Genant *et al.* proposed and later modified a method for scoring hand and foot radiographs.[124] The scoring system considers erosive changes at 16 sites in the hand and six in the foot, and JSN at 11 and six sites, respectively. Erosions are scored according to an eight-point scale with 0.5 increments, where 0 indicates normal, 0+ questionable or subtle change, 1 mild, 1+ mild/worse, 2 moderate, 2+ moderate/worse, 3 severe, and 3+ severe/worse damage. Joint space narrowing is scored according to a nine-point scale with 0.5 increments, where 0–3+ scores correspond to those of erosions and 4 indicates ankylosis or dislocation. The score for erosion and those for JSN for both hands range from 0 to 98 and 0 to 104, respectively. After separately summing the two scores for both hands, each is normalized to a scale from 0 to 100.

In 1989, van der Heijde modified Sharp's method by suggesting an evaluation of erosions in 16 joints for each hand and wrist and six joints for each foot on a scale from 1 to 5. One point is scored if erosions are discrete and five when complete collapse of the bone is observed. The score for erosion ranges from 0 to 160 in the hands and from 0 to 120 in the feet, where the maximum erosion score for a joint in the foot is 10. Joint space narrowing is assessed in 15 joints for each hand and wrist and six joints for each foot. JSN is combined with a score for subluxation and scored 0 for a normal joint; 1 for focal or doubtful; 2 for generalized, less than 50% of the original joint space; 3 for generalized, more than 50% of the original joint space or subluxation; and 4 for bony ankylosis or complete luxation. The score for JSN ranges from 0 to 120 in the hands and from 0 to 48 in the feet.

In 1999, van der Heijde[130] described a simplified method of scoring radiographs based on the Sharp/van der Heijde score that assesses the same joints, but instead of grading, the number of joints with erosions and JSN are simply summed.[130] The Larsen score, developed in 1974, is based on a comparison with a set of standard films. It differentiates six stages from 0 (normal) to 5, reflecting gradual, progressive deterioration and provides an overall measure of joint damage in 15 joints of the wrist and 10 joints of the feet. This method was modified several times between 1974 and 1999.[125,126] In 1995, Larsen[126] devised a way to evaluate radiographs in long-term studies.[126] The main differences from the original method are the deletion of scores for the thumbs and first metacarpophalangeal joint for the frequent interference of degenerative changes; subdivision of the wrist into four quadrants; deletion of soft tissue swelling and osteoporosis; distinction between erosions of different sizes. The grading scale ranges from 0 to 5, with 0 indicating intact bony outlines and normal joint space; 1, erosion rewer than 1 mm in diameter or JSN; 2, one or several small erosions (diameter more than 1 mm); 3, marked erosions; 4, severe erosions (usually no joint space left and the original bony outlines are only partly preserved); and 5, mutilating changes (the original bony outlines have been destroyed). The total score ranges from 0 to 160. The scoring systems have been validated in many clinical trials.

The Ratingen score, developed in 1998 as a variation of the Larsen score,[127] restricts scoring of an individual joint to definite changes of erosion and joint destruction. The extension of the erosion into the bone is not considered. The amount of joint surface destruction is defined by the length of the clearly visible interruption of the cortical plate in relation to the total joint surface and graded as 1 when there are one or several definite erosions with destruction of less than 20% of the total surface; 2 when joint surface destruction is between 21 and 40%; 3 when the surface destruction is between 41 and 60%; 4 when it is between 61 and 80%; and 5 when it is more than 80%. Adding the scores from 38 areas gives a total score ranging from 0 to 190. In 2003, a new modification to Larsen's scoring system was developed by Matsuno *et al.*,[128] which considers erosions

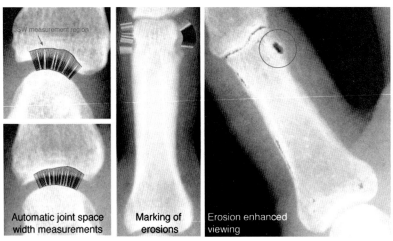

Figure 3. *Left:* automatic joint space width measurement at the MCP joint. *Center:* automatic erosion spotting. *Right:* erosion visualization.

more precisely. In 2000, Wolfe *et al.*[222] proposed a new approach for evaluation of the severity of RA, the short erosion scale, a modification of the Larsen method (1995), which considers 12 joints: three of four regions of the wrist as defined by Larsen (medial-proximal, medial-distal, and lateral-proximal) and the second, third, and fifth metacarpophalageals (MCPs). Each joint is graded as in the 1995 Larsen system.

Comparisons of various scoring systems have been published.[7,129,130] In general, compared to the Larsen method, the Sharp/van der Heijde method has a better sensitivity to change, although it is considerably more time-consuming. There is still no universally accepted technique and modifications to the existing schemes are often proposed. Considerable interobserver variation, especially when dealing with multicenter trials, must be taken into account when applying any of these methods.[131]

Computer-Aided RA Assessment. Several computer-aided programs for semiautomatic measurements of joint space have been introduced.[1,132–135] These systems differ in their degree of automation, reproducibility of results, precision, and the number of joints examined. Recently, methods for fully automatic measurement of joint space width in hand radiographs, automatic erosion spotting,

and the visualization of pathological deviations from healthy bone texture caused by RA have been proposed.[1,136]

Both methods rely on active shape models to delineate the bone contours.[137] The models are trained on data annotated by experts and can detect anatomical structures (e.g., bones) in new data. They provide information about position consistency during follow-up examinations thereby enabling erosion tracking for the analysis of the local development of the disease effects, or the definition of measurement zones on prototype bones, for the quantification of the joint space width. Figure 3 illustrates automatic joint space width measurement at the MCP joint, automatic erosion spotting, and erosion visualization.[1,136]

The reported smallest detectable difference for the joint space width measurement ranged from 0.08 to 0.31 mm, which corresponds to a coefficient of variation of 2 to 7%. The automatic erosion detection of full erosions provides for an area under the receiver operating characteristic (ROC) curve of 0.92 with regard to expert annotation. These new concepts introduce a measurement technique (independent of plain film radiograph limitations) at comparable technical outcome and precision as for manual or semiautomatic methods.

Scoring Ultrasound Data

Musculoskeletal US is versatile and has been shown to be more sensitive than conventional radiography in the detection of erosions without X-ray exposure.[138] Ultrasound performance in RA is somewhat uneven. When compared with clinical examination, conventional radiography, and contrast-enhanced MRI in a variety of inflammatory arthritides, US appears to be more sensitive than radiography for detecting inflammatory soft tissue lesions and structural damage in individuals with effectively normal radiographs (Larsen score grade 0–1). On the other hand, MRI is considered more sensitive in the detection of synovitis. Bone edema and loss of articular cartilage are not detected with US, whereas on MRI virtually all of the synovium can be evaluated with high resolution.[139] Bone erosions can be detected with high accuracy[140] on superficial bone surfaces, whereas, for example, a substantial carpal bone surface is inaccessible to US.[138]

As sonographic findings of grayscale changes, synovial thickening, joint fluid, and erosions may remain after joint inflammation has subsided, they seem to be ill-suited as characteristics for monitoring treatment response.[141] Nevertheless, several groups have developed scoring systems for all three categories in finger joints.[142–144]

Scheel *et al.*[143] suggested assessing finger joint synovitis by focusing on the palmar side and applying semiquantitative grading instead of quantitative measurements. They also recommended using the "sum of three fingers" method in longitudinal trials. In their study, no significant differences between individual PIP joints or individual MCP joints were observed. They concluded that all the fingers within each of these joint groups should be treated equally for statistical calculations. The estimated optimal cutoff point for distinguishing between healthy and disease-affected joints was 0.6 mm for both MCP joints (sensitivity 94%, specificity 89%) and PIP joints (sensitivity 90%, specificity 88%). Another conclusion was that there was no significant difference between semiquantitative US scores and quantitative US measurements, with the best results for joint combinations achieved using the "sum of four fingers" (second through fifth MCP and PIP joints) and the "sum of three fingers" (second through fourth MCP and PIP joints) methods.

Ellegaard *et al.*[144] published a study in which various scoring systems for US were tested on a larger group of healthy controls (24 men and women between ages 30 and 54) to determine to what extent synovial tissue is seen on grayscale US in healthy joints. Each person was scanned in 69 positions. The images were graded on a scale from 0 to 4 with two scoring systems, where scores 0–1 were defined as normal and 2–4 as pathological. With scoring system I, only markedly hypoechoic synovium was graded. With scoring system II, marked hypoechogenicity was not a criterion. According to the results, with systems I and II, respectively, 89 and 95% of the joints had at least one pathological score. The authors concluded that the number of healthy joints that were graded with pathological scores with both scoring systems was unacceptably high, which indicates that many of the scores interpreted as pathological in patients with RA may just be normal findings, with increasing numbers in older patients.

Most of the scoring systems are semiquantitative with three to five classes. Normally, scoring is performed as a visual evaluation, where higher numbers indicate more pathology. Not all investigators believe that it is possible to distinguish between synovial hypertrophy and joint fluid with acceptable accuracy, so some centers do not attempt to do so, but rather combine the two as synovial hypertrophy. This latter approach is often called a synovitis score, which is somewhat inaccurate because thickened synovium need not be inflamed. Furthermore, it has not been defined when synovium is pathologically thickened and therefore it is possible that the proposed scoring systems will score unacceptably high in normals.[144] Scoring systems

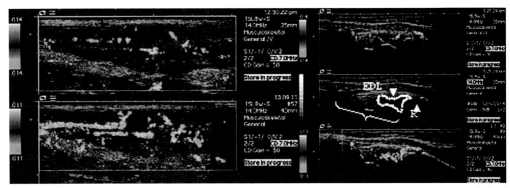

Figure 4. Effect of machine upgrade. The images compare two Acuson Sequoia units—one with the latest upgrade and one without. *Left:* Longitudinal images of Achilles tendonitis without (*top*) and with (*bottom*) upgrade. The two images are almost identical in position, which can be seen on the gray-scale part as well as with color. The machine with the upgrade has higher color Doppler sensitivity. Top image shows fragmented vessels that are much more confluent in bottom image. Bottom image appears most hyperemic. *Right:* Longitudinal images of the radiocarpal joint in a 12-year-old patient with juvenile rheumatoid arthritis. Top image is without upgrade; middle with the upgrade. [With permission from Torp-Pedersen and Terslev.[146]]

have not yet been developed for larger joints such as the wrist or the knee.

The development of Doppler techniques for assessment of the blood flow in the vascular synovium, which reflects inflammatory activity, has enhanced the diagnostic power of US and its value in the detection and grading of synovial inflammation.[145,146] Terslev *et al.* demonstrated that Doppler US and postcontrast MRI arrive at comparable results in terms of estimation of synovial inflammatory activity.[141] However, there was no apparent correlation between MRI or US estimates of inflammation and values obtained for the visual activity score, health assessment questionnaire, duration of early morning stiffness, erythrocyte sedimentation rate (ESR), or c-reactive protein (CRP).[147]

Doppler has been used increasingly in the detection and grading of synovial inflammation,[146] where its main advantage is its ability to quickly assess variations in the inflammation as well as immediate response to therapy. Depending on the quality of the equipment, Doppler may be able to detect some normal synovial flow as well as all pathologic flow (modern high-end equipment) or, conversely, only some of the pathologic flow and none of the normal flow (medium- or low-end equipment).

Figure 4 illustrates the effect of machine upgrade. Owing to the variation in equipment quality, there is no general agreement on how to define the flow in pathologic and healthy tissue.[148] In some centers the mere presence of Doppler activity is regarded as proof of hyperemia and in others certain threshold levels must be exceeded before pathological hyperemia is diagnosed.

Several scoring systems associated with Doppler imaging have been developed. As with grayscale scoring, most are semiquantitative with four classes. Scoring is done visually, and in all systems the higher grades are defined as different percentages of synovial area being covered with color. There seems to be a consensus for the following system: 0, no Doppler activity in the synovium; 1, one or two single spots; 2, confluent areas covering up to half of the synovial area; and 3, confluent areas covering more than half of the synovial area. The synovium is not always easy to distinguish from the surrounding tissues and it has only been tested on finger joints. Generally, classification is performed based on the features in the image and not by biology. The size of the classes is unknown and scores are highly dependent on the scanning equipment and the experience of the operator.

A similar but continuous system is the color fraction (CF). The synovium is traced on a computer and the CF is the number of color pixels divided by the total number of pixels. The CF is a continuous variable and is theoretically better suited for showing differences in synovial perfusion. A weakness of the CF is that shrinkage in synovial volume (as a treatment response) will elevate the CF and counteract a fall caused by a reduction in flow. The CF has the same problems with the synovial tracing and might not be accurate in some patients. The best performance in a reliability study was evident when the CF was made with a trace defined by including normal anatomy with the synovial trace.

Several studies have tested the relationship between traditional clinical signs of synovitis and synovial disease as determined by US, using grayscale synovial hypertrophy and Doppler scores, both pre- and postcontrast.[149] Most find moderate agreement among the clinical signs of disease,[141] but much work must be done before it will be possible to use a valid US Doppler score for monitoring disease activity in RA.[148,150,151] No standardized scoring methods have yet been developed, although guidelines for gray-scale US have been suggested.[152] Doppler grading of arthritis is not a fully investigated discipline. Further work is needed to define the quality of the US equipment as well as the machine settings.

Scoring MRI Data

Today, MRI is considered to be the most sensitive imaging modality for musculoskeletal disease assessment. It provides a larger field of view and higher tissue contrast, and it permits visualizing of bone and soft tissue in three orthogonal planes. MRI examinations are performed using high- and low-field scanning equipment; routine sequences include T1-weighted images, which provide good anatomical detail; T2 fast spin-echo (FSE) images, where fluid/edema and fat produce a high signal; T2-weighted fat-suppressed images, where bone edema is highlighted, short tau inversion recovery (STIR) im-

ages; and T1 images postintravenous injection of the contrast gadolinium-based agents.

MRI has a much higher prognostic value compared to conventional radiography owing to its ability to identify new bone erosions, on average, 1 year before these erosions are visible on X-ray images[153] and to show synovitis and bone edema changes, which can be used to identify progressive erosive disease even when clinical activity is suppressed. Interobserver variability has been studied extensively by several research groups. Basic interpretation of RA changes on MRI among readers is relatively consistent. The major issue is the time needed for data analysis and interpretation. A large number of scoring systems, both quantitative and qualitative, have been developed in recent years in order to monitor both the evolution and the treatment of musculoskeletal diseases.[154-159]

OMERACT-RAMRIS

A relatively short time ago, the OMERACT-MRI collaboration was set up to address issues concerning the reading of MRI data, which resulted in the introduction of a scoring system known as OMERACT-RAMRIS (rheumatoid arthritis magnetic resonance imaging scoring system).[153,160] Synovitis, bone marrow edema, and erosions were defined and quantified using the EULAR-OMERACT-RAMRIS reference atlas, which contains standardized reference images of the MCP and carpal joints and requirements for examination techniques along with detailed protocols.[161-163]

According to RAMRIS, the degree of synovitis is scored on a scale from 0 to 3 for every examined joint area depending on an arbitrary grading of the synovitis from no synovitis to mild, moderate, and severe (worst). The synovitis is scored in the distal radioulnar, radiocarpal, intercarpal–carpometacarpal, and second to fourth MCP joints. Bone changes are scored in the carpal, distal radius, distal ulna, and metacarpal bases. Erosions are graded on a scale from 0 to 10 with intervals of 10% volume involvement, and bone marrow edema is scored on a scale from 0 to 3 with intervals of 33% volume involvement. Long bones are scored to a depth of 1 cm from the articular surface.

Recently, the group has suggested a scoring system for the evaluation of both tenosynovitis and psoriatic arthritis.[164] The reliability of this scoring system has been assessed in multiple studies, which all show low intrareader variation, but low interreader correlation.[165] There is still a debate over the relative reliability of wrist and MCP scores.[162,166]

Several studies applied the OMERACT scoring system to diagnosis, assessment of the disease activity, and response to treatment evaluation.[165] OMERACT scores appear to be sensitive to early erosions, but not to long-term progression.[167,168] Scores for edema in the MCP joints, synovitis, and bone edema have been shown to correlate with RA symptoms and potentially can be used for disease diagnosis. OMERACT scores appear to be reliable and moderately sensitive for RA assessment. The disadvantages of such measurements are the time involved and the potential for human bias.

Volume Measurements

The volume of synovium, bone erosion, synovial fluid, and cartilage can be measured directly, in cubic or square millimeters in contrast-enhanced or unenhanced images. Such measurements correlate well with disease activity and have been used as biomarkers. The simplest way to estimate the volume is to outline the anatomy on the postcontrast images and measure the volume. Another approach is to consider the subtraction images and calculate the number of pixels whose intensity level is above a certain threshold value, which of course requires definition of an optimal threshold level. Principal component analyses and k-means techniques have also been employed for data segmentation[169]; however, these methods require initialization and knowledge of the underlying physical procedure, which are often user defined and data dependent.

The reproducibility of synovial volume measurements has been analyzed.[170–172] Intraobserver, interobserver, and interscan errors were approximately 5% in the knee and wrist and reproducibility errors were 18%.[170] Studies have shown that small changes in synovial volume are better detected with volume measurements than with OMERACT scoring. Some work has been done in regard to erosion volume,[3,173] synovial fluid,[1710,1701] and cartilage volume.[174] The reproducibility of these methods is good, but interobserver agreement is poor, with little evidence of benefit from either training or thinner slices.[165]

It should be taken into account that volume measurements can be influenced by the dose of the contrast-enhancing agent and acquisition parameters. The acquisition protocol as well as patient motion during the examination can affect the edges or borders of tissues of interest and outlining the volume is time-consuming and subjective. With the use of efficient software algorithms, the speed of volume measurements as well as the accuracy can be significantly increased.

Scoring Contrast-Enhanced Dynamic MRI Data

Some of the most compelling evidence suggests that contrast-enhanced dynamic MRI (DCE-MRI) is likely to be a more useful marker for disease activity than measured synovial volume.[175–179] In recent years, DCE-MRI has become a commonly used method for diagnosis and monitoring of inflammatory diseases,[180–184] and it has evolved as an important technique for evaluating various diseases of the musculoskeletal system.[185–187] The gadolinium is preferentially taken up at sites of inflammation such as synovitis and edema, allowing further delineation between healthy and perfused tissues. DCE-MRI provides information about tissue vascularity, perfusion, and capillary permeability, and so permits assessment of the degree of inflammation and posttreatment progress evaluation.[188]

In DCE-MRI, a temporal variation of the MRI signal intensity occurs following intravenous administration of the contrast agent, normally Gd-DTPA. The time course of signal changes corresponds to the underlying changes in local bulk tissue concentration of the agent, which in turn depends on the degree of inflammatory activity. This information about tissue behavior has led to the development of a number of qualitative and quantitative scoring methods. A simple, but subjective, qualitative technique is the "naive review method," in which an observer examines the contrast enhancement sequentially on all images of the dynamic sequence. However, detection of small areas of enhancement or areas with discrete enhancement (especially in the wrist studies) can be difficult.

Early qualitative analysis methods were based on image subtraction, in which the pre-contrast image is subtracted from all subsequent images of the dynamic study.[187,188] The subtracted images are then viewed one by one. With such methods, it is possible to detect the most highly enhanced tissues (for biopsy or injections). However, estimation of measures such as the magnitude of enhancement and time of onset of enhancement or recognition of the late-enhancing tissues such as fat on the early subtracted images is difficult.

Pharmacokinetic Methods

Quantitative analysis of DCE-MRI data can be performed using two fundamentally different groups of methods: pharmacokinetic[189–191] and heuristic.[2,192–197] Pharmacokinetic methods[189–191] provide a framework that can be used to link the physics of MRI signal acquisition and the underlying pathophysiology that governs contrast agent kinetics. They rely on a common set of assumptions regarding the properties of the principal compartments and their interactions but adopt different representations for temporal variations of the contrast agent concentration in the blood plasma. Implementation of these methods in clinical settings is difficult, especially when high spatial resolution and multislice coverage are required.[198]

In some studies[189,190] the contrast agent concentration in the blood plasma is represented as a theoretical function in response to an injection, which is often idealized as a delta function. Such a representation fits the experimental data well when the temporal resolution of the DCE-MRI is low and the acquisition time is long. With higher resolution the characteristic shape of the contrast agent uptake in the tissue of interest resembles a sigmoid, which cannot be accurately described by these methods.[179] Furthermore, long acquisition times incur more noise as a result of movement and may provoke patient discomfort.

In clinical practice, it is impossible to assess the accuracy with which pharmacokinetic variables reflect the true underlying changes in the concentration of the contrast agent.[180] The accuracy of the estimates depend on the pharmacokinetic model used and the signal-to-noise ratio in any individual case. This is a particular problem in applications where noise is the dominant, or only, cause of variation in contrast agent concentration.[180] Comparative analyses of these methods can be found elsewhere.[179,198]

Semiautomated Heuristic Methods

Alternatively, contrast enhancement can be quantified in terms of heuristic parameters such as maximum enhancement (ME), initial rate of enhancement (IRE), and time of onset of enhancement (T_{onset}). These heuristic parameters have been seen to correlate with pharmacokinetic measurements of inflammation.[176–178] In contrast to pharmacokinetic parameters, heuristic estimation is relatively straightforward and fast. Most such analyses have examined individual signal intensity curves derived from user-defined regions of interest (ROI) analyses or on voxel-by-voxel basis. Currently, for the MCP joints and wrist studies dynamic curves are calculated from an approximately 2–3 mm^2 ROI positioned in the area of maximal visual enhancement.[199] Measurements of IRE and

ME contain both spatial and temporal information,[200] which means that the validity of an ROI analysis relies on the position and size of the ROI, as its misplacement might result in a 20–30% difference in measurements.[199,200] This reflects an interpretive vulnerability and implies poor reproducibility of the techniques that describe the shape of the enhancement curves.[180]

In spite of these limitations, DCE-MRI was able to differentiate RA patients with high and intermediate disease activity from those in remission and from normal controls. The degree of enhancement of the synovial membrane correlated significantly with several clinical markers (number of tender and swollen joints, Ritchie's index, health assessment questionnaire) and laboratory (ESR, CRP) parameters, and with the disease activity score, a composite index of disease activity. This technique can also be used to evaluate possible differences among different types of arthritis.[201]

A semiautomated approach proposed for DCE-MRI data of the analysis of MCP joints[196] was the first attempt to perform quantitative analyses objectively. It uses the commercially available software ANALYZE[202] for manual segmentation and identification of tissues of interest. Signal intensity versus time curves are normalized over a mean baseline computed from the first three values, and their geometrical properties such as height and slope are considered. The normalized signal is

$$b = \sum_{t=1}^{3} \frac{I(t)}{3}, \hat{I}(t) = \frac{I(t)}{b}, t = 1 \ldots T. \quad (1)$$

In Eq. (1) T is the number of dynamic frames in the temporal slice; no enhancement is expected in the first three, so they are often taken as a baseline.

To assess the extent of RA, ME, IRE, and T_{onset} are computed from the enhancement curves. The parameters are estimated by passing an averaging window of length $n = 5$ (a number found empirically for the MCP data[196]) over the signal intensity versus time curve and determining the gradient of the linear best fit in each window.[196] The maximal such gradient is taken as IRE, and the instant at which this occurs is recorded as the time of onset of enhancement T_{onset}. ME is found as a maximum of mean intensity values calculated in each window.

At this stage, pixels in which signal intensity vs. time curves exhibit $T_{onset} > 60$ s or ME < 1.2 are regarded as unlikely to be of clinical interest as either the uptake has not been appreciable or the behavior is outside of the expected time interval.[196] This permits the measurement of N_{total}, the total number of enhancing pixels, which allows for assessment of a patient's condition. The disadvantage of this method is that the manual selection of thresholding requires participation of a human operator, which makes the results subjective. Moreover, the size of the moving window depends heavily on the degree of noise present in the data, the scanning equipment, and the time-course of the arrival of the contrast agent,[196,203] and has to be adjusted to process the data acquired by a particular scanner or at fixed acquisition settings (as different scanners generate data of different noise levels). This implies manual intervention, which makes the results subjective. This method has not been evaluated for clinical use.

Computer-Aided Heuristic Approach

A fully automated method for quantitative analysis of DCE-MRI data was recently proposed.[2,197] The method incorporates automated efficient preprocessing techniques that allow for the segmentation of the areas of no interest, such as background and markers, and efficient alignment of three-dimensional volumes within the DCE-MRI study, thus reducing the artifacts caused by patient's motion.

Further, pixels in a temporal slice are classified according to the behavior of normalized signal intensity versus time curves, which may be explained by underlying phases of the data acquisition. Starting from a baseline, the perfused tissues absorb the contrast agent and their

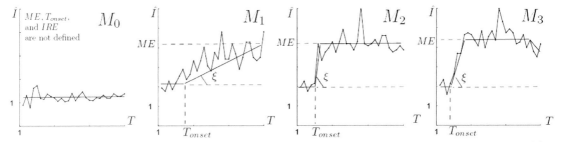

Figure 5. Estimation of heuristics for each approximation model: M_0–M_3. ME has not been reached for model M_1. ξ is the slope of the normalized signal intensity versus time curve $\hat{I}$ that is taken as IRE.

intensity increases (wash-in phase); the intensity usually increases up to a certain point and then exhibits a plateau (of variable width) followed by a wash-out phase (gradual signal intensity decrease). This knowledge of the underlying temporal pattern of the contrast agent uptake was used to classify and approximate signal intensity versus time curves as an aid to noise reduction.

The authors suggest classifying all tissues into four classes:

- M_0: Negligible enhancement. Some tissues within cortical and trabecular bone, inactive joints, skin, and areas unaffected by disease do not absorb Gd-DTPA and are not expected to show intensity enhancement in the later frames of temporal slices.
- M_1: Base/wash-in. There is often a proportion of curves in which the maximal intensity has not been reached by the end of the scanning procedure, indicating constant leakage into locally available extracellular space. The Gd-DPTA absorption and signal intensity versus time curves enhancement continues after the scanning has been completed.
- M_2: Base/wash-in/plateau. Full absorption of the Gd-DTPA by the tissues.
- M_3: Base/wash-in/plateau/wash-out. The wash-out phase is observed at the end of the scanning procedure.

To decide on the "best" model for a particular voxel, a statistical test was employed.[204] When individual curves are approximated by one of the models, it is the parameters of maximum enhancement, initial rate of enhancement, and time of onset of enhancement that are extracted rather than the raw data. This, in addition to the motion correction algorithm employed earlier, reduces the influence of noise. When parameters are estimated for each pixel, they can be presented in the form of parametric maps that depict activation events.

In parametric mapping of Gd-DTPA uptake, each voxel is color coded according to the model it has assumed: M_0, no color; M_1, red; M_2, green; and M_3, blue. Voxels allocated within blood vessels usually assume M_3, indicating the presence of the wash-out phase. An affected area is split into several clusters of blue and green, with some areas being colored red, which allows identification of tissues in which there was no peak in signal intensity during the acquisition of DCE-MRI data. Such imaging allows assessment of the Gd-DTPA kinetics and tissue behavior classification based on the temporal pattern of the contrast agent uptake. Brighter colors (white-yellow) correspond to perfused tissue with high values of ME and IRE; darker colors (dark-red) indicate tissue with mild perfusion. Parametric maps provide information of the spread and magnitude of RA (Fig. 5).

Figure 6 illustrates the Gd-DTPA uptake map and parametric maps of ME and IRE superimposed on the postcontrast DCE-MRI image acquired from the wrist joint of an active RA patient. Owing to the preprocessing techniques employed,[60,205] artifactual enhancement has been minimized in parametric

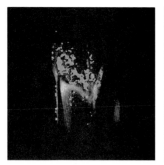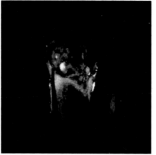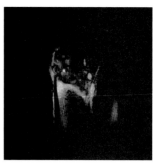

Figure 6. Gd-DTPA uptake and parametric maps of the maximum enhancement and rate of wash-in superimposed on the postcontrast image of the wrist joint acquired from a patient with active RA, using an ESAOTE 0.2-T scanner. The Gd-DTPA uptake map provides information on the classification of the tissues: blue, presence of wash-out; green, intensity plateau; red, continues uptake. Tissues with high maximum enhancement and rate of wash-in are plotted in white-yellow colors and tissues with low parameters are shown in dark red.

maps constructed with this technique and they show preferable characteristics (such as sharpness), permitting easier differentiation of structures of interest.

The technique allows clear discrimination of the tissues based on their degree of perfusion. Distribution of the colored pixels in the parametric maps gives reliable information on the relevant and expected areas of high inflammatory activity. Parametric maps give the reader information on areas where the patient has the most perfusion and provide more comprehensive information regarding localized disease activity. This is valuable for disease diagnosis and guidance of intra-articular therapy. Fully automated counting of the enhanced voxels is used as a statistic for quantification of inflammation. The method was tested on the data acquired with low (0.2- to 0.6-T) and high (1-T, 1.5-T) field scanners from joints representing both healthy controls and active RA patients.[197] The first release of software dedicated to RA data processing, DYNAMIKA™, is available at www.image-analysis.org. Assessment of the algorithm for clinical use in a small pilot study was published[197] and is a work in progress.

Parametric Mapping from the Patient

Region-of-interest-based methods provide a compact representation of the results, but they lack spatial resolution and are prone to partial volume averaging errors. To visualize the extent of inflammation, both heuristic and kinetic parameters can be presented in the form of parametric maps, which are two-dimensional images depicting these parameters. Thus, a parametric map is a two-dimensional representation of a chosen property of interest (e.g., ME, IRE) superimposed on the anatomy image.

The first mention of parametric maps can be dated back to the late 1980s–early 1990s, when they were first used for DCE-MRI data analysis acquired in preclinical contrast agent trials. Later in the 1990s, clinical trials were performed on patients,[189–191,195] culminating in the modern definition of such maps.[206–210]

The value of the parametric mapping technique lies in the speed and ease of interpretation of DCE-MRI data sets and its simple display, suitable for clinical interpretation even by nonexperts. Parametric maps can depict quantitative enhancement information as a color map exactly coregistered with anatomic images on a pixel-by-pixel basis. This type of display has a number of advantages, including an appreciation of the heterogeneity of enhancement and elimination of the need for selective placement of user-defined ROIs. The risk of missing important diagnostic information and of creating ROIs that contain more than one tissue type is thus reduced. Figure 7 illustrates parametric maps constructed for dynamic temporal slices

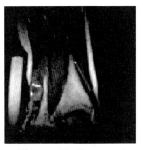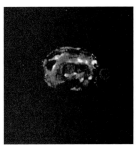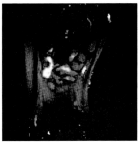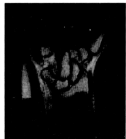

Figure 7. Parametric maps of maximum enhancement acquired from an RA patient's tendon, wrist, and hand. *Far right:* parametric map constructed for a dynamic slice acquired from a healthy control. Brighter colors (white-yellow) correspond to higher activity, dark red colors to lower.

acquired from a tendon, MCP joint, and wrist of an RA patient and the wrist of a healthy control with DYNAMIKA^{TM}.[197] The benefits of parametric mapping are obvious; however, the technique is not widely adopted in medical practice. There are no established standards for assessment of quality of the parametric maps that might delineate the degree of noise that is acceptable and how well a parametric map reflects activation events.

Summary

Disease activity in RA can be quantitatively expressed in terms of inflammatory activity or joint damage. Several damage scores have been developed, each having specific characteristics for reproducibility and sensitivity to change.

The most commonly used methods for assessment of X-ray data are Sharp, Larsen, and van der Heijde/Sharp scores, and their variants. The Sharp-based techniques provide separate scores for erosions and for joint space narrowing; the Larsen and its variants provide an overall score. Analysis of posteroanterior radiographs of the hand and foot and the use of multiple trained readers is standard. Reported intra- and interrater reliability values are generally higher than 0.70 and the sensitivity to change (normally measured with a standardized response mean) is higher than 0.8.[129]

Conclusions based upon disease activity and progression data derived from X-ray analysis might be problematic.[166,211,212] First, soft tissue changes cannot be classified adequately since they are not sufficiently well depicted on conventional radiographs, so advanced stages of RA are overrepresented when graded with conventional radiography.[213] Second, methods for scoring radiographic damage concentrate on the hands and feet, whereas damage in larger joints may be of equal importance for a patient's functional ability.[214]

Several prospective follow-up imaging studies performed to compare radiography, US, and MRI findings demonstrate that US and MRI are more sensitive for visualization of inflammatory and destructive changes in joints and have major potential for improved examination compared to X-ray. Both US and MRI are in good agreement with clinical findings.[215–217]

Doppler US is an emerging technology that may provide a noninvasive assessment of disease processes by measuring the vascularity of the musculoskeletal system. Doppler technique with and without an echo-enhancing contrast agent may be helpful for evaluation and quantification of disease activity.[141,218] Currently, this technology is being used mainly to evaluate patients with RA. Evaluation of pannus, pannus differentiation (hypervascular, hypovascular, and avascular), and assessment of intraarticular vascularization can be performed. Several authors have made use of quantitative and semiquantitative analyses of synovial volume, more or less effectively linking it to disease activity. In RA, the clinical evaluation showed only weak to moderate correlation. This, however, may be due to the failure of clinical examination to detect mild synovitis as opposed to the highly sensitive US Doppler. The measurement process with the Doppler technique is time-consuming and highly subjective, being dependent on both the opinion of the operator and the equipment used, so the technique might not be appropriate for routine use.

Ultrasound measurements are still in need of thorough scientific principles of design with selected statistical methods to describe and quantify the findings. In US studies, both acquisition and data interpretation phases have to be evaluated, particularly in regard to their reliability and responsiveness.[151] Without confidence in these measurement characteristics, the utility of Doppler US is compromised.

MRI is well suited to providing quantitative measurements in RA because of its ability to visualize bone and soft tissues in three dimensions. The OMERACT scoring system has been validated and allows straightforward evaluation of bone erosions, bone marrow edema, and synovial volume, all of which predict erosion progression.[165] The disadvantage of such quantification is that it relies heavily on the experience of the reader and is time-consuming. Certain artifacts occurring in the images might be easily interpreted by an experienced reader, but would present difficulties for the less experienced observer.[219] There is also no visual representation of the scoring results. Volume measurements are often performed directly by manually outlining the inflamed synovium or erosions, which is a very time-consuming operation that would greatly benefit from development of semiautomated and automated techniques.

DCE-MRI has emerged as a promising modality for evaluation of disease activity and response to treatment. Using new methods for quantification of the results such as kinetic[198] and heuristic[2] modeling can allow for semi- and fully automated assessment of disease activity. The advantage of the new methods is that they often include preprocessing techniques, which

are designed to reduce artifacts due to the patient's movements, permit automated extraction of tissues of interest, and, ultimately, quantification of disease activity. This ensures high sensitivity and reproducibility of the results, removes human bias from evaluation, and saves time and resources.

A number of studies suggest that measurements made from the enhancement curve are sensitive to various physiological parameters, including synovial perfusion and capillary permeability. Consequently, they are expected to be good markers for inflammation in RA.

Conclusion

A major goal driving the development of new imaging techniques and scoring methods is to identify the most appropriate treatment for RA and OA. Traditional imaging in the form of plain film radiography has historically been used in RA and OA research. There are many published studies regarding the efficacy of disease-modifying drugs that have considered radiographic damage in the form of erosions without employing imaging other than radiographs as surrogate markers of structural efficacy. Recently, it has been demonstrated that erosions are seen in 10–26% of patients within 3 months of disease onset and are present in 75% of patients within 2 years.[220] Unfortunately, in RA, changes appear on the radiograph with a delay up to a year and only after a considerable loss of bone.[221]

In the light of rapidly evolving research in OA and RA, new imaging techniques such as MRI and US are being used in diagnostic imaging and drug development processes. More studies are now employing sophisticated imaging outcome measures such as Doppler US or DCE-MRI to quantify changes in synovial perfusion. The development of this more advanced imaging has enabled the investigation of the pathological interrelationship between synovitis and bone damage. Qualitative and quantitative analyses of inflammatory synovial tissue, bone marrow edema in rheumatic arthritis, and cartilage thickness in OA are ongoing.

Traditional scoring systems developed for X-ray are not directly applicable to the new data coming out of MRI and US studies. Accepted scoring methods designed for MRI and US are predominantly qualitative and are based on visual assessment of the data with further grading according to a given scale. Such analyses can provide adequate information on the spread and magnitude of the inflammation, but suffer from a lack of objectivity and reproducibility. Emerging quantitative computed-aided methods represent a new approach to monitoring disease activity and evaluating the effect of treatment.

Obviously, extraction of quantitative measurements is not trivial. Several scoring systems for MRI and US have been suggested over the years. Some of them, such as region-of-interest or volume-of-interest methods, lack spatial resolution and are prone to partial volume averaging errors, whereas others, such as OMERACT, Doppler, and volume measurements, are time-consuming and can be influenced by the opinion of the reader. There is compelling evidence that novel pixel-by-pixel-based scoring techniques, such as parametric mapping and kinetic modeling, have great potential for automating scoring processes and delivering objective results. The aim of these new systems is to counteract the limits of traditional evaluation, which is prone to high personnel costs and human errors. Furthermore, replacing time-consuming, tedious scoring techniques with computer-aided methods can potentially save time and resources. More importantly, automated methods are far more objective.

Conflicts of Interest

The authors declare no conflicts of interest.

References

1. Peloschek, P., G. Langs, M. Weber, *et al.* 2007. An automatic model-based system for joint space measurements on hand radiographs: Initial experience. *Radiology* **245:** 855–862.

2. Kubassova, O., R.D. Boyle & A. Radjenovic. 2007. Quantitative analysis of dynamic contrast-enhanced MRI datasets of the metacarpophalangeal joints. *Acad. Radiol.* **14:** 1189–1200.

3. Lorenzo, P., M.T. Bayliss & D. Heinegard. 2004. Altered patterns and synthesis of extracellular matrix macromolecules in early osteoarthritis. *Matrix Biol.* **23:** 381–391.

4. Felson, D.T. 2004. An update on the pathogenesis and epidemiology of osteoarthritis. *Radiol. Clin. N. Am.* **42:** 1–9.

5. Baraliakos, X., J. Davis, W. Tsuji & J. Braun. 2005. Magnetic resonance imaging examinations of the spine in patients with ankylosing spondylitis before and after therapy with the tumor necrosis factor alpha receptor fusion protein etanercept [abstract]. *Arthritis Res. Ther.* **7:** P27.

6. van der Heijde, D., L. Simon, J. Smolen, *et al.* 2002. How to report radiographic data in randomized clinical trials in rheumatoid arthritis: Guidelines from a roundtable discussion. *Arthritis Rheum.* **47:** 215–218.

7. Sharp, J.T., F. Wolfe, M. Lassere, *et al.* 2004. Variability of precision in scoring radiographic abnormalities in rheumatoid arthritis by experienced readers. *J. Rheumatol.* **31:** 1062–1072.

8. Sharp, J.T., M.D. Lidsky, L.C. Collins & J. Moreland. 1971. Methods of scoring the progression of radiologic changes in rheumatoid arthritis. Correlation of radiologic, clinical and laboratory abnormalities. *Arthritis Rheum.* **14:** 706–720.

9. Kellgren, J.H. & J.S. Lawrence. 1957. Radiological assessment of osteo-arthrosis. *Ann. Rheum. Dis.* **16:** 494–502.

10. Hirsch, R., R.J. Fernandes, S.R. Pillemer, *et al.* 1998. Hip osteoarthritis prevalence estimates by three radiographic scoring systems. *Arthritis Rheum.* **41:** 361–368.

11. Madsen, O.R., O. Schaadt, H. Bliddal, *et al.* 1994. Bone mineral distribution of the proximal tibia in gonarthrosis assessed in vivo by photon absorption. *Osteoarthr. Cartilage* **2:** 141–147.

12. Bagge, E., A. Bjelle & A. Svanborg. 1992. Radiographic osteoarthritis in the elderly. A cohort comparison and a longitudinal study of the '70-year old people in Goteborg'. *Clin. Rheumatol.* **11:** 486–491.

13. Cooper, C. 1995. Radiographic atlases for the assessment of osteoarthritis. *Osteoarthr. Cartilage* **3**(A): 1–2.

14. Gunther, K.P. & Y. Sun. 1999. Reliability of radiographic assessment in hip and knee osteoarthritis. *Osteoarthr. Cartilage* **7:** 239–246.

15. Schiphof, D., M. Boers & S.M.A. Bierma-Zeinstra. 2008. Differences in descriptions of Kellgren and Lawrence grades of knee osteoarthritis. *Ann. Rheum. Dis.* Published online, ahead of print: http://ard.bmj.com/cgi/content/abstract/ard.2007.079020v1.

16. Recht, M.P., J. Kramer, S. Marcelis, *et al.* 1993. Abnormalities of articular cartilage in the knee: Analysis of available MR techniques. *Radiology* **187:** 473–478.

17. Recht, M.P., D.W. Piraino, G.A. Paletta, *et al.* 1996. Accuracy of fat-suppressed three-dimensional spoiled gradient-echo FLASH MR imaging in the detection of patellofemoral articular cartilage abnormalities. *Radiology* **198:** 209–212.

18. Felson, D.T., S. McLaughlin, J. Goggins, *et al.* 2003. Bone marrow edema and its relation to progression of knee osteoarthritis. *Ann. Intern. Med.* **139:** 330–336.

19. Eckstein, F., D. Burstein & T.M. Link. 2006. Quantitative MRI of cartilage and bone: Degenerative changes in osteoarthritis. *NMR Biomed.* **19:** 822–854.

20. Bredella, M.A., P.F. Tirman, C.G. Peterfy, *et al.* 1999. Accuracy of T2-weighted fast spin-echo MR imaging with fat saturation in detecting cartilage defects in the knee: Comparison with arthroscopy in 130 patients. *AJR Am. J. Roentgenol.* **172:** 1073–1080.

21. Biswal, S., T. Hastie, T.P. Andriacchi, *et al.* 2002. Risk factors for progressive cartilage loss in the knee: A longitudinal magnetic resonance imaging study in forty-three patients. *Arthritis Rheum.* **46:** 2884–2892.

22. Peterfy, C.G., A. Guermazi, S. Zaim, *et al.* 2004. Whole-organ magnetic resonance imaging score (WORMS) of the knee in osteoarthritis. *Osteoarthr. Cartilage* **12:** 177–190.

23. Ding, C., P. Garnero, F. Cicuttini, *et al.* 2005. Knee cartilage defects: Association with early radiographic osteoarthritis, decreased cartilage volume, increased joint surface area and type II collagen breakdown. *Osteoarthr. Cartilage* **13:** 198–205.

24. Ding, C., F. Cicuttini, F. Scott, *et al.* 2005. Association between age and knee structural change: A cross-sectional MRI based study. *Ann. Rheum. Dis.* **64:** 549–555.

25. Ding, C., F. Cicuttini, F. Scott, *et al.* 2005. Knee structural alteration and BMI: A cross-sectional study. *Obes. Res.* **13:** 350–361.

26. Disler, D.G., T.R. McCauley, C.G. Kelman, *et al.* 1996. Fat-suppressed three-dimensional spoiled gradient-echo MR imaging of hyaline cartilage defects in the knee: Comparison with standard MR imaging and arthroscopy. *AJR Am. J. Roentgenol.* **167:** 127–132.

27. Recht, M.P., D.W. Goodwin, C.S. Winalski & L.M. White. 2005. MRI of articular cartilage: Revisiting current status and future directions. *AJR Am. J. Roentgenol.* **185:** 899–914.

28. Broderick, L.S., D.A. Turner, D.L. Renfrew, *et al.* 1994. Severity of articular cartilage abnormality in patients with osteoarthritis: Evaluation with fast spin-echo MR vs arthroscopy. *AJR Am. J. Roentgenol.* **162:** 99–103.

29. Kawahara, Y., M. Uetani, N. Nakaharaand, *et al.* 1998. Fast spin-echo MR of the articular cartilage in the osteoarthrotic knee. Correlation of MR and arthroscopic findings. *Acta Radiol. Diagn.* **39:** 120–125.

30. Masi, J.N., C.A. Sell, C. Phan, *et al.* 2005. Cartilage MR imaging at 3.0 versus that at 1.5 T: Preliminary results in a porcine model. *Radiology* **236:** 140–150.

31. Guermazi, A., S. Zaim, B. Taouli, *et al.* 2003. MR findings in knee osteoarthritis. *Eur. Radiol.* **13:** 1370–1386.

32. Wang, Y., C. Ding, A.E. Wluka, *et al.* 2006. Factors affecting progression of knee cartilage defects in normal subjects over 2 years. *Rheumatology* **45:** 79–84.

33. Peyron, J.C. 1986. Osteoarthritis: The epidemiologic viewpoint. *Clin. Orthop.* **213:** 13–19.

34. Sarzi-Puttini, P., M.A. Cimmino, R. Scarpa, *et al.* 2005. Osteoarthritis: An overview of the disease and its treatment strategies. *Semin. Arthritis Rheum.* **35:** 1–10.

35. Roemer, F.W., A. Guermazi, J.A. Lynch, *et al.* 2005. Short tau inversion recovery and proton density-weighted fat suppressed sequences for the evaluation of osteoarthritis of the knee with a 1.0T dedicated extremity MRI: Development of a time-efficient sequence protocol. *Eur. Radiol.* **15:** 978–987.

36. Kornaat, P.R., R.Y. Ceulemans, H.M. Kroon, *et al.* 2005. MRI assessment of knee osteoarthritis: Knee osteoarthritis scoring system (KOSS)—interobserver and intra-observer reproducibility of a compartment-based scoring system. *Skeletal Radiol.* **34:** 95–102.

37. Conaghan, P.G., D. Hunter, A. Tennant, *et al.* 2004. Evaluation an MRI scoring system for osteoarthritis of the knee using modern psychometric approaches [abstract]. *Osteoarthr. Cartilage* **12**(B): S118.

38. Eckstein, F. 2004. Noninvasive study of human cartilage structure by MRI. *Methods Mol. Med.* **101:** 191–217.

39. Hunter, D.J., G.H. Lo, D. Gale, *et al.* 2008. The reliability of a new scoring system for knee osteoarthritis MRI and the validity of bone marrow lesion assessment: BLOKS (Boston-Leeds osteoarthritis knee score). *Ann. Rheum. Dis.* **67:** 206–211.

40. Cohen, B.Z.A., D.M. McCarthy, S.D. Kwark, *et al.* 1999. Knee cartilage topography, thickness and contact areas from MRI: In-vitro calibration and in-vivo measurements. *Osteoarthr. Cartilage* **7:** 95–109.

41. Ateshian, G.A., L.J. Soslowsky & V.C. Mow. 1991. Quantitation of articular surface topography and cartilage thickness in knee joints using stereophotogrammetry. *J. Biomech.* **24:** 761–776.

42. Millington, S., G. Markus, R. Wozelka, *et al.* 2006. Quantification of ankle articular cartilage topography and thickness using a high resolution stereophotography system. *Osteoarthr. Cartilage* **15:** 205–211.

43. Hohe, J., G. Ateshian, M. Reiser, *et al.* 2002. Surface size, curvature analysis and assessment of knee joint incongruity with MRI in vivo. *Magn. Reson. Imaging* **47:** 554–561.

44. Cohen, Z.A., H. Roglic, R.P. Grelsamer, *et al.* 2001. Patellofemoral stresses during open and closed kinetic chain exercises. An analysis using computer simulation. *Am. J. Sport Med.* **29:** 480–487.

45. Cohen, Z.A., J.H. Henry, D.M. McCarthy, *et al.* 2003. Computer simulations of patellofemoral joint surgery: Patient-specific models for tuberosity transfer. *Am. J. Sport Med.* **31:** 87–98.

46. Eckstein, F., G. Ateshian, R. Burgkart, *et al.* 2006. Proposal for a nomenclature for magnetic resonance imaging based measures of articular cartilage in osteoarthritis. *Osteoarthr. Cartilage* **14:** 974–983.

47. Peterfy, C.G., C.F. van Dijke, D.L. Janzen, *et al.* 1994. Quantification of articular cartilage in the knee with pulsed saturation transfer subtraction and fat-suppressed MR imaging: Optimization and validation. *Radiology* **192:** 485–491.

48. Eckstein, F., I.A. Gavazzen, H. Sittek, *et al.* 1996. Determination of knee joint cartilage thickness using three-dimensional magnetic resonance chondro-crassometry (3D MR-CCM). *Magnet. Reson. Med.* **36:** 256–265.

49. Piplani, M.A., D.G. Disler, T.R. McCauley, *et al.* 1996. Articular cartilage volume in the knee: Semiautomated determination from three-dimensional reformations of MR images. *Radiology* **198:** 855–859.

50. Eckstein, F., M. Schnier, M. Haubner, *et al.* 1998. Accuracy of cartilage volume and thickness measurements with magnetic resonance imaging. *Clin. Orthop. Relat. R.* **352:** 137–148.

51. Kshirsagar, A.A., P.J. Watson, J.A. Tyler & L.D. Hall. 1998. Measurement of localized cartilage volume and thickness of human knee joints by computer analysis of three-dimensional magnetic resonance images. *Invest. Radiol.* **33:** 289–299.

52. Solloway, S., C. Hutchinson, J. Waterton & C. Taylor. 1997. The use of active shape models for making thickness measurements of articular cartilage from MR images. *Magnet. Reson. Med.* **37:** 943–952.

53. Kauffmann, C., P. Gravel, B. Godbout, *et al.* 2003. Computer-aided method for quantification of cartilage thickness and volume changes using MRI: Validation study using a synthetic model. *IEEE T. Bio-Med. Eng.* **50:** 978–988.

54. Burgkart, R., C. Glaser, A. Hyhlik-Dürr, *et al.* 2001. Magnetic resonance imaging-based assessment of cartilage loss in severe osteoarthritis: Accuracy, precision and diagnostic value. *Arthritis Rheum.* **44:** 2072–2077.

55. Lynch, J.A., S. Zaim, J. Zhao, *et al.* 2000. Cartilage segmentation of 3D MRI scans of the osteoarthritic knee combining user knowledge and active contours. In *SPIE Proceedings on Medical Imaging*: 925–935.

56. Stammberger, T., F. Eckstein, M. Michaelis, *et al.* 1999. Interobserver reproducibility of quantitative cartilage measurements: Comparison of B-spline snakes and manual segmentation. *Magn. Reson. Imaging* **17:** 1033–1042.

57. Vincent, L. & P. Soille. 1991. Watersheds in digital spaces: An efficient algorithm based on immersion simulations. *IEEE T. Pattern Anal.* **13:** 583–598.

58. Fillard, P., X. Pennec, V. Arsigny & N. Ayache. 2007. Clinical DT-MRI estimation, smoothing, and fiber tracking with log-Euclidean metrics. *Med. Imaging* **26:** 1472–1482.

59. Eggers, H., T. Knopp & D. Potts. 2007. Field inhomogeneity correction based on gridding reconstruction for magnetic resonance imaging. *Med. Imaging* **26:** 374–384.

60. Periaswamy, S. & H. Farid. 2006. Medical image registration with partial data. *Med. Image Anal.* **10:** 452–464.

61. Felfoul, O., J.B. Mathieu, G. Beaudoin & S. Martel. 2008. In vivo MR-tracking based on magnetic signature selective excitation. *Med. Imaging* **27:** 28–35.

62. Link, T.M., R. Stahl & K. Woertler. 2007. Cartilage imaging: Motivation, techniques, current and future significance. *Eur. Radiol.* **17:** 1135–1146.

63. Dunn, T.C., Y. Lu, H. Jin, *et al.* 2004. T_2 relaxation time of cartilage at MR imaging: Comparison with severity of knee osteoarthritis. *Radiology* **232:** 592–598.

64. Glaser, C. 2005. New techniques for cartilage imaging: T_2 relaxation time and diffusion-weighted MR imaging. *Radiol. Clin. North Am.* **43:** 641–653.

65. Mosher, T.J., H.E. Smith, C. Collins, *et al.* 2005. Change in knee cartilage T_2 at MR imaging after running: A feasibility study. *Radiology* **234:** 245–249.

66. Stahl, R., G. Blumenkrantz, J. Carballido-Gamio, *et al.* 2007. MRI-derived T_2 relaxation times and cartilage morphometry of the tibio-femoral joint in

subjects with and without osteoarthritis during a 1-year follow-up. *Osteoarthr. Cartilage* **15:** 1225–1234.

67. Koff, M.F., K.K. Amrami & K.R. Kaufman. 2007. Clinical evaluation of T_2 values of patellar cartilage in patients with osteoarthritis. *Osteoarthr. Cartilage* **15:** 198–204.

68. Bashir, A., M.L. Gray, R.D. Boutin & D. Burstein. 1997. Glycosaminoglycan in articular cartilage: In vivo assessment with delayed Gd-DTPA-enhanced MR imaging. *Radiology* **205:** 551–558.

69. Boesen, M., K.E. Jensen, E. Qvistgaard, *et al.* 2006. Delayed gadolinium-enhanced magnetic resonance imaging (dGEMRIC) of hip joint cartilage: Better cartilage delineation after intra-articular than intravenous gadolinium injection. *Acta Radiol.* **47:** 391–396.

70. Kwack, K.S., J.H. Cho, M.M. Kim, *et al.* 2008. Comparison study of intraarticular and intravenous gadolinium-enhanced magnetic resonance imaging of cartilage in a canine model. *Acta Radiol.* **49:** 65–74.

71. Bashir, A., M.L. Gray & D. Burstein. 1996. Gd-DTPA as a measure of cartilage degradation. *Magnet. Reson. Med.* **36:** 665–673.

72. Tiderius, C.J., J. Svensson, P. Leander, *et al.* 2004. dGEMRIC (delayed gadolinium-enhanced MRI of cartilage) indicates adaptive capacity of human knee cartilage. *Magnet. Reson. Med.* **51:** 286–290.

73. Tiderius, C.J., L.E. Olsson, F. Nyquist & L. Dahlberg. 2005. Cartilage glycosaminoglycan loss in the acute phase after an anterior cruciate ligament injury: Delayed gadolinium-enhanced magnetic resonance imaging of cartilage and synovial fluid analysis. *Arthritis Rheum.* **52:** 120–127.

74. Williams, A., L. Sharma, C.A. McKenzie, *et al.* 2005. Delayed gadolinium-enhanced magnetic resonance imaging of cartilage in knee osteoarthritis: Findings at different radiographic stages of disease and relationship to malalignment. *Arthritis Rheum.* **52:** 3528–3535.

75. Williams, A., B. Mikulis, N. Krishnan, *et al.* 2007. Suitability of T1 Gd as the 'dGEMRIC index' at 1.5T and 3.0T. *Magnet. Reson. Med.* **58:** 830–834.

76. Williams, A., S.K. Shetty, D. Burstein, *et al.* 2008. Delayed gadolinium enhanced MRI of cartilage (dGEMRIC) of the first carpometacarpal (1CMC) joint: A feasibility study. *Osteoarthr. Cartilage* **16:** 530–532.

77. Williams, A., A. Gillis, C. McKenzie, *et al.* 2004. Glycosaminoglycan distribution in cartilage as determined by delayed gadolinium-enhanced MRI of cartilage (dGEMRIC): Potential clinical applications. *AJR Am. J. Roentgenol.* **182:** 167–172.

78. Burstein, D., J.H. Velyvis, K.T. Scott, *et al.* 2001. Protocol issues for delayed Gd(DTPA)-enhanced MRI (dGEMRIC) for clinical evaluation of articular cartilage. *Magnet. Reson. Med.* **45:** 36–41.

79. Kim, Y.J., D. Jaramillo, M.B. Millis, *et al.* 2003. Assessment of early osteoarthritis in hip dysplasia with delayed gadolinium-enhanced magnetic resonance imaging of cartilage. *J. Bone Joint Surg.* **85:** 1987–1992.

80. Tiderius, C.J., L.E. Olsson, P. Leander, *et al.* 2003. Delayed gadolinium-enhanced MRI of cartilage (dGEMRIC) in early knee osteoarthritis. *Magnet. Reson. Med.* **49:** 488–492.

81. Hohe, J., S. Faber, T. Stammberger, *et al.* 2000. A technique for 3D in vivo quantification of proton density and magnetization transfer coefficients of knee joint cartilage. *Osteoarthr. Cartilage* **8:** 426–433.

82. Hohe, J., S. Faber, M. Reiser, *et al.* 2002. Three-dimensional analysis and visualization of regional MR signal intensity distribution of articular cartilage. *Med. Eng. Phys.* **24:** 219–227.

83. Kimelman, T., A. Vu, P. Storey, *et al.* 2006. Three-dimensional T_1 mapping for dGEMRIC at 3.0T using the Look Locker method. *Invest. Radiol.* **41:** 198–203.

84. McKenzie, C.A., A. Williams, P.V. Prasad & D. Burstein. 2006. Three-dimensional delayed gadolinium-enhanced MRI of cartilage (dGEMRIC) at 1.5T and 3.0T. *Magn. Reson. Imaging* **24:** 928–933.

85. Trattnig, S., T.C. Mamisch, K. Pinker, *et al.* 2008. Differentiating normal hyaline cartilage from post-surgical repair tissue using fast gradient echo imaging in delayed gadolinium-enhanced MRI (dGEMRIC) at 3 Tesla. *Eur. Radiol.* **18:** 1251–1259.

86. Trattnig, S., S. Marlovits, S. Gebetsroither, *et al.* 2007. Three-dimensional delayed gadolinium-enhanced MRI of cartilage (dGEMRIC) for in vivo evaluation of reparative cartilage after matrix-associated autologous chondrocyte transplantation at 3.0 T: Preliminary results. *Magn. Reson. Imaging* **26:** 974–982.

87. Qvistgaard, E., S. Torp-Pedersen, R. Christensen & H. Bliddal. 2006. Reproducibility and inter-reader agreement of a scoring system for ultrasound evaluation of hip osteoarthritis. *Ann. Rheum. Dis.* **65:** 1613–1619.

88. Hattori, K., K. Mori, T. Habata, *et al.* 2003. Measurement of the mechanical condition of articular cartilage with an ultrasonic probe: Quantitative evaluation using wavelet transformation. *Clin. Biomech.* **18:** 553–557.

89. Disler, D.G., E. Raymond, D.A. May, *et al.* 2000. Articular cartilage defects: In vitro evaluation of accuracy and interobserver reliability for detection and grading with US. *Radiology* **215:** 846–851.

90. Laasanen, M.S., S. Saarakkala, J. Toyras, *et al*. 2005. Site-specific ultrasound reflection properties and superficial collagen content of bovine knee articular cartilage. *Phys. Med. Biol.* **50:** 3221–3233.

91. Laasanen, M.S., J. Toyras, A. Vasara, *et al*. 2006. Quantitative ultrasound imaging of spontaneous repair of porcine cartilage. *Osteoarthr. Cartilage* **14:** 258–263.

92. Saarakkala, S., M.S. Laasanen, J.S. Jurvelin & J. Toyras. 2006. Quantitative ultrasound imaging detects degenerative changes in articular cartilage surface and subchondral bone. *Phys. Med. Biol.* **51:** 5333–5346.

93. Spriet, M.P., C.A. Girard, S.F. Foster, *et al*. 2005. Validation of a 40 MHz B-scan ultrasound biomicroscope for the evaluation of osteoarthritis lesions in an animal model. *Osteoarthr. Cartilage* **13:** 171–179.

94. Laasanen, M.S., J. Toyras, A.I. Vasara, *et al*. 2003. Mechano-acoustic diagnosis of cartilage degeneration and repair. *J. Bone Joint Surg.* **85:** 78–84.

95. Dougados, M., X. Ayral, V. Listrat, *et al*. 1994. The SFA system for assessing articular cartilage lesions at arthroscopy of the knee. *Arthroscopy* **10:** 69–77.

96. Brismar, B.H., T. Wredmark, T. Movin, *et al*. 2002. Observer reliability in the arthroscopic classification of osteoarthritis of the knee. *J. Bone Joint Surg.* **84B:** 42–47.

97. Li, X., S. Martin, C. Pitris, *et al*. 2004. High-resolution optical coherence tomographic imaging of osteoarthritic cartilage during open knee surgery. *Arthritis Res. Ther.* **26:** 627–635.

98. Garon, M., A. Legare, R. Guardo, *et al*. 2002. Streaming potentials maps are spatially resolved indicators of amplitude, frequency and ionic strength dependant responses of articular cartilage to load. *J. Biomech.* **35:** 207–216.

99. Bae, W., C. Lewis, M. Levenston & R. Sah. 2006. Indentation testing of human articular cartilage: Effects of probe tip geometry and indentation depth on intra-tissue strain. *J. Biomech.* **39:** 1039–1047.

100. Jaffre, B., A. Watrin, D. Loeuille, *et al*. 2003. Effects of antiinflammatory drugs on arthritic cartilage: A high-frequency quantitative ultrasound study in rats. *Arthritis Rheum.* **48:** 1594–1601.

101. Laasanen, M.S., J. Toyras, J. Hirvonen, *et al*. 2003. Novel mechano-acoustic technique and instrument for diagnosis of cartilage degeneration. *Physiol. Meas.* **23:** 491–503.

102. Suh, J.-K.F., I. Youn & F.H. Fu. 2001. An in situ calibration of an ultrasound transducer: A potential application for an ultrasonic indentation test of articular cartilage. *J Biomech.* **34:** 1347–1353.

103. Silman, A.J. & J.E. Pearson. 2002. Epidemiology and genetics of rheumatoid arthritis. *J. Arthritis Res. Ther.* **4:** S265–S272.

104. Gabriel, S.E. 2001. The epidemiology of rheumatoid arthritis. *Radiol. Clin. North Am.* **27:** 269–281.

105. Arnett, F.C., S.M. Edworthy, D.A. Bloch, *et al*. 1988. The American Rheumatism Association 1987 revised criteria for the classification of rheumatoid arthritis. *Arthritis Rheum.* **31:** 315–324.

106. Prevoo, M.L.L., P.L.C.M. van Riel, M.A. Van't Hof, *et al*. 1993. Validity and reliability of joint indices: A longitudinal study in patients with recent onset rheumatoid arthritis. *Rheumatology* **32:** 589–594.

107. Hart, L.E., P. Tugwell, W.W. Buchanan, *et al*. 1985. Grading of tenderness as a source of interrater error in the Ritchie articular index. *J. Rheumatol.* **12:** 716–717.

108. Scott, D.L., E.H.S. Choy, A. Greeves, *et al*. 1996. Standardising joint assessment in rheumatoid arthritis. *Clin. Rheumatol.* **15:** 579–582.

109. Hernandez-Cruz, B. & M.H. Cardiel. 1998. Intraobserver reliability of commonly used outcome measures in rheumatoid arthritis. *Clin. Exp. Rheumatol.* **16:** 459–462.

110. Fuchs, H.A., R.H. Brooks, L.F. Callahan & T. Pincus. 1989. A simplified twenty-eight-joint quantitative articular index in rheumatoid arthritis. *Arthritis Rheum.* **35:** 531–537.

111. Smolen, J.S., G. Eberl, F.C. Breedveld, *et al*. 1995. Validity and reliability of the twenty-eight-joint count for the assessment of rheumatoid arthritis activity. *Arthritis Rheum.* **38:** 38–43.

112. Symmons, D.P.M., A.B. Hassell, K.A.N. Gunatillaka, *et al*. 1995. Development and preliminary assessment of a simple measure of overall status in rheumatoid arthritis (OSRA) for routine clinical use. *Int. J. Med.* **88:** 429–437.

113. Cranney, A., R. Goldstein, B. Pham, *et al*. 1999. A measure of limited joint motion and deformity correlates with HLA-DRB1 and DQB1 alleles in patients with rheumatoid arthritis. *Ann. Rheum. Dis.* **58:** 703–708.

114. Spiegel, T.M., J.N. Spiegel & H.E. Paulus. 1987. The joint alignment and motion scale: A simple measure of joint deformity in patients with rheumatoid arthritis. *J. Rheumatol.* **14:** 887–892.

115. Ferraz, M.B., L.M. Oliviera, P.M.P. Araujo, *et al*. 1990. EPM-ROM scale: An evaluative instrument to be used in rheumatoid arthritis trials. *Clin. Exp. Rheumatol.* **8:** 491–494.

116. Zijlstra, T.R., H.J. Bernelot-Moens & M.A.S. Bukhari. 2002. The rheumatoid arthritis articular damage score: First steps in developing a clinical index of long term damage in RA. *Ann. Rheum. Dis.* **61:** 20–23.

117. Thorsen, H., T.M. Hansen, S.P. McKenna, *et al*. 2001. Adaptation into Danish of the Stanford health assessment questionnaire (HAQ) and the

rheumatoid arthritis quality of life scale (RAQoL). *Scand. J. Rheumatol.* **30:** 103–109.

118. Welsing, P.M., A.M.M. van Gestel, H.L.M. Swinkels, *et al.* 2001. The relationship between disease activity, joint destruction, and functional capacity over the course of rheumatoid arthritis. *Arthritis Rheum.* **44:** 2009–2017.

119. Danneskiold-Samsøe, B. & G. Grimby. 1986. Isokinetic and isometric muscle strength in patients with rheumatoid arthritis: The relationship to clinical parameters and the influence of corticosteroid. *Clin. Radiol.* **5:** 459–467.

120. Schiottz-Christensen, B., K. Lyngberg, N. Keiding, *et al.* 2001. Use of isokinetic muscle strength as a measure of severity of rheumatoid arthritis: A comparison of this assessment method for RA with other assessment methods for the disease. *Clin. Radiol.* **20:** 423–427.

121. Scott, D.L., C. Antoni, E.H. Choy & P.C.L.M. van Riel. 2003. Joint counts in routine practice. *Rheumatology* **42:** 919–923.

122. Sharp, J.T., D.Y. Young, G.B. Bluhm, *et al.* 1985. How many joints in the hands and wrists should be included in a score of radiologic abnormalities used to assess rheumatoid arthritis? *Arthritis Rheum.* **28:** 1326–1335.

123. Sharp, J.T., G.B. Bluhm, A. Brook, *et al.* 1985. Reproducibility of multiple-observer scoring of radiologic abnormalities in the hands and wrists of patients with rheumatoid arthritis. *Arthritis Rheum.* **28:** 16–24.

124. Genant, H.K., Y. Jiang, C. Peterfy, *et al.* 1998. Assessment of rheumatoid arthritis using a modified scoring method on digitized and original radiographs. *Arthritis Rheum.* **41:** 1583–1590.

125. Edmonds, J., A. Saudan, M. Lassere & D.L. Scott. 1999. Introduction to reading radiographs by the Scott modification of the Larsen method. *J. Rheumatol.* **26:** 740–742.

126. Rau, R. & G. Herborn. 1995. A modified version of Larsen's scoring method to assess radiologic changes in rheumatoid arthritis. *J. Rheumatol.* **22:** 1976–1982.

127. Rau, R., S. Wassenberg, G. Herborn, *et al.* 1998. A new method of scoring radiographic change in rheumatoid arthritis. *J. Rheumatol.* **25:** 2094–2106.

128. Matsuno, H., K. Yudoh, T. Hanyu, *et al.* 2003. Quantitative assessment of hand radiographs of rheumatoid arthritis: Interobserver variation in a multicenter radiographic study. *J. Orthop. Sci.* **8:** 467–473.

129. Boini, S. & F. Guillemin. 2001. Radiographic scoring methods as outcome measures in rheumatoid arthritis: Properties and advantages. *Ann. Rheum. Dis.* **60:** 817–827.

130. Van der Heijde, D. 2000. How to read radiographs according to the Sharp/van der Heijde method. *J. Rheumatol.* **27:** 261–263.

131. Swinkels, H.L., R.F. Laan, M.A. Van't Hof, *et al.* 2001. Modified sharp method: Factors influencing reproducibility and variability. *Semin. Arthritis Rheu.* **31:** 176–190.

132. Wassenberg, S., G. Herborn, S. Fischer & R. Rau. 1994. Comparison of Larsen's and Sharp's method of scoring radiographs in rheumatoid arthritis. *Arthritis Rheum.* **37:** S250.

133. Bottcher, J., A. Pfeil, A. Rosholm, *et al.* 2006. Computerized quantification of joint space narrowing and periarticular demineralization in patients with rheumatoid arthritis based on digital x-ray radiogrammetry. *Invest. Radiol.* **41:** 36–44.

134. Finckh, A., P. de Pablo, J.N. Katz, *et al.* 2006. Performance of an automated computer-based scoring method to assess joint space narrowing in rheumatoid arthritis: A longitudinal study. *Arthritis Rheum.* **54:** 1444–1450.

135. Goligher, E.C., J. Duryea, M.H. Liang, *et al.* 2006. Radiographic joint space width in the fingers of patients with rheumatoid arthritis of less than one year's duration. *Arthritis Rheum.* **54:** 1440–1443.

136. Langs, G., P. Peloschek, H. Bischof & F. Kainberger. 2007. Model-based erosion spotting and visualization in rheumatoid arthritis. *Acad. Radiol.* **14:** 1179–1188.

137. Cootes, T., C. Taylor, D. Cooper & J. Graham. 1995. Active shape models—their training and application. *Comput. Vis. Image Und.* **61:** 38–59.

138. Wakefield, R.J., W.W. Gibbon, P.G. Conaghan, *et al.* 2000. The value of sonography in the detection of bone erosions in patients with rheumatoid arthritis. *Arthritis Rheum.* **43:** 2762–2770.

139. Backhaus, M., G.R. Burmester, D. Sandrock, *et al.* 2002. Prospective two year follow up study comparing novel and conventional imaging procedures in patients with arthritic finger joints. *Ann. Rheum. Dis.* **61:** 895–904.

140. Grassi, W., E. Filippucci, A. Farina, *et al.* 2001. Ultrasonography in the evaluation of bone erosions. *Ann. Rheum. Dis.* **60:** 98–103.

141. Terslev, L., S. Torp-Pedersen, E. Qvistgaard, *et al.* 2003. Estimation of inflammation by Doppler ultrasound: Quantitative changes after intra-articular treatment in rheumatoid arthritis. *Ann. Rheum. Dis.* **62:** 1049–1053.

142. Balint, P.V., D. Kane, H. Wilson, *et al.* 2002. Ultrasonography of entheseal insertions in the lower limb in spondyloarthropathy. *Ann. Rheum. Dis.* **61:** 905–910.

143. Scheel, A.K., K.G.A. Hermann, E. Kahler, *et al.* 2005. A novel ultrasonographic synovitis scoring

system suitable for analyzing finger joint inflammation in rheumatoid arthritis. *Arthritis Rheum.* **52:** 733–743.

144. Ellegaard, K., S. Torp-Pedersen, C.C. Holm, *et al.* 2007. Ultrasound in finger joints: Findings in normal subjects and pitfalls in the diagnosis of synovial disease. *Ultraschall Med.* **28:** 401–408.

145. Strunk, J., P. Klingenberger, K. Strube, *et al.* 2005. Three-dimensional Doppler sonographic vascular imaging in regions with increased MR enhancement in inflamed wrists of patients with rheumatoid arthritis. *Joint Bone Spine* **73:** 518–522.

146. Torp-Pedersen, S.T. & L. Terslev. 2008. Settings and artefacts relevant in colour/power Doppler ultrasound in rheumatology. *Ann. Rheum. Dis.* **67:** 143–149.

147. Freestona, J. & P. Emery. 2007. The role of MRI and ultrasound as surrogate markers of structural efficacy of treatments in rheumatoid arthritis. *Joint Bone Spine* **74:** 227–229.

148. Szkudlarek, M., M. Court-Payen, S. Jacobsen, *et al.* 2003. Interobserver agreement in ultrasonography of the finger and toe joints in rheumatoid arthritis. *Arthritis Rheum.* **48:** 955–962.

149. Wakefield, R.J., W.W. Gibbon & P. Emery. 1999. The current status of ultrasonography in rheumatology. *Rheumatology* **38:** 195–198.

150. Rees, J.D., J. Pilcher, C. Heron & P.D.W. Kiely. 2007. A comparison of clinical vs ultrasound determined synovitis in rheumatoid arthritis utilizing gray-scale, power Doppler and the intravenous microbubble contrast agent 'Sono-Vue'. *Rheumatology* **3:** 454–459.

151. Joshua, F., J. Edmonds & M. Lassere. 2006. Power Doppler ultrasound in musculoskeletal disease: A systematic review. *Semin. Arthritis Rheu.* **36:** 99–108.

152. Backhaus, M., G.-R. Burmester, T. Gerber, *et al.* 2001. Guidelines for musculoskeletal ultrasound in rheumatology. *Ann. Rheum. Dis.* **60:** 641–649.

153. Østergaard, M., C. Peterfy, P. Conaghan, *et al.* 2003. OMERACT rheumatoid arthritis magnetic resonance imaging studies: Core set of MRI acquisitions, joint pathology definitions, and the OMERACT RA-MRI scoring system. *J. Rheumatol.* **30:** 1385–1386.

154. Gilkeson, G., R. Polisson, H. Sinclair, *et al.* 1988. Early detection of carpal erosions in patients with rheumatoid arthritis: A pilot study of magnetic resonance imaging. *J. Rheumatol.* **15:** 1361–1366.

155. Jones, A., M. Regan, J. Ledingham, *et al.* 1993. Importance of placement of intra-articular steroid injections. *Br. Med. J.* **307:** 1329–1330.

156. Bliddal, H. 1999. Placement of intra-articular injections verified by mini air-arthrography. *Ann. Rheum. Dis.* **58:** 641–643.

157. Berna-Serna, J.D., F. Martinez, M. Reus, *et al.* 2006. Wrist arthrography: A simple method. *Eur. Radiol.* **16:** 469–472.

158. Hayashi, N., Y. Watanabe, T. Masumoto, *et al.* 2004. Utilization of low-field MR scanners. *Magnet. Reson. Med.* **3:** 27–38.

159. Bird, P., B. Ejbjerg, M. Lassere, *et al.* 2007. A multireader reliability study comparing conventional high-field magnetic resonance imaging with extremity low-field MRI in rheumatoid arthritis. *J. Rheumatol.* **34:** 854–856.

160. Ejbjerg, B., F. McQueen, M. Lassere, *et al.* 2005. An introduction to the EULAR-OMERACT rheumatoid arthritis MRI reference image atlas. *Ann. Rheum. Dis.* **64:** i23–i47.

161. Ejbjerg, B., F. McQueen, M. Lassere, *et al.* 2005. The EULAR-OMERACT rheumatoid arthritis MRI reference image atlas: The wrist joint. *Ann. Rheum. Dis.* **64:** 23–47.

162. Bird, P., P. Conaghan, B. Ejbjerg, *et al.* 2005. The development of the EULAR-OMERACT rheumatoid arthritis MRI reference image atlas. *Ann. Rheum. Dis.* **64:** i8–i10.

163. Conaghan, P., P. Bird, B. Ejbjerg, *et al.* 2005. The EULAR-OMERACT rheumatoid arthritis MRI reference image atlas: The metacarpophalangeal joints. *Ann. Rheum. Dis.* **64:** i11–i21.

164. McQueen, F., M. Lassere, P. Bird, *et al.* 2007. Developing a magnetic resonance imaging scoring system for peripheral psoriatic arthritis. *J. Rheumatol.* **34:** 859–861.

165. Hodgson, R.J., P. O'Connor & R. Moots. 2008. MRI of rheumatoid arthritis: Image quantitation for the assessment of disease activity, progression and response to therapy. *Rheumatology* **47:** 13–21.

166. Conaghan, P.G., P. O'Connor, D. McGonagle, *et al.* 2003. Elucidation of the relationship between synovitis and bone damage: A randomized magnetic resonance imaging study of individual joints in patients with early rheumatoid arthritis. *Arthritis Rheum.* **48:** 64–71.

167. Østergaard, M., A. Duer, H. Nielsen, *et al.* 2005. Magnetic resonance imaging for accelerated assessment of drug effect and prediction of subsequent radiographic progression in rheumatoid arthritis: A study of patients receiving combined anakinra and methotrexate treatment. *Ann. Rheum. Dis.* **64:** 1503–1506.

168. Palosaari, K., J. Vuotila, R. Takalo, *et al.* 2006. Bone oedema predicts erosive progression on wrist MRI in early RA: A 2-yr observational MRI and NC scintigraphy study. *Rheumatology* **45:** 1542–1548.

169. Klarlund, M., M. Østergaard, E. Rostrup, *et al.* 1999. Dynamic MRI and principal component analysis of finger joints in rheumatoid arthritis,

polyarthritis, and healthy controls. International Society for MRI in Medicine: http://cds.ismrm.org/ismrm-1999/PDF2/409.pdf (last access on 03.05.07).

170. Østergaard, M., M. Stoltenberg, O. Henriksen & I. Lorenzen. 1996. Quantitative assessment of synovial inflammation by dynamic gadolinium-enhanced magnetic resonance imaging: A study of the effect of intra-articular methylprednisolone on the rate of early synovial enhancement. *Rheumatology* **35:** 50–59.

171. Østergaard, M., M. Stoltenberg, P. Gideon, *et al.* 1996. Changes in synovial membrane and joint effusion volumes after intraarticular methylprednisolone. Quantitative assessment of inflammatory and destructive changes in arthritis by MRI. *J. Rheumatol.* **23:** 1151–1161.

172. Savnik, A., H. Bliddal, J.R. Nyengaard & H.S. Thomsen. 2002. MRI of the arthritic finger joints: Synovial membrane volume determination, a manual vs a stereologic method. *Eur. Radiol.* **12:** 94–98.

173. Bird, P., M. Lassere, R. Shnier & J. Edmonds. 2003. Computerized measurement of magnetic resonance imaging erosion volumes in patients with rheumatoid arthritis: A comparison with existing magnetic resonance imaging scoring systems and standard clinical outcome measures. *Arthritis Rheum.* **48:** 614–624.

174. Verstraete, K.L., F. Almqvist, P. Verdonk, *et al.* 2004. Magnetic resonance imaging of cartilage and cartilage repair. *Clin. Radiol.* **59:** 674–689.

175. McQueen, F.M. 2000. Magnetic resonance imaging in early inflammatory arthritis: What is its role? *Rheumatology* **39:** 700–706.

176. Tamai, K., M. Yamato, T. Yamaguchi & W. Ohno. 1994. Dynamic magnetic resonance imaging for the evaluation of synovitis in patients with rheumatoid arthritis. *Arthritis Rheum.* **37:** 1151–1157.

177. Gaffney, K., J. Cookson, D. Blake, *et al.* 1995. Quantification of rheumatoid synovitis by magnetic resonance imaging. *Arthritis Rheum.* **38:** 1610–1617.

178. Konig, H., J. Sieper & K.J. Wolf. 1990. Rheumatoid arthritis: Evaluation of hypervascular and fibrous pannus with dynamic MR imaging enhanced with Gd-DTPA. *J. Radiol.* **16:** 473–477.

179. Tofts, P.S., G. Brix, D.L. Buckley, *et al.* 1999. Estimating kinetic parameters from dynamic contrast-enhanced T(1)-weighted MRI of a diffusable tracer: Standardized quantities and symbols. *Magn. Reson. Imaging* **10:** 223–232.

180. Jackson, A. 2004. Analysis of dynamic contrast enhanced MRI. *Br. J. Radiol.* **77:** 154–166.

181. Padhani, A.R. 2002. Dynamic contrast-enhanced MRI in clinical oncology: Current status and future directions. *Magn. Reson. Imaging* **16:** 407–422.

182. Reddick, W.E., J.S. Taylor & B.D. Fletcher. 1999. Dynamic MR imaging (DEMRI) of microcirculation in bone sarcoma. *Magn. Reson. Imaging* **10:** 277–285.

183. Reece, R.J., M.C. Kraan, A. Radjenovic, *et al.* 1999. Dynamic gadolinium enhanced MR monitoring of inflammatory changes in rheumatoid arthritis with the new DMARD leflunomide versus methotrexate. *Arthritis Rheum.* **42:** 364–365.

184. Laarhoven, H.W.M., M. Rijpkema, C.J.A. Punt, *et al.* 2006. Method for quantitation of dynamic MRI contrast agent uptake in colorectal liver metastases. *Magn. Reson. Imaging* **18:** 315–320.

185. Brown, J., D. Buckley, A. Coulthard, *et al.* 2000. Magnetic resonance imaging screening in women at genetic risk of breast cancer: Imaging and analysis protocol for the UK multicentre study. *Magn. Reson. Imaging* **18:** 765–776.

186. Warner, E., D.B. Plewes, K.A. Hill, *et al.* 2004. Surveillance of BRCA1 and BRCA2 mutation carriers with magnetic resonance imaging, ultrasound, mammography, and clinical breast examination. *JAMA* **292:** 1317–1325.

187. Erlemann, R., M.F. Reiser, P.E. Peters, *et al.* 1989. Musculoskeletal neoplasms: Static and dynamic Gd-DTPA-enhanced MR imaging. *J. Radiol.* **171:** 767–773.

188. Verstraete, K.L., Y.D. Deene, H. Roels, *et al.* 1994. Benign and malignant musculoskeletal lesions: Dynamic contrast-enhanced MR imaging–parametric 'first-pass' images depict tissue vascularization and perfusion. *J. Radiol.* **192:** 835–843.

189. Tofts, P.S. & A.G. Kermode. 1991. Measurement of the blood-brain barrier permeability and leakage space using DEMRI. *Magn. Reson. Med.* **17:** 357–367.

190. Brix, G., W. Semmler, R. Port, *et al.* 1991. Pharmacokinetic parameters in CNS Gd-DTPA enhanced MR imaging. *J. Comput. Assist. Tomo.* **15:** 621–628.

191. Larsson, H.B., M. Stubgaard, J.L. Frederiksen, *et al.* 1990. Quantitation of blood-brain barrier defect by magnetic resonance imaging and Gadolinium-DTPA in patients with multiple sclerosis and brain tumors. *Magnet. Reson. Med.* **16:** 117–131.

192. D'Arcy, J.A., D.J. Collins, I.J. Rowland, *et al.* 2002. Applications of sliding window reconstruction with Cartesian sampling for dynamic contrast enhanced MRI. *J. NMR Biomed.* **15:** 174–183.

193. Heywang, S.H., A. Wolf, E. Pruss, *et al.* 1989. MR imaging of the breast with Gd-DTPA: Use and limitations. *Eur. Radiol.* **171:** 95–103.

194. Kaiser, W.A. & E. Zeitler. 1989. MR imaging of the breast: Fast imaging sequences with and without Gd-DTPA. Preliminary observations. *Eur. Radiol.* **170:** 681–686.

195. Kuhl, C.K., P. Mielcareck, S. Klaschik, *et al*. 1999. Dynamic breast MR imaging: Are signal intensity time course data useful for differential diagnosis of enhancing lesions? *Eur. Radiol.* **211:** 101–110.

196. Radjenovic, A. 2003. *Measurement of physiological variables by dynamic Gd-DTPA enhanced MRI*. Ph.D. Thesis, School of Medicine, University of Leeds, Leeds, UK.

197. Kubassova, O., M. Boesen, R.D. Boyle, *et al*. 2007. Fast and robust analysis of dynamic contrast enhanced MRI datasets. In *Proceedings of International Conference on Medical Image Computing and Computer Assisted Intervention* **2:** 261–269.

198. Radjenovic, A., J.P. Ridgway & M.A. Smith. 2006. A method for pharmacokinetic modelling of dynamic contrast enhanced MRI studies of rapidly enhancing lesions acquired in a clinical setting. *Phys. Med. Biol.* **51:** 187–197.

199. Cimmino, M.A., S. Innocenti, F. Livrone, *et al*. 2003. Dynamic gadolinium-enhanced MRI of the wrist in patients with rheumatoid arthritis. *Arthritis Rheum.* **48:** 674–680.

200. McQueen, F. 2004. Comments on the article by Cimmino *et al*.: Dynamic gadolinium-enhanced MRI of the wrist in patients with rheumatoid arthritis. *Arthritis Rheum.* **50:** 674–680.

201. Cimmino, M.A., M. Parodi, S. Innocenti, *et al*. 2005. Dynamic magnetic resonance imaging of the wrist in psoriatic arthritis reveals imaging patterns similar to those of rheumatoid arthritis. *Arthritis Res. Ther.* **7:** R725–R731.

202. Robb, A., D.P. Hanson, R.A. Karwoski, *et al*. 1989. ANALYZE: A comprehensive, operator-interactive software package for multidimensional medical image display and analysis. *Int. J. Comp. Med. Imaging Graphics* **13:** 433–454.

203. Hodgson, R.J., S. Connoly, T. Barnes, *et al*. 2007. Pharmacokinetic modelling of DCE-MRI of the hand and wrist in rheumatoid arthritis and the response to anti-TNF alpha therapy. *Magnet. Reson. Med.* **58:** 482–489.

204. Chakravarti, I.M., G.H. Laha & J. Roy. 1967. *Handbook of Methods of Applied Statistics*. Vol. 1: 8th ed. John Wiley and Sons. New York.

205. Kubassova, O., R.D. Boyle & M. Pyatnizkiy. 2005. Bone segmentation in metacarpophalangeal MR data. In *Proceedings of the Third International Conference on Advances in Pattern Recognition* **2:** 726–735.

206. Tofts, P.S. & E.P. du Boulay. 1990. Towards quantitative measurements of relaxation times and other parameters in the brain. *J. Neuroradiol.* **32:** 407–415.

207. Tofts, P.S., B.A. Rerkowitz & M. Schnall. 1995. Quantitative analysis of dynamic Gd-DTPA enhancement in breast tumors using a permeability model. *Magnet. Reson. Med.* **33:** 564–568.

208. Panting, J.R., P.D. Gatehouse, Z.G. Yang, *et al*. 2001. Echo-planar magnetic resonance myocardial perfusion imaging: Parametric map analysis and comparison with thallium SPECT. *Magn. Reson. Imaging* **13:** 192–200.

209. Sùilleabhain, K. 2004. Dynamic contrast-enhanced MRI predicts response to antiangiogenesis agents. *Online J. OncoLog* 49. http://www2.mdanderson.org/depts/oncolog/articles/04/6-jun/6-04-2.html (last access on 03.05.07).

210. Tofts, P.S. 1997. Modelling tracer kinetics in dynamic Gd-DTPA MR imaging. *Magn. Reson. Imaging* **7:** 91–101.

211. Foley-Nolan, D., J.P. Stack, M. Ryan, *et al*. 1991. MRI in the assessment of rheumatoid arthritis–a comparison with plain film radiographs. *Br. J. Rheumatol.* **30:** 101–106.

212. Alasaarela, E., I. Suramo, O. Tervonen, *et al*. 1998. Evaluation of humeral head erosions in rheumatoid arthritis: A comparison of ultrasonography, magnetic resonance imaging, computed tomography and plain radiography. *Br. J. Rheumatol.* **37:** 1152–1156.

213. Sommer, O.J., A. Kladosek, V. Weiler, *et al*. 2005. Rheumatoid arthritis: A practical guide to state-of-the-art imaging, image interpretation, and clinical implications. *Radiographics* **25:** 381–398.

214. Kuper, H.H., M.A. van Leeuwen, P.L. van Riel, *et al*. 1997. Radiographic damage in large joints in early rheumatoid arthritis: Relationship with radiographic damage in hands and feet, disease activity, and physical disability. *Rheumatology* **36:** 855–860.

215. Wiell, C., M. Szkudlarek, M. Hasselquist, *et al*. 2007. Ultrasonography, magnetic resonance imaging, radiography, and clinical assessment of inflammatory and destructive changes in fingers and toes of patients with psoriatic arthritis. *Arthritis Res. Ther.* **9:** R119. [A correction for this article has been published in *Arthritis Res. Ther.* 10: 402.]

216. Scheel, A.K., K.G. Hermann, S. Ohrndorf, *et al*. 2006. Prospective 7 year follow up imaging study comparing radiography, ultrasonography, and magnetic resonance imaging in rheumatoid arthritis finger joints. *Ann. Rheum. Dis.* **65:** 595–600.

217. Sugimoto, H., A. Takeda & K. Hyodoh. 2000. Early-stage rheumatoid arthritis: Prospective study of the effectiveness of MR imaging for diagnosis. *J. Radiol.* **216:** 569–575.

218. Terslev, L. & S.T. Torp-Pedersen. 2008. Settings and artefacts relevant in colour/power Doppler ultrasound in rheumatology. *Ann. Rheum. Dis.* **67:** 143–149.

219. McQueen, F., M. Østergaard, C. Peterfy, *et al*.

2005. Pitfalls in scoring MR images of rheumatoid arthritis wrist and metacarpophalangeal joints. *Ann. Rheum. Dis.* **64:** 48–55.

220. Kirwan, J.R. Systemic low-dose glucocorticoid treatment in rheumatoid arthritis. *Rheum. Dis. Clin. N. Am.* **27:** 389–403.

221. Ejbjerg, B.J., A. Vestergaard, S. Jacobsen, *et al.* 2006. Conventional radiography requires a MRI-estimated bone volume loss of 20% to 30% to allow certain detection of bone erosions in rheumatoid arthritis metacarpophalangeal joints. *Arthritis Res. Ther.* **8:** R59.

222. Wolfe, F., D.M. van der Heijde & A. Larsen. 2000. Assessing radiographic status of rheumatoid arthritis: introduction of a short erosion scale. *J. Rheumatol.* **27:** 2090–2099.

Complexities of MRI and False Positive Findings

Sanjeev Khanna and John V. Crues, III

Radnet–Pronet, Los Angeles, California, USA

MRI is a robust technology that allows for superior contrast of muscles, tissues, and bones within the body, which enables visualization of soft tissue pathology that cannot be seen with CT or plain film radiography. In order to appreciate the subtle (and sometimes not so subtle) intricacies of MRI, one must have a basic knowledge of the MRI physics involved to acquire an image, which leads to better recognition and a clearer understanding of some of the more important artifacts seen with MRI, including incomplete fat suppression, chemical shift, magnetic susceptibility, magic angle, partial volume, wraparound, and motion artifact. There are, however, many complexities and pitfalls in imaging the rheumatoid wrist. Normal anatomy such as capsular insertion sites and nutrient vessels can mimic erosion sites. The magic angle phenomenon can mimic tendon tears. Alignment abnormalities can be simulated based on wrist positioning. By having a solid understanding of the physics of magnetic resonance, anatomy, and the disease processes involved, many of these pitfalls can be avoided.

Key words: MRI; pitfalls; artifact; erosions; MRI physics; fat suppression; tendons; masses; chemical shift; imaging

Introduction

In order to appreciate and comprehend the complexities of MRI, one must first understand the basic principles of MRI physics. There are many excellent basic texts that detail the intricacies of MRI physics,[1] and it is beyond the scope and interest of this chapter to delve too deeply into these fundamentals. Notwithstanding, it is imperative to have a basic knowledge of MRI physics in order to obtain maximal image quality and information from each examination.

Basic MRI

In order to create MRI scans, one must place protons (hydrogen nuclei) within a magnetic field ($\mathbf{B}_0$). This causes the protons to pre-cess around the direction of $\mathbf{B}_0$ and creates an energy difference between the protons whose magnetic moments are aligned with and opposite to the magnetic field, so a slightly greater number of protons are aligned parallel with $\mathbf{B}_0$. The vector sum of all the individual proton magnetic moments results in a nonzero magnetic moment for the object being imaged, that is, the body becomes a magnet. When the protons are exposed to an external electromagnetic field ($\mathbf{B}_1$) with a frequency equal to the proton precession frequency, the protons absorb energy from the $\mathbf{B}_1$ field, flipping from parallel to antiparallel to the applied magnetic field. This energy, which is absorbed by the protons, is later released and detected by radiofrequency coils placed close to the body and used to create stunning images of the body's internal structures. This process requires briefly placing magnetic field gradients on the body to obtain spatial information, so that a computer can determine where in the body the energy is being released, which enables it to generate a two- or three-dimensional map. This spatial map of the

Address for correspondence: Sanjeev Khanna, M.D., 1411 7th St. #314, Santa Monica, CA, USA 90401. Voice: +773-398-2741. jeev3rad@yahoo.com

MRI and Ultrasound in Diagnosis and Management: Ann. N.Y. Acad. Sci. 1154: 239–258 (2009).
doi: 10.1111/j.1749-6632.2009.04393.x © 2009 New York Academy of Sciences.

location of signal source from within the body is the image used for medical diagnoses.

The quality of the image is partly determined by the signal-to-noise ratio (SNR), which is directly proportional to the magnetic field strength, so higher field strength usually allows for more detail within the image.

Spatial resolution refers to the observer's ability to distinguish two objects as separate and distinct and is determined by the size of the smallest three-dimensional volumetric units making up the image. Decreasing voxel size increases the ability to discern small structures. However, this comes at a price, as noise increases with decreases in voxel size.[2] Therefore, increases in spatial resolution can be useless if there is insufficient signal to support an interpretable image, which is the primary reason that high-field imaging is said to provide better spatial resolution.

Image contrast refers to the ability to discriminate the signal intensities between tissues. Tissue contrast is determined by the T1, T2, T2*, flow, and spin density parameters. One is able to accentuate the tissue characteristics by maximizing these parameters. Image contrast is paramount in detecting and characterizing lesions.

Magnetic field strength is measured in Tesla units (T). MRI machines are considered high field if they operate at 1.0 T or higher; mid-field MRI is 0.5 to 1.0 T; and low-field is 0.5 T and below. High-field MRI units allow for the acquisition of improved spatial resolution and decreases in examination time; however, it is debatable whether they provide more diagnostic information benefiting the patient. Merl *et al.* performed a prospective study evaluating 122 patients with suspected shoulder pathology using low-field and high-field MRI.[3] They found no difference in the diagnosis of impingement, rotator cuff lesions, or labral abnormalities. Zlatkin *et al.* performed a retrospective study on 160 patients, comparing surgical findings with low-field MRI,[4] and found the sensitivity and specificity for rotator cuff tears to be 90 and 93%, respectively. Taouli

and colleagues compared high-field MRI, low-field MRI, and radiography of the wrists and hands of 18 patients with rheumatoid arthritis to detect and grade bone erosions, joint space narrowing, and synovitis.[5] They found that high-field and low-field MRI showed similar results, that is, using high-field spin-echo MRI as the reference standard, the sensitivity, specificity, and accuracy of low-field three-dimensional gradient echo MRI for erosions were 94, 93, and 94%, respectively.[6]

Conversely, Magee and colleagues prospectively interpreted shoulder MRIs from 40 patients who had a complete shoulder MRI examination on a 0.2-T system and limited imaging on a 1.5-T unit.[7] Proton density axial and fat-saturated T2-weighted coronal and sagittal sequences were performed. Each radiologist interpreted the open unit (low field strength) images first and the high-field images second and compared the results from 28 patients who also underwent arthroscopy with the MRI interpretations. They found full-thickness supraspinatus tendon tears in four patients that could be diagnosed definitively on the high-field unit but not on the open unit and three labral tears and two superior labral anteroposterior lesions that could be depicted definitively on the high-field unit but not on the open unit. Thus they concluded that high-field MRI allowed for more accurate diagnosis compared to low-field units.

Unfortunately, there is no simple right answer. The best choice depends on a series of factors including cost, applications, accessibility, patient preference, patient tolerance, and competitive motivations. Most radiologists would agree that high-field MRI scans provide for better-quality images, but whether this provides more diagnostic information for specific disease processes is subject to debate.[8,9]

MRI Sequences

The primary advantage of MRI over all other imaging technologies is the robust

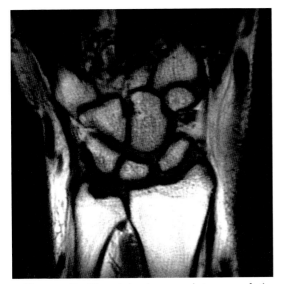

Figure 1. T1-weighted coronal image of the wrist: This image demonstrates the normal high-fat signal bone marrow. The cortex of the bones is homogeneously low in signal.

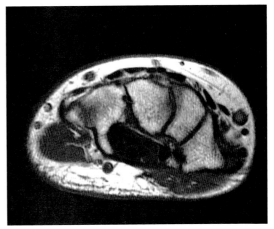

Figure 2. Fast spin-echo T2-weighted axial image through the wrist: This image shows high signal within the fat and low signal within the tendons and tendon sheaths. Abnormal fluid would be high in signal intensity on this image.

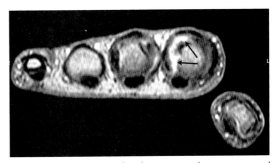

Figure 3. T1-weighted image with contrast and fat suppression. Contrast enhancement increases the sensitivity for synovitis (arrows).

diversity of contrast that can be obtained between biological tissues using different MRI pulse sequences. Pulse sequences vary by changing the nature and timing of **B**$_1$ pulses and magnetic field gradients during image acquisition. Different sequences are often labeled using MRI jargon that roughly relates to the main source of contrast in the images. T1, T2, proton density, fast spin echo, gradient echo, inversion recovery, and T1 relaxation/recovery with or without fat suppression are just a few of the plethora of pulse sequences widely available for rheumatologic imaging. Simply put, T1-weighted images are obtained by emphasizing the T1 relaxation times and deemphasizing the T2 relaxation times. This allows for tissues that have a relatively short T1 relaxation time to appear bright on T1 images (fat) and those that have a relatively long T1 relaxation time to appear dark (CSF, urine) (Fig. 1).[1]

Conversely, T2-weighted images are obtained by minimizing the contributions from T1 relaxation times and emphasizing T2 relaxation times (Fig. 2).[10] Proton-density-weighted images can be thought of as intermediately weighted, and images are obtained by minimiz-

ing the effects of T1 and T2 relaxation.[10] Intermediately weighted images are useful for depicting structures such as bone or fibrous tissue contrasted with a background of soft tissue or fluid with a higher signal intensity.[1] Placing a specific radiofrequency pulse that saturates fat within the image before acquiring the data is very useful with T1-weighted images to increase the sensitivity for contrast enhancement (i.e., synovitis; Fig. 3). When used with proton-density sequences, fat suppression increases sensitivity for bone marrow edema and soft tissue injuries (Fig. 4).

MRI image information can be acquired by using two-dimensional or three-dimensional acquisition techniques. Unlike

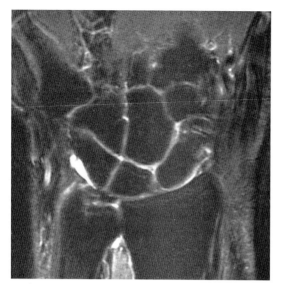

Figure 4. Coronal proton density with fat suppression. These images increase the sensitivity to marrow edema, as edema is bright on these sequences and the high signal within normal bone marrow is suppressed.

two-dimensional images, three-dimensional acquisitions are thin and contiguous without any gaps between the slices. This can minimize partial-volume artifacts (discussed below), but three-dimensional techniques require more acquisition time than two-dimensional techniques, which severely limits their use with standard pulse sequences. However, we believe that one three-dimensional gradient-echo sequence is essential in the evaluation of erosive disease in rheumatoid arthritis. Voxels with dimensions of less than 1 mm in all three planes are necessary to accurately follow small changes in erosion sizes when determining response to therapy (Fig. 5A and B).[11]

Inversion recovery sequences, in particular short tau inversion recovery (STIR), are very useful for wrist/hand imaging and musculoskeletal imaging in general. The contrast for STIR images appears reversed as compared to standard T1 images (Fig. 6), which allows for effective fat suppression and lesion identification through the additive effects of T1 and T2 contrast. STIR images make lesions that are embedded in fat, that is, bone marrow, more conspicuous by suppressing the fat signal from

the underlying bone and allowing the lesion's own signal to stand out. However, STIR images cannot distinguish among blood products, contrast enhancement, and fat. The signals from all three are suppressed.[10]

Pitfalls in MRI

With the introduction of clinical MRI in the 1980s, X-ray occult bone injuries were detected as regions within the bone marrow of low signal intensity on T1-weighted images and high signal intensity on T2-weighted images (Fig. 7A and B).[12] These areas were shown to be marrow edema from trabecular bone injuries. MRI's sensitivity for these lesions was improved with the introduction of fat-suppressed proton-density, fat-suppressed T2, and STIR imaging. Acute bone marrow edema on MRI has been described as having a feathery appearance with poorly defined margins.[13] Similar appearing regions of high signal intensity can be seen within the subcortical bone at joint margins as precursor lesions before X-ray-defined bone erosions can be detected.[14] High-signal lesions seen as precursors to bone erosions tend to be more sharply delineated than typical edema caused by trauma, and recent pathological evidence has shown these lesions to be water that contains inflammatory cells in place of the normal fat-containing cells within normal marrow.[15]

Consequently, it appears more accurate to refer to these lesions as osteitis, rather than bone marrow edema. Instead of being simply a precursor to bone erosions, it is likely that these areas of osteitis represent the first stage of inflammation, which is the fundamental pathology that causes bone erosions in rheumatoid arthritis (Fig. 8A and B). If the inflammation is not controlled at this early stage of the erosive process, the trabecular bone is destroyed, a process that may be irreversible (Fig. 9A and B). Ongoing inflammation then destroys the overlying cortex and the lesions become detectable by X-ray imaging techniques. Though the erosion

A

B

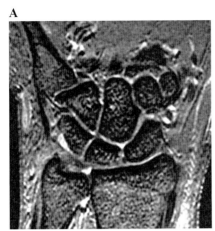 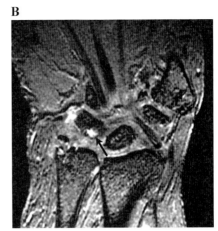

Figure 5. (**A**) Coronal three-dimensional gradient echo. This sequence allows the acquisition of thin contiguous slices, which are not practical with two-dimensional sequences. The normal bone at high field is inhomogeneous owing to trabecular susceptibility artifacts. The bone marrow is more uniform in signal intensity on these sequences at low-field imaging. (**B**) A triquetral erosion is seen on the three-dimensional gradient-echo sequence (arrow). Small erosions may be missed on thicker slices and subtle changes in size may not be accurately detected on thicker two-dimensional images with spaces between the slices.

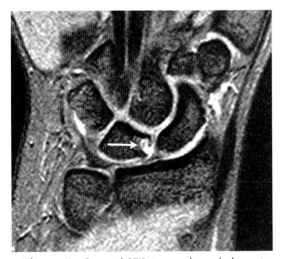

Figure 6. Coronal STIR image through the wrist. Note how the signal seems reversed as compared to the T1 coronal image seen in Figure 1. The bone erosion is well visualized (white arrow).

process begins with osteitis, many authors reserve the term erosion for lesions containing cortical destruction.[16,17] The destruction of the trabecular bone and cortex is well visualized on MRI as low signal on T1-weighted images and high signal on fluid-sensitive images involving the subcortical bone and cortex.

In the study by Benton,[16] the strongest predictor of functional outcome at 6 years was the presence of focal high-signal lesions on fluid-sensitive sequences, which they referred to as MRI bone marrow edema. These lesions were probably osteitis rather than interstitial free water and therefore potentially reversible before the development of erosions with effective therapy. Less effective therapy can result in clinical improvement but continued progression of erosive disease.[18] As noted by C.G. Peterfly and colleagues, bone marrow edema of the carpus may be useful for predicting which patients are more likely to progress and for monitoring antierosive treatments.[14,19] Furthermore, the resolution of bone marrow edema before erosions can develop provides direct evidence that the erosive process has stopped at that particular site, which allows for evaluation of the therapeutic effect of the medication.[14]

Erosion Pitfalls

The anatomy of the carpal and metacarpal bones is complex. Many small bones, miniscule

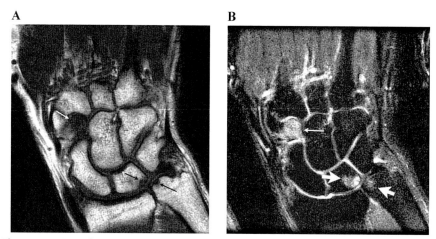

Figure 7. (**A**) Chronic traumatic marrow edema. The ulnar side of the lunate and the distal ulna demonstrate decreased signal on the T1-weighted images and high signal on the STIR images. (**B**) Ulnar abutment (thick white arrows). The trapezoid also shows edema (thin white arrow). The margins of the abnormal signal are sharply delineated, indicative of chronic injury.

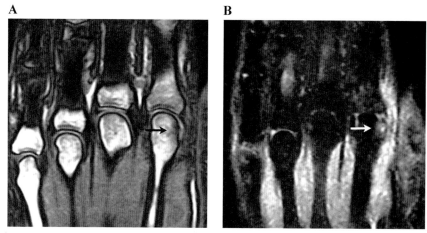

Figure 8. (**A**) Osteitis. The T1-weighted coronal image indicates indistinct low signal within the marrow adjacent to the margins of the MCP joint (arrow). This represents osteitis, the first stage of inflammation causing bone erosions in rheumatoid arthritis. (**B**) Osteitis. The STIR image demonstrates high-signal (arrow) osteitis involving the radial aspect of the second metacarpal head.

ligaments, tiny tendons, nerves, muscles, and vessels work in harmony in a normally functioning wrist. Recognizing the normal anatomy, let alone the pathological disease processes, is challenging enough. In this section, we review normal anatomy that can mimic rheumatologic disease processes in the rheumatoid wrist.

Ejberg *et al.* described mild synovitis and small bone erosions in 2% of healthy subjects (7/420 patients).[20] These small bone erosions most commonly involved the capitate and lunate bones. However, rarely did these lesions in asymptomatic subjects demonstrate contrast enhancement or bone marrow edema, signs that may be useful for distinguishing arthritic from normal joints. The capitate has both volar and dorsal grooves, which if not recognized for what they are can be easily misinterpreted as

A

B

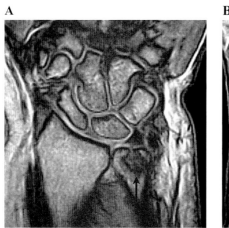
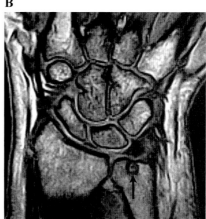

Figure 9. (**A**) Decrease in erosion size. The coronal GRE image demonstrates an erosion of the distal ulna (arrow). (**B**) A similar image to that shown in Figure 9A but 14 months later, after the patient had been placed on a TNF-alpha inhibitor, shows substantial decrease in the size of the erosion (arrow).

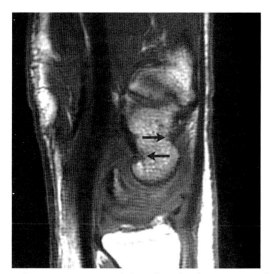

Figure 10. Normal dorsal and volar grooves of the capitate. A common false positive diagnosis of bone erosion is mistaking the normal cortical contours of the volar and dorsal aspect of the capitate as erosions.

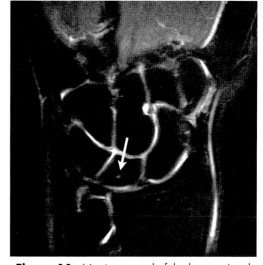

Figure 11. Nutrient vessel of the lunate. Another potential normal variant that can simulate erosions are nutrient vessel foramina, especially those involving the dorsal aspect of the lunate (arrow).

abnormal (Fig. 10). Defects in the cortex where the nutrient artery enters can appear similar to erosions, especially on the dorsal aspect of the lunate (Fig. 11).[17] Normal cortical irregularities are commonly seen involving the base of the second metacarpal bone (Fig. 12A and B) and the bare area of the triquetrum (Fig. 13).[21] Most normal variants do not have an abnor-

mal MRI signal within the marrow space of the bone, but normal bone marrow signal is also characteristic of chronic erosive disease.

The intrinsic muscles of the hand are located on the palmar aspect, subdivided into thenar, hypothenar, and lumbrical muscles.[22] These insert into the carpal bones and help to maintain proper motion and stability of the wrist. The

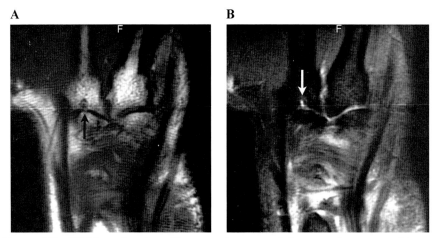

Figure 12. (**A**) Normal variant. The normal contour of the second metacarpal base can simulate an erosion (arrows): T1-weighted image. (**B**) Normal variant. The normal contour of the second metacarpal base can simulate an erosion (arrows): STIR coronal image.

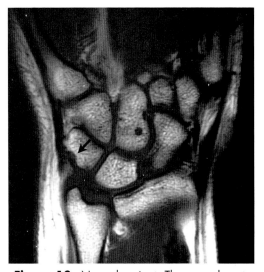

Figure 13. Normal variant. The normal contour of the triquetrum can simulate an erosion. This may involve either the bare area (arrow) or proximal pole.

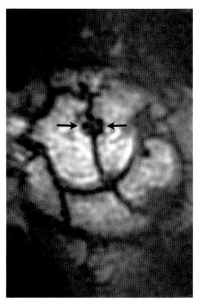

Figure 14. Normal variant. The hamate–capitate interosseous ligament attachment site can simulate erosions (arrows).

ligamentous anatomy of the wrist is also complex. The volar, dorsal, and interosseous ligaments also help to stabilize the carpus.[23] The intrinsic interosseous ligamentous attachment sites can mimic erosions (Fig. 14). One way to differentiate erosions from ligament attachment sites is that bone marrow edema should not be present at the ligamentous insertion sites.[17] Regions of bone at capsular insertion sites can also be associated with focal cortical

indentations at the margins of the metacarpal heads.

In addition to normal variants, trauma—especially chronic repetitive trauma—can mimic erosive disease on MRI studies, but these lesions can usually be differentiated from erosive disease based upon the location of the abnormality. Trauma often involves the

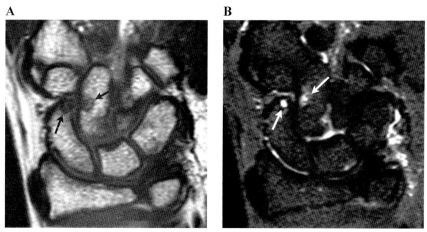

Figure 15. (A) Scaphocapitate impingement. Chronic repetitive impaction of the distal scaphoid on the capitate presents as low-signal areas of the distal scaphoid and capitate on T1-weighted images (arrows). **(B)** Scaphocapitate impingement. These areas may be high in signal intensity on STIR or PDFS images (arrows).

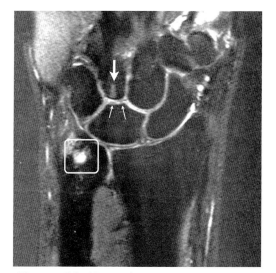

Figure 16. Hamatolunate impingement. Note the area of increased signal along the proximal hamate bone (large arrow) in addition to the abnormal medial fossa (small arrows) of a type 2 lunate. Incidental erosion of the distal ulna is seen (box).

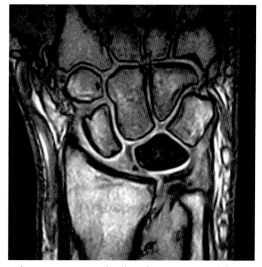

Figure 17. Kienbock's disease. Signal loss on this three-dimensional GRE coronal image within the lunate is characteristic of Kienbock's disease.

subchondral bone of the joints, leading to degenerative joint disease. Common locations of chronic repetitive trauma simulating erosions include: scaphocapitate impingement (Fig. 15A and B), hamatolunate impingement (Fig. 16), and the ulnar abutment syndrome (Fig. 7B). Kienbock's disease from repetitive trauma to the lunate can also mimic erosive disease (Fig. 17). These trauma-related focal bone abnormalities typically present with MRI findings of high signal on fluid-sensitive techniques from edema or granulation tissue, which appear similar to osteitis on all MRI sequences. Acute fractures present with decreased signal on T1-weighted images replacing the normal

A   B

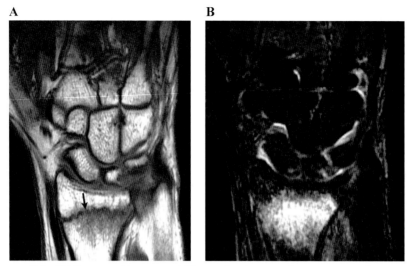

Figure 18. (A) Fracture. The coronal T1-weighted image demonstrates a low-signal line traversing the distal radius, representing a fracture line (arrow). **(B)** Fracture. The STIR coronal image through the same area demonstrates the associated bone marrow edema surrounding the fracture line.

bright bone marrow signal. A distinct low-signal line is seen if the bone is broken (Fig. 18A and B). Acute bone injuries tend to present with much larger bone injuries than inflammatory erosions and usually involve the subchondral bone at the points of force transfer, whereas inflammatory erosions primarily involve the margin of a joint at the capsular attachment.

Tendons and Ligaments

In addition to bone erosions, tendons and ligaments are also commonly involved in the inflammation of rheumatoid arthritis. The anatomical structures that comprise the TFC complex (triangular fibrocartilage) are not universally agreed upon. However, most descriptions include the triangular fibrocartilage, the meniscus homologue, the ulnar collateral ligament, the dorsal and volar radioulnar ligaments, and the sheath of the extensor carpi ulnaris tendon.[24] The TFC proper is a thick disclike low-signal band of tissue that covers the ulnar head (Fig. 19). It arises from the hyaline cartilage on the ulnar aspect of the radius and

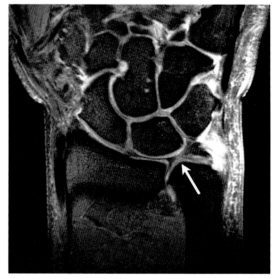

Figure 19. Normal TFC. Note the low signal of the TFC with its characteristic "bow-tie" configuration on this 3.0-T image.

inserts into the fovea (the junction between the ulnar head and the ulnar styloid). Tears in the TFC can be traumatic or degenerative in nature. Traumatic tears may be associated with a fracture of the ulnar styloid and a disruption of the radioulnar ligaments.[25] Degenerative tears

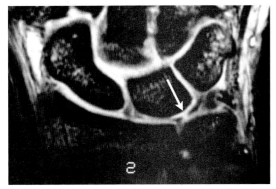

Figure 20. Tear in the TFC. Note the break in the normal "bow-tie" configuration as the fluid signal separates the TFC through a central tear (arrow).

are common in rheumatoid arthritis, characterized by diffuse increased signal intensity, generalized thinning of the TFC, and perforation in the central avascular region (Fig. 20). The TFC can also have a striated appearance as it attaches onto the fovea. An actual tear in the TFC can be differentiated from this normal appearance by noting fluid signal, not just intermediate signal, interrupting the normal attachment site.[26]

MRI is very useful for evaluating tendinosis and tenosynovitis in the wrist. Tendinosis refers to the enlargement or increased signal within the tendon itself, usually as a consequence of chronic microscopic tears and the healing response within a tendon or ligament (Fig. 21A and B). Tenosynovitis refers to inflammation of the synovial-lined tendon sheath and presents on MRI. Fluid circumferentially encases the tendon and distends the tendon sheath (Fig. 22A and B).[25] Tendinosis/tenosynovitis commonly affects the extensor carpi ulnaris (ECU; Fig. 21B), the first extensor compartment (De Quervain's tenosynovitis; Fig. 23), and the flexor tendons (Fig. 24). An avoidable pitfall in evaluating for tenosynovitis is visualizing fluid signal within the tendon sheath with only the T2 images. One must compare the T1 images to make sure that the "fluid" is not actually fat signal, which can also appear bright on the T2 sequences (Fig. 25A and B).

Carpal Instability and Alignment Abnormalities

The main patterns of carpal instability related to the proximal carpal row include dorsal intercalated segmental instability (DISI) and volar intercalated segmental instability (VISI). DISI presents on MRI as a dorsal tilt of the lunate with respect to the capitate on sagittal images (Fig. 26) and typically results from lateral structural injuries to the wrist, often involving dissociation of the scapholunate articulation or scapholunate ligament tears. VISI typically arises from medial structural injuries to the wrist, often involving dissociation of the lunotriquetral articulation. On MRI, VISI presents with a volar tilt of the lunate on sagittal images (Fig. 27). Zanetti *et al.*[27] found that the lunate appears more dorsally tilted on MRI scans as compared with the normal lateral radiographs, so care must be taken not to overcall DISI on MRIs. This tilt was present in neutrally positioned wrists and exacerbated with ulnar deviation and was absent in radial deviation.

Masses

Fortunately, more than 98% of wrist masses are benign.[24] The most common wrist mass is the ganglion cyst.[25] Most ganglion cysts arise as out-pouchings from the capsule of the carpal joints or tendon sheaths; therefore, they display the characteristic appearance of cysts on MRI with homogeneously low T1 and high T2 signal. Some 70% of all wrist ganglia occur dorsally in the region of the scapholunate ligament. The next most common location is located volarly. These can arise from the radioscaphoid, scapholunate, scaphotrapezial, or metacarpotrapezial joint.[25] It is often possible to see the cyst arising directly from the joint space, tendon itself, or the tendon sheath (Fig. 28A and B). Although rare, in the setting of suggestive clinical findings, the differential diagnosis should also include a neuroma. Gadolinium can differentiate between

A   B

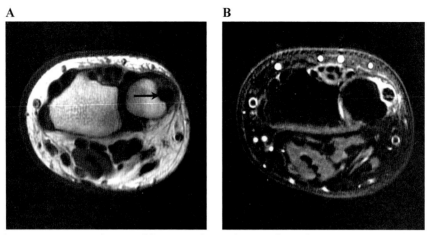

Figure 21. (**A**) Tendinosis of the ECU. The tendon is enlarged owing to microscopic tears or tendinosis within the tendon (arrow). Mild thickening is seen in the synovium of the tendon sheath, consistent with mild tenosynovitis on this T1-weighted image. (**B**) Tendinosis of the ECU. The PDFS image shows high-signal-intensity tissue surrounding the ECU.

A   B

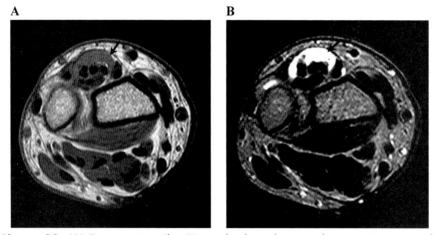

Figure 22. (**A**) Tenosynovitis. This T1-weighted axial image demonstrates intermediate signal surrounding the extensor tendons (arrow). (**B**) High-signal fluid is seen surrounding the extensor tendons on the axial T2-weighted images (arrow).

the two as neuromas enhance and the ganglion cysts do not.[28] Other lesions that have a characteristic appearance on MRI include typical lipomas (Fig. 29), hemangiomas (Fig. 30A and B), pigmented villonodular synovitis (PVNS; Fig. 31), and desmoid tumors.[29]

MRI Artifacts

In addition to becoming familiar with the appearance of normal and abnormal anatomy displayed on the detailed images provided by MRI, the interpreter must recognize common artifacts seen on MRIs of the musculoskeletal system. Some of the more important artifacts seen in MRIs of rheumatoid arthritis include: incomplete fat suppression, chemical shift, magnetic susceptibility, magic angle, partial volume, wraparound, and motion.

One of the advantages of high-field imaging is that the precession frequency of fat and water are sufficiently separated that the fat signal can be independently suppressed, increasing

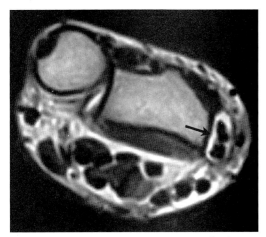

Figure 23. De Quervain's synovitis. Fluid is seen surrounding the first extensor compartment tendons, consistent with tenosynovitis (arrow).

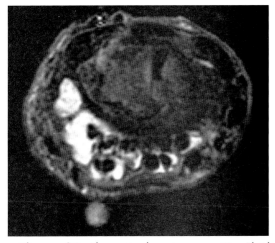

Figure 24. Flexor tendons tenosynovitis. Fluid is seen surrounding the flexor tendons on this T2-weighted image.

the sensitivity for detecting contrast enhancement on T1-weighted images and edema on fluid-sensitive sequences. If the suppression is uniform across the image, then the resultant scan can be diagnostically useful. If the fat suppression is nonuniform across the image, then artifacts from this may masquerade as disease (Fig. 32A and B). Incomplete fat suppression results from inhomogeneity within the magnetic field ($\mathbf{B}_0$), inadequate shimming, ferro-

magnetic materials within the magnetic field, or inhomogeneous RF excitation.[30] Such suboptimal scans can occur when the anatomic structures being imaged are asymmetric and far from the isocenter of the magnet, such as patients lying within the magnet with their wrists at their sides.[31] The incomplete fat suppression in the bone marrow of the carpal bones can simulate a disease process such as bone marrow edema or contusion.[30]

The fact that fat and water resonate at different frequencies creates an additional artifact, especially when imaging at high fields. The most common image reconstruction algorithm for the calculation the final images uses Fourier transform techniques. With these techniques, spatial location is encoded by the use of magnetic field gradients with location in space associated with the frequency at which the nuclei are resonating. Since fat and water resonate at slightly different frequencies when in the same magnetic field, fat and water in the same location within the body are mapped at slightly different locations on the images in the frequency-encoded direction. This artifact can cause obscuration of interfaces between adjacent fat-based and water-based tissues, such as bone marrow (fat-based) and articular cartilage (water-based) (Fig. 33).

Magnetic susceptibility refers to the ability of a material to become magnetized in a magnetic field. If adjacent structures with different magnetic susceptibilities are present within the image, then the magnetic field difference created between the objects when they are placed in the $\mathbf{B}_0$ field can create artifacts. Ferromagnetic materials (such orthopedic hardware) can cause severe degradation of images owing to distortion of the magnetic field (Fig. 34), which may prevent acquisition of diagnostic quality images.[30]

The magic angle phenomenon occurs when ligaments, tendons, menisci, labrum, or any other tissue containing collagen is oriented at 55° to the magnetic field. The increased signal intensity can mimic tendinosis, partial tears, or complete tears (Fig. 35).[32]

A

B

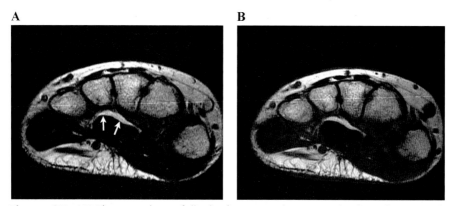

Figure 25. (**A**) Flexor tendon pitfall. The fast spin-echo T2-weighted axial images show increased signal intensity deep to the flexor tendons (arrows). This can be mistaken for fluid. (**B**) Flexor tendon pitfall. The T1-weighted axial images show the "fluid" seen on the T2 images to be high in signal on the T1-weighted images. This is fat and not tenosynovitis.

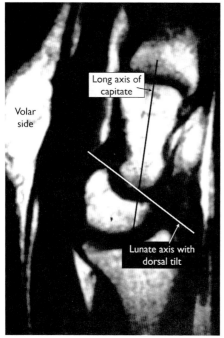

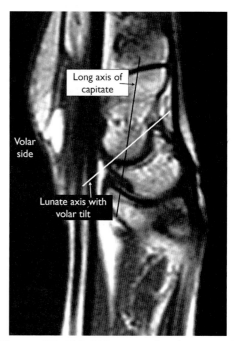

Figure 26. DISI instability. Dorsal intercalated segmental instability presents on MRI as a dorsal tilt of the lunate with respect to the capitate on sagittal images.

Figure 27. VISI. Volar intercalated segmental instability presents as a volar tilt of the lunate on sagittal images.

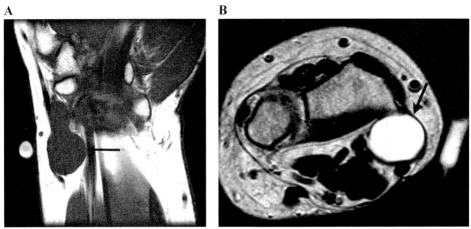

Figure 28. (A) Ganglion cyst. Cysts present as lobular low-signal sharply defined fluid collection on the T1 coronal images (arrow). **(B)** Ganglion cyst. Note the bright signal of the ganglion cyst on the T2 axial image (arrow).

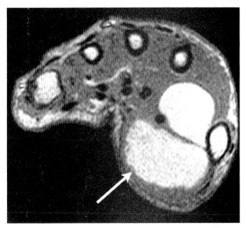

Figure 29. Lipoma: The lipid within lipomas demonstrates characteristic high signal intensity on T1-weighted images (arrow). Lipomas uniformly suppress on fat-suppressed images.

Partial Volume Artifact

Artifacts from partial volume averaging occur when the structure being imaged is only partially contained within the voxel. This can lead to adjacent tissues of different signal intensities averaging their respective signal intensities, leading to blurring or indistinct margins. Partial volume averaging of bones and soft tissues in the wrist can mimic erosions with sharply defined margins and low-signal cortex. This can be seen on the three-dimensional GRE images and can be clarified by an examination in the perpendicular plane.[17] However, volume averaging is much more of a problem with traditional two-dimensional Fourier transformation images with thicker-slice images. The most reliable way to minimize partial volume artifacts is to minimize the size of the voxel in all three dimensions, and much of the current development in MRI of joints concerns development of efficient pulse sequences that minimize the voxel size.[9]

Wraparound Artifact

Wraparound artifact occurs when the field of view is smaller than the body part being imaged. This leads to image data outside the field of view being "wrapped around" to the opposite side of the image (Fig. 36).[1]

MRI is very sensitive to motion, and images can be severely degraded by patient movement during the several minutes required to acquire a sequence. Most study protocols contain multiple sequences, and it can be very difficult for patients suffering from arthritis to remain still for extended periods of time.

A

B

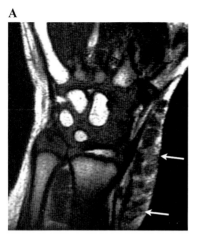
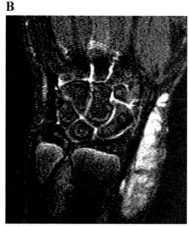

Figure 30. (A) Hemangioma. The inhomogeneous soft tissue mass along the radial aspect of the wrist shows typical characteristics of a hemangioma (arrows). The increased signal on the T1 image represents fat within the mass. A phlebolith within the mass was seen on X-ray (not shown). **(B)** Hemangioma. Note the bright hypervascular tissue of the hemangioma on the STIR image.

Comfortable positioning is essential. Some authors have found that smaller-extremity MRI machines may be better tolerated in this patient population.[33]

Synovitis

Synovitis is a hallmark of rheumatoid arthritis.[34] The secretion of degrading enzymes breaks down the articular cartilage and causes bone destruction. In the synovial joint, articulating bones are covered by cartilage, except at the site of insertion of the fibrous capsule. In this bare area the synovium is in direct contact with the bone at the margin of the joint, increasing its susceptibility to bone destruction induced by synovitis.[35] Several studies have discussed the correlation of synovial volume determined by MRI with the onset of bone erosion, and others have shown MRI to be superior to plain film radiography in assessing synovial disease.[36–38] However, many difficulties hamper the ability to evaluate synovitis with MRI. Thickened synovial tissue can be difficult to differentiate from synovial fluid on standard T1- and T2-weighted and fat-suppressed sequences.

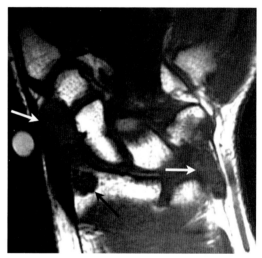

Figure 31. PVNS. Diffuse low signal intensity on T1-weighted images involving proliferative synovial tissue is characteristic of pigmented villonodular synovitis due to hemosiderin deposition (white arrows). An erosion involves the distal radius (black arrow).

Moreover, in chronic rheumatoid arthritis suppression of the inflammation is not associated with the synovial volume returning to normal; thus, synovial volume is not an ideal measure of the activity of inflammation in

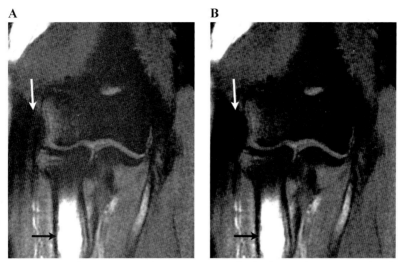

Figure 32. (**A**) Inhomogeneous fat suppression. The high signal intensity within the proximal radius is due to inhomogeneous fat suppression from magnetic field inhomogeneity (black arrow). Water suppression causes abnormal low signal within the lateral soft tissues (white arrow). (**B**) Inhomogeneous fat suppression. Uniform fat suppression is present in the same patient on the STIR images. Note the common extensor tendon tear (tennis elbow; white arrow), which was suppressed on the PDFS inhomogeneous image in Figure 32A.

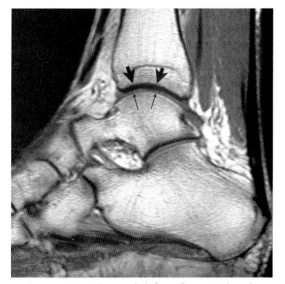

Figure 33. Chemical shift artifact. Lipid and water resonate at slightly different frequencies; consequently fat is shifted superiorly and water inferiorly in the vertical (frequency-encoded) direction. This causes an artificial black line between marrow fat and articular cartilage at the distal tibia (fat arrows) and obscuration of the subchondral bone of the talar dome (thin arrows).

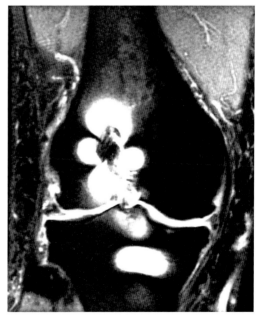

Figure 34. Metal artifact. Metal materials (such orthopedic hardware) can cause severe degradation of images due to distortion of the fields.

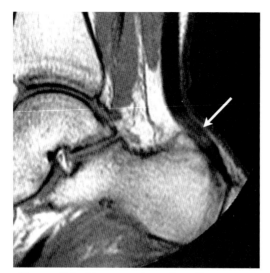

Figure 35. Magic angle artifact. The magic angle phenomenon occurs when ligaments, tendons, menisci, labrum, or any other tissue containing ordered molecules (collagen) are oriented at 55° to the magnetic field. Increased signal intensity is seen in the distal Achilles tendon as it becomes angled at 55° to the main magnetic field near its insertion into the calcaneous (arrow). This is due to magic angle artifact, not insertional tendinosis.

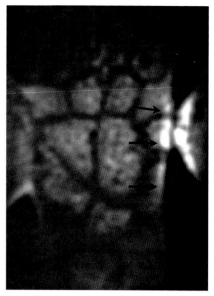

Figure 36. Wraparound artifact. When the acquisition field of view is too small, aliasing in the Fourier transform technique causes data from outside the field of view to be "wrapped around" to the opposite side of the image. In this example tissue from the proximal wrist from outside the field of view overlaps to the right side of the image (arrows) in this three-dimensional gradient-echo image.

long-standing disease. The rate of enhancement of the synovium within 1 min of intravenous injection of contrast correlates better with the severity of inflammation than synovial volume alone.[34] Dynamic contrast-enhanced MRI is a very promising tool for assessing synovitis and risk for erosive disease in inflammatory arthropathies (see Fig. 3).

Summary

In conclusion, MRI is a robust multiplanar technology that offers superior visualization of bones and superior soft tissue contrast without the use of ionizing radiation. In order to maximize the quality and information from each examination, it is imperative to have a basic understanding of MRI physics. Once a basic understanding is achieved, it is much easier to avoid the most common pitfalls encountered. In the future, as our understanding of rheumatoid arthritis continues to evolve, MRI's role as

a tool for diagnosis, management, and treatment will also continue to evolve.

References

1. Mitchell, D. & M. Cohen. 2003. *MRI Principles.* W.B. Saunders. Philadelphia.
2. Bradley, W.G., K.E. Kortman & J.V. Crues. 1985. Central nervous system high-resolution magnetic resonance imaging: Effect of increasing spatial resolution on resolving power. *Radiology* **156:** 93–98.
3. Merl, T., M. Scholz, P. Gerhadt, *et al.* 1999. Results of a prospective multicenter center study for the evaluation of a diagnostic quality of an open whole-body low-field MRI unit. A comparison with high-field MRI measured by the applicable gold standard. *Eur. J. Radiol.* **30:** 43–53.
4. Zlatkin, M.B., C. Hoffman & F.G. Shellock. 2004. Assessment of the rotator cuff and glenoid labrum using an extremity MR system: MR results compared to surgical findings from a multi-center study. *J. Magn. Reson. Imaging* **19:** 623–631.
5. Taouli, B., S. Zaim, C.G. Peterfy, *et al.* 2004. Rheumatoid arthritis of the hand and wrist:

Comparison of three imaging techniques. *AJR Am. J. Roentgenol.* **182:** 937–943.

6. Ejbjerg, B., E. Narvestad, S. Jacobsen, *et al.* 2005. Optimized, low cost, low field dedicated extremity MRI is highly specific and sensitive for synovitis and bone erosions in rheumatoid arthritis wrist and finger joints: A comparison with conventional high-field MRI and radiography. *Ann. Rheum. Dis.* **64:** 1280–1287.

7. Magee, T., M. Shapiro & D. Williams. 2003. Comparison of high-field-strength versus low-field-strength MRI of the shoulder. *AJR Am. J. Roentgenol.* **181:** 1211–1215.

8. Ghazinoor, S., J.V.I. Crues & C. Crowley. 2007. Low-field musculoskeletal MRI. *J. Magn. Reson. Imaging* **25:** 234–244.

9. Kuo, R., M. Panchal, L. Tanenbaum & J.V.I. Crues. 2007. 3.0 Tesla imaging of the musculoskeletal system. *J. Magn. Reson. Imaging* **25:** 245–261.

10. Mugler, J. 2005. Basic principles. In *Clinical Magnetic Resonance Imaging.* R. Edelman, J. Hesselink, M. Zlatkin & J. Crues, Eds.: 23–57. W.B. Saunders. Philadelphia.

11. Chen, T., J. Crues, M. Ali & O. Troum. 2006. Magnetic resonance imaging is more sensitive than radiographs in detecting change in size of erosions in rheumatoid arthritis. *J. Rheumatol.* **33:** 1957–1967.

12. Blum, G.M., P.F.J. Tirman & J.V. Crues, III. 1993. Osseous and cartilaginous trauma. In *MRI of the Knee,* 2nd ed. J.H. Mink, M.A. Reicher, J.V. Crues, III, & A.L. Deutsch, Eds.: 295–332. Raven Press. New York.

13. McQueen, F. 2007. A vital clue to deciphering bone pathology: MRI bone oedema in rheumatoid arthritis and osteoarthritis. *Ann. Rheum. Dis.* **66:** 1549–1552.

14. Peterfy, C.G. 2004. MRI of the wrist in early rheumatoid arthritis. *Ann. Rheum. Dis.* **63:** 473–477.

15. Jimenez-Boj, E., I. Noebauer, F. Kainberger, *et al.* 2006. Nome marrow edema in MRI scans of patients with rheumatoid arthritis is caused by inflammatory infiltrates in the bone marrow. *Arthritis Rheum.* **54:** S550.

16. Benton, N., N. Stewart, J. Crabbe, *et al.* 2004. MRI of the wrist in early rheumatoid arthritis can be used to predict functional outcome at 6 years. *Ann. Rheum. Dis.* **63:** 555–561.

17. McQueen, F., M. Østergaard, C.G. Peterfy, *et al.* 2005. Pitfalls in scoring MR images of rheumatoid arthritis wrist and metacarpophalangeal joints. *Ann. Rheum. Dis.* **64:** i48–i55.

18. McQueen, F.M., N. Stewart, J. Crabbe, *et al.* 1999. Magnetic resonance imaging of the wrist in early rheumatoid arthritis reveals progression of erosions despite clinical improvement. *Ann. Rheum. Dis.* **58:** 156–163.

19. Conaghan, P.G., F. McQueen, C.G. Peterfy, *et al.* 2005. The evidence for magnetic resonance imaging as an outcome measure in proof-of-concept rheumatoid arthritis studies. *J. Rheumatol.* **32:** 2465–2469.

20. Ejbjerg, B., E. Narvestad, E. Rostrup, *et al.* 2004. Magnetic resonance imaging of wrist and finger joints in healthy subjects occasionally shows changes resembling erosions and synovitis as seen in rheumatoid arthritis. *Arthritis Rheum.* **50:** 1097–1106.

21. Robertson, P.L., P.J. Page & G.J. McColl. 2006. Inflammatory arthritis-like and other MR findings in wrists of asymptomatic subjects. *Skeletal Radiol.* **35:** 754–764.

22. Moore, K. 1992. *Clinically Oriented Anatomy,* 3rd ed. Lippincott Williams and Wilkens. Philadelphia.

23. Berquist, T. 2001. Hand and wrist. In *MRI of the Musculoskeletal System,* 4th ed. T. Berquist, Ed.: 773–841. Lippincott Williams & Wilkins. Philadelphia.

24. Zlatkin, M. 2005. Wrist and hand. In *Clinical Magnetic Resonance Imaging.* R. Edelman, J. Hesselink, M. Zlatkin & J. Crues, Eds.: 3309–3365. W.B. Saunders. Philadelphia.

25. Oneson, S., L. Scales, S. Erickson & M. Timins. 1996. MR imaging of the painful wrist. *Radiographics* **16:** 997–1008.

26. Timins, M., S. O'Connor, S. Erickson & S. Oneson. 1996. MR imaging of the wrist: Normal findings that may simulate disease. *Radiographics* **16:** 987–995.

27. Zanetti, M., J. Hodler & L. Gilula. 1998. Assessment of dorsal or ventral intercalated segmental instability configurations of the wrist: Reliability of sagittal MR images. *Radiology* **206:** 339–345.

28. Seymour, R. & P.G. White. 1998. Magnetic resonance of the painful wrist. *Br. J. Radiol.* **71:** 1323–1330.

29. Dalinka, M. 1994. MR imaging of the wrist. *AJR Am. J. Roentgenol.* **164:** 1–9.

30. Storey, P. 2005. Artifacts and solutions. In *Clinical Magnetic Resonance Imaging.* R. Edelman, J. Hesselink, M. Zlatkin & J. Crues, Eds.: 577–629.: W.B. Saunders. Philadelphia.

31. Berquist, T. & R. Morin. 2001. General technical considerations in musculoskeletal magnetic resonance imaging. In *MRI of the Musculoskeletal System.* T. Berquist, Ed.: 63–97. Lippincott Williams & Wilkins. Philadelphia.

32. Erickson, S., I. Cox, J. Hyde, *et al.* 1991. Effect of tendon orientation on MR imaging signal intensity: A manifestation of the "magic angle" phenomenon. *Radiology* **181:** 389–392.

33. Gaylis, N., S. Needell & D. Rudensky. 2007. Comparison of in-office magnetic resonance imaging versus conventional radiography in detecting changes in erosions after one year of infliximab therapy in

patients with rheumatoid arthritis. *Mod. Rheumatol.* **17:** 273–278.

34. Cimmino, M.A., S. Innocenti, F. Livrone, *et al*. 2003. Dynamic gadolinium-enhanced magnetic resonance imaging of the wrist in patients with rheumatoid arthritis can discriminate active from inactive disease. *Arthritis Rheum.* **48:** 1207–1213.

35. Sommer, O.J., A. Kladosek, V. Weiler, *et al*. 2005. Rheumatoid arthritis: A practical guide to state-of-the-art imaging, image interpretation, and clinical implications. *Radiographics* **25:** 381–398.

36. Østergaard, M., M. Hansen, M. Stoltenberg, *et al*. 1999. Magnetic resonance imaging determined syn-ovial membrane volume as a marker of disease activity and a predictor of progressive joint destruction in the wrists of patients with rheumatoid arthritis. *Arthritis Rheum.* **42:** 918–929.

37. Savnik, A., H. Bliddal, J.R. Nyengaard & H.S. Thomsen. 2002. MRI of the arthritic finger joints: Synovial membrane volume determination, a manual vs. a stereologic method. *Eur. Radiol.* **12:** 94–98.

38. Østergaard, M., A. Duer, U. Moller & B. Ejbjerg. 2004. Magnetic resonance imaging of peripheral joints in rheumatic diseases. *Best Pract. Res. Cl. Rh.* **18:** 861–879.

Index of Contributors